Financial Management
for Health-System Pharmacists

Financial Management for Health-System Pharmacists

Andrew L. Wilson, Pharm.D., FASHP
Senior Manager
Health Sciences Advisory Services
Ernst & Young LLP
Richmond, VA

American Society of Health-System Pharmacists
Bethesda, MD

Any correspondence regarding this publication should be sent to the publisher, American Society of Health-System Pharmacists, 7272 Wisconsin Avenue, Bethesda, MD 20814, attention: Special Publishing.

The information presented herein reflects the opinions of the contributors and advisors. It should not be interpreted as an official policy of ASHP or as an endorsement of any product. The information contained in this program, and the companion workbook, are to be used as guidance.

Because of ongoing research and improvements in technology, the information and its applications contained in this text are constantly evolving and are subject to the professional judgment and interpretation of the practitioner due to the uniqueness of each pharmacy's role. The editors, contributors, and ASHP have made reasonable efforts to ensure the accuracy and appropriateness of the information presented in this document. However, any user of this information is advised that the editors, contributors, advisors, and ASHP are not responsible for the continued currency of the information, for any errors or omissions, and/or for any consequences arising from the use of the information in the document in any and all practice settings. Any reader of this document is cautioned that ASHP makes no representation, guarantee, or warranty, express or implied, as to the accuracy and appropriateness of the information contained in this document and will bear no responsibility or liability for the results or consequences of its use.

Director, Special Publishing: Jack Bruggeman
Senior Editorial Project Manager: Dana Battaglia
Editorial Resources Manager: Katy Thompson, Publication Services, Inc.
Cover Design: Jim DeVall, DeVall Advertising
Page Design: Carol Barrer

Library of Congress Cataloging-in-Publication Data

Financial management for health-system pharmacists / [edited] by Andrew L. Wilson.
     p. ; cm.
  Includes bibliographical references and index.
  ISBN 978-1-58528-163-3
1. Hospital pharmacies—Economic aspects. 2. Hospital pharmacies—Finance. I. Wilson, Andrew L. II. American Society of Health-System Pharmacists.
  [DNLM: 1. Pharmacy Service, Hospital—economics. 2. Financial Management—methods. 3. Pharmacy Service, Hospital—organization & administration. WX 179 F4918 2008]
  RA975.5.P5F56 2008
  362.17'820681—dc22

                                       2008036534

ISBN: 978-1-58528-163-3

Table of Contents

Foreword

As a pharmacy leader you have a major responsibility to your organization to appropriately manage the financial resources with which you are entrusted. While this financial responsibility probably is not why you choose to practice in health system pharmacy, it is critical to the on-going success and viability of your organization. The pharmacy revenue and expenditure is a significant part of the total health system's financial resources that are needed to ensure the current and future clinical care that your community expects.

This book is an excellent way for you to support your effective financial stewardship. Most health systems have evolved complex, computerized financial systems that produce a variety of different reports which can seem daunting to understand. As a pharmacist you already have the analytical and mathematical skills to handle this responsibility. Managing the financial aspects of a health system's pharmacy is not different than your personal finances, in that you shouldn't spend more than you have and you need to plan effectively to support the future as well as today. In you job as a health system pharmacy manager you are just dealing with a lot more zeros at the end of the pharmacy numbers.

You will find in this book two levels of chapters; a high level view of the total financial system and how its parts interrelate, and a second level that contains very detailed chapters describing each aspect of the system. Using the background of the high level chapters, you can set out to ask your health system's finance department to explain their systems and the available reports. I would also suggest you develop a thorough understanding of the budget cycle, including revenue, expense and capital budget. Developing a thorough understanding and a management plan for the reports you receive is critical to your stewardship of the hospital's resources. Since the pharmacy computer system provides the data for the budgets and reports, knowing how the drug database and charge master are set up and managing the frequency of updating allows you to "make sense" of the data and ensure it's accuracy. Think through this output and understand how it is used in the organization's financial system because it often drives staffing levels and benchmarking through its productivity aspects. Be certain that you verify all of your department's financial data to identify error, problems and disconnects and make corrections if, for example, the hospital did not receive the correct contract price for a pharmaceutical. Don't neglect the accuracy of drug charging and be certain to develop an understanding of reimbursement, as this becomes the pharmacy revenue which contributes to the organization's operating income. The detail level chapters provide the opportunity to "fine tune" the various aspects of this financial responsibility. As you discharge your financial responsibility look for additional opportunities to enhance the accuracy of your data and maximize the pharmacy revenue.

Your senior leadership, pharmacy staff, and patients are depending on you.

Sara J. White, MS, FASHP
Pharmacy Leadership Coach
Director of Pharmacy (retired)
Mountain View, CA

Preface

As healthcare continues to consume an ever larger portion of the United States' gross national product each year patients, health plans, employers, government agencies and others focus on the elements of care that drive increasing costs. While the ultimate focus of all parties is on the effectiveness and utility of care, and on patient outcomes, the basis for understanding the resources consumed in the delivery of medications and the value of pharmaceutical care is a sound financial management system, well tended by a thoughtful management team.

Pharmacy leadership's attention has been appropriately focused on direct patient care services, medication safety, competency, compliance, automation and a host of critical issues that leverage the education, skills, knowledge and compassion of pharmacists. The continuing focus on quality of care and on building a safe medication use system provides the context for the development of sound management practices and processes. Marshalling the resources to support this objective requires a thorough, disciplined and accurate record of the costs and inputs consumed in care delivery. Each of the key initiatives above is characterized by the need for resources to support the capital and operating costs of new technology, upgraded facilities and equipment, and trained professional and technical staff.

A well prepared, financially savvy pharmacy leader not only understands the concepts and structure associated with these financial systems, but also develops, manages and maintains the systems processes and reporting within the organization for which he or she is responsible. The growing size and scope of pharmacy resources required, the sheer cost of salaries, drugs, automation and information systems required in a complex, modern health system pharmacy require a more thoughtful and diligent approach than in that taken in the past.

Within this framework, Financial Management for Health System Pharmacists has been developed to provide, context, knowledge and specific detailed recommendations for the financial management of a health system pharmacy. A thoughtful reading of this text is only the starting point for the pharmacy leader seeking to provide this aspect of organizational support and leadership. Applying the principles and practices outlined by the authors, and working each day to develop and maintain this crucial aspect of pharmacy systems will ensure that pharmacists and the pharmacy profession support their contribution to the health care system, and assist in creating the future for their health systems, their peers and coworkers, themselves, and most importantly for our patients.

Andrew L. Wilson, Pharm.D., FASHP
Richmond, VA

Contributors

John A. Armitstead, M.S., R.Ph., FASHP
Director of Pharmacy Services
Assistant Dean for Medical Center
Pharmacy Services
University of Kentucky HealthCare
Lexington, KY

Paul W. Bush, Pharm.D., M.B.A., FASHP
Director of Pharmacy Services
Medical University of South Carolina
Medical Center
Clinical Associate Dean
South Carolina College of Pharmacy
Charleston, SC

Teresa Centers
Director, Fiscal Planning and Analysis
UK HealthCare
Lexington, KY

Paul J. Conlon, B.S., M.B.A.
Manager for Pharmacy Budget & Finance
University Healthcare
Department of Pharmacy Services
Salt Lake City, UT

Sharon Murphy Enright, B.S. Pharm., M.B.A.
Senior Manager
Health Care Advisory Services
Richmond, VA

Kristin Fox-Smith
Pharmacy Billing Manager
University of Utah Hospital & Clinics
Salt Lake City, UT

Ann R. Hamlin, R.Ph.
Associate Director of Pharmacy - Finance
University of Kentucky Hospital
Lexington, KY

Noel C. Hodges, R.Ph., M.B.A.
Division Director of Pharmacy
HCA Supply Chain Services
Central Atlantic Division
Richmond, VA

James M. Hoffman, Pharm.D., M.S., BCPS
Medication Outcomes & Safety Officer
St. Jude Children's Research Hospital
Memphis, TN

Philip E. Johnson, M.S., R.Ph., FASHP
Director of Pharmacy
Moffitt Cancer Center
Tampa, FL

James A. Jorgenson, R.Ph., M.S., FASHP
Executive Director for Pharmacy Services
Clarian Health Partners
Department of Pharmacy
Indianapolis, IN

Michael R. McDaniel, R.Ph., M.B.A., FASHP
Director of Pharmacy Services
Huntsville Hospital
Huntsville, AL

Alan H. Mutnick, Pharm.D., FASHP
Corporate Director, Clinical Services
Catholic Healthcare Partners
Cincinnati, OH

Michael J. Oinonen, Pharm.D., MPH
Director, CDB/CRM and Data Quality
Clinical Data & Informatics
University HealthSystem Consortium
Oak Brook, IL

Fred J. Pane, R.Ph.
Senior Director of Pharmacy Affairs
Premier Inc.
Charlotte, NC

Ronald P. Powell, Jr.
Central Atlantic Division
HCA Supply Chain Services
Richmond, VA

Steve Rough, M.S., R.Ph.
Director of Pharmacy
University of Wisconsin Hospital and Clinics
Madison, WI

Wayne Russell, Pharm.D., FASHP
Senior Director Pharmacy Contracting
Premier Inc.
Charlotte, NC

Alice Schuman, MPH, CMA
Assistant Director, Business Operations
University of Michigan Health System
Ann Arbor, MI

Nilay D. Shah, Ph.D.
Assistant Professor of Health Services Research
Associate Consultant
Division of Health Care Policy and Research
Mayo Clinic
Rochester, MN

Chad S. Stashek, Pharm.D., M.S.
Inpatient Operations Manager,
Pharmacy Services
Oregon Health & Science University
Portland, OR

James G. Stevenson, Pharm.D., FASHP
Director of Pharmacy Services
University of Michigan Health System
Associate Dean for Clinical Sciences
College of Pharmacy
Ann Arbor, MI

Lee C. Vermeulen, R.Ph., M.S., FCCP
Director, Center for Drug Policy
Department of Pharmacy
University of Wisconsin Hospitals and Clinics
Madison, WI

Roy J. Ward, Jr.
Chief Financial Officer (retired)
Henrico Doctors' Hospital
Richmond, VA

Andrew L. Wilson, Pharm.D., FASHP
Senior Manager
Health Sciences Advisory Services
Ernst & Young LLP
Richmond, VA

Doug Wong, Pharm.D.
Director, Pharmacy Business Solutions
Pharmacy Healthcare Solutions, Ltd.
Fort Washington, PA

Peter K. Wong, Ph.D., M.S., M.B.A., R.Ph.
Vice president, Quality & Safety
Sisters of Charity of Leavenworth Health System
Lenexa, KS

Billy Woodward, R.Ph.
Renaissance Pharmacy Services, LLC
Temple, TX

Review of Financial Management and Cost Accounting Principles

Ronald P. Powell, Jr.
Noel C. Hodges

Purpose of This Chapter

This chapter will provide an overview of the health-care industry and hospital financial accounting and reporting issues. The reader will gain insight to the industry and to the accounting and reporting issues facing hospitals today. This chapter will provide the framework for more detailed discussions in subsequent chapters.

The "Business" of Health Care

Make no mistake, health care is business—big business. At over 15 percent of the gross national product (GNP), health-care spending continues to rise sharply. This creates tremendous pressure on hospital leaders to manage their organizations—whether organized as community-based/not-for-profit, for-profit, or academic medical centers—more effectively than many other businesses. Operating efficiently and generating a return on investment is crucial for all hospitals, regardless of ownership, to provide replacement equipment and new technology to keep up with the demands of consumers. For some hospitals, another important aspect of efficient operations is making interest payments on bonds and other indebtedness or making dividend payments to shareholders. For other hospitals, especially rural facilities, efficient operations simply equates to survival.

Mission and Community Focus

Hospitals are guided by a mission and a focus on the community. This characteristic distinguishes hospitals from most other businesses. Today's health-care managers, including pharmacy directors, must balance between making solid business decisions and providing services or programs for the community. With limited resources, health-care leaders often must choose carefully how resources are used and which needs the hospital can reasonably meet.

Another area that distinguishes hospitals from most other businesses is the number of stakeholders involved. How many other businesses provide services to customers (patients) as ordered by independent practitioners (physicians not typically employed by the hospital) and paid for by a third party? Many of the supplies used by hospitals are dictated by the preferences of physicians who have no responsibility for the cost of those supplies. Other stakeholders include the employed caregivers, the lenders, the owners, the vendors, and the community. These various relationships create a complex operational environment not found in other businesses.

Efficient hospital operations, defined by an excess of revenues over expenses, are often equated to margin. Some argue that generating margin is somehow inherently wrong in health care. However, margin (or return on investment) is needed to replace aging equipment and facilities and to provide new technology for tomorrow's health-care needs. These uses of margin support the mission of the hospital. It has been said that "without margin, there is no mission."

Governance

Most hospitals are organized either as community-based or not-for-profit facilities, for-profit facilities, or academic medical centers.

Community-based/not-for-profit facilities are generally organized as tax-exempt under the Internal Revenue Service regulations (501 (c)(3)). Their primary purpose is to provide community benefit through various programs and services. Access to capital is mainly through donations (which are usually tax deductible to the donor), bonds and other debt instruments, and efficient operations.

For-profit facilities are generally organized as taxable entities. In addition to their mission as an organization, their primary focus is on generating a return for the shareholder or owner(s). Access to capital is mainly through the sale of stock, debt instruments, and efficient operations.

Both not-for-profit and for-profit entities have similar pressures in providing for the needs of the community. Both entities are required to see patients in the emergency room regardless of their ability to pay. Other than public perception, one of the largest distinguishing factors between the two is access to capital and the payment of taxes.

Academic medical centers are similar to the community/not-for-profit facilities, except that a major part of their mission is teaching new health-care professionals and funding research. These additional activities carry a higher cost structure, which is often offset in some measure by other funding sources, such as grants, state legislative funding, and so forth.

All hospitals, regardless of organization, are governed by a board of trustees. There are many different names for this board, including board of directors. Generally, this board oversees all hospital operations. Board composition commonly consists of members of the hospital's senior management team and representatives from the medical staff and the community.

Senior leadership may include the chief executive officer or president, the chief financial officer or vice president of finance, the chief nursing officer, and other administrative officers. Titles will vary depending upon the facility's style and organization. These leaders are accountable to the board for the strategic and tactical decisions made for the operation of the facility.

Department leaders, such as the pharmacy director, are responsible for the day-to-day operational decisions made in the facility. Department leaders often provide input to strategic plans and work with senior leadership to develop implementation plans for the future.

Environmental Factors

Hospital operations are subject to regulatory oversight by numerous agencies and accreditation bodies. The Joint Commission on Accreditation of Healthcare Organizations (JCAHO), the state pharmacy board, the Centers for Medicare and Medicaid Services (CMS), and the state health department are examples of a few of the many regulatory organizations that seek to reshape the way health care will be delivered in the future. Consumer, payer, and employer groups have also been formed in recent years to address the issue of rising health-care costs and how to improve health-care outcomes. All of these organizations will affect the Pharmacy Director's role in managing the hospital of the future.

The rising cost of caring for the indigent, uninsured, and underinsured is threatening the financial life of many of America's hospitals. The number of Americans living below 200 percent of the Federal Poverty Level (as published by the federal government each spring) continues to increase. Although some citizens seek health care in free clinics, many use hospital emergency rooms. This comes at a high cost and, for most, is an inappropriate setting for health care.

Because of the increasing cost of health insurance premiums, many employees have found coverage to be either unaffordable or unavailable. Many Americans have decided to risk uninsurance to channel financial resources into other areas of their lives. Others have become temporarily uninsured between jobs. In order to reduce health insurance premiums, some employers have offered health plans with high deductibles, which is the amount that beneficiaries must pay before their health insurance will begin to pay, or high copayments, which is the total amount that the beneficiary must pay. Although these plans reduce monthly premium costs, they may become financially stressful when services are needed.

Providing care for indigent, uninsured, and underinsured Americans is challenging the resources of the health-care system. All hospitals are wrestling with this issue. Charity care write-offs and debt expense are among the top financial problems for hospitals. It will take a collaboration of hospitals, safety net providers, communities, payers, and government to solve the issue. Pharmacy directors can play a significant role in creating pharmacy solutions for indigent patients. Many pharmaceutical manufacturers offer programs that provide drugs for patients who cannot afford their medications. Assisting the hospital and the patient with access to these programs is a valuable role of today's pharmacy director.

Overview of the Fiscal Services Department

Fiscal Services is the collective name for a number of different departments often led by the chief financial officer. In some facilities, fiscal services simply refers to the accounting department. Table 1.1 lists the various departments often associated with the chief financial officer, their responsibilities, and who is typically in charge of the department. Titles and specific positions vary among hospitals.

The chief financial officer (CFO) or vice president often reports to the chief executive officer or president and is responsible for the financial operation of the hospital. The CFO must ensure the integrity of the financial reporting, financial systems, and financial health of the organization. In addition, the CFO ensures compliance with a number of different

Table 1.1. Typical Departments within Fiscal Services

Department	Responsibilities	Typical Person In Charge
Accounting	Handles all general ledger accounting, monthly reporting, and subsidiary ledger accounting for the hospital; typically responsible for maintaining fixed asset records, reconciling all general ledger accounts monthly, and assisting department leaders with understanding monthly reports	Controller
Business Office	Handles all aspects of billing and collections for patient accounts	Business Office Director or Patient Accounts Director
Payroll	Handles all payroll functions for the hospital	Payroll Manager or Supervisor
Accounts Payable	Handles all payments to vendors for the hospital	Accounts Payable Manager or Supervisor
Purchasing and Materials Management	Handles all procurement and materials warehousing and distribution for the hospital	Materials Manager and Purchasing Manager or Supervisor
Decision Support	Analyzes financial and clinical data across the hospital and supports strategic decision making	Director of Decision Support or Financial Analyst
Development	Organizes and conducts fund raising for community-based/not-for-profit hospitals	Director of Development
Treasury	In larger organizations or health-care systems, a separate treasury function will manage investments and cash accounts	Treasurer or Director of Treasury
Cost Reporting	Prepares annual cost reports for Medicare and other governmental payers as required and keeps the organization current on changing regulations	Director of Reimbursement or Cost Reporting Supervisor
Managed Care	Negotiates and maintains managed care contracts	Director of Managed Care

financial regulations, especially in the area of billing and cost reporting. In the past, the CFO was viewed as a "behind the scenes" administrator whose role was somewhat transparent to department leaders and managers. However, CFOs are part of the strategic decision-making in most of today's hospitals. CFOs must have an appreciation for the full complexities of hospital operations to fully align the financial objectives with the strategic objectives of the organization. Pharmacy directors will be well served by forging a relationship with the CFO and understanding the financial implications of their daily operational decisions.

Another key financial player is the controller. The controller handles the day-to-day accounting and reporting issues for the hospital. The controller is often the go-to person hospital staff turn to with questions about how to accomplish specific financial and accounting tasks.

The Accounting Cycle

The accounting cycle can best be explained by quickly reviewing the revenue cycle, the expense cycle, "capital" items, the budget, and the monthly close and reporting process.

The Revenue Cycle

Revenues are generated when services are provided to patients. See the Income Statement section for a more detailed description of revenues and net revenue. All hospitals have a system in place to "capture charges" for the services provided. In most cases, this system is automated. However, in some hospitals or departments, the system may be manual. Whether automated or manual, charges are entered into the patient accounting system (billing system). Bills are generated after the patient is discharged. There is typically a short lag between the discharge and when the bill is produced (often referred to as "dropped") to ensure that all charges were adequately captured and billed in accordance with regulations or payer requirements. Hospitals generally bill the patient's insurance carrier on behalf of the patient and keep the patient informed as to the status of the claim. Once the insurance carrier (or governmental payer such as Medicare) adjudicates the claim, the hospital will write off discounts as appropriate and bill the patient for any patient portion due (copayment or deductible) as identified by the carrier.

The revenue cycle is affected by the clinical department's successful capture of charges for the services provided, the complexities of the negotiated contracts with the carrier, and the timeliness of the payments received from the carrier and the patient. Quick turnaround of accounts receivable (amounts billed to carriers and patients but uncollected at month-end) is crucial to provide ongoing cash flow to the organization.

The patient accounting system is generally automated and linked with the general ledger accounting system. In some cases, the interface between the two may be manual.

The Expense Cycle

Expenses are the result of commitments for costs incurred in the provision of patient services or the operation of the hospital. Successful hospitals have a defined process to bind the organization to financial commitments. A typical process starts with a purchase request or requisition to be completed by the department leader. This document includes information on the proposed purchase, including vendor, amount, a description of item to be purchased, the general ledger account code, the budgeted amount, and the business justification for the purchase. The purchase requisition is generally submitted to senior leadership or administration for review and approval. Upon approval, the purchase requisition is sent to the hospital's purchasing department, where a formal purchase order is completed and the purchase order is communicated to the vendor. In some organizations, the department leader handles communication with the vendor after approval is obtained from administration. Once the items are appropriately received by the hospital and an invoice is received, the accounts payable department will match the invoice with the original purchase order and requisition. If the amounts match, the invoice will be paid. If not, the documents are often returned to the originating department to resolve the discrepancy. Accounts payable will typically not pay a vendor's invoice until all discrepancies are adequately resolved.

Like the patient accounting system, the purchasing and accounts payable systems are most often automated and linked with the general ledger accounting system. In some cases, the interface between the systems may be manual.

"Capital" Items

Certain high-dollar items with a useful life of greater than one year are generally referred to as "capital" items. They derive this name because they are reported on the balance sheet as an asset rather than on the income statement as an expense. These items generally require additional review and consideration. Quite often, the analysis required to support the expenditure includes a return on investment calculation. The approval process is often similar to that described under "The Expense Cycle" above. Departmental leadership should consult with the CFO to understand the specific requirements for capital purchases.

The Budget

The budget is the annual roadmap for the organization to obtain its strategic objectives. In most organizations, development of the budget is a lengthy, complicated process that involves close analysis of historical trends and future projections. Typical budget planning can begin six or eight months prior to the end of the hospital's fiscal year. Some hospitals prepare the budget primarily through the work of the CFO, the controller, and decision support analysts. Others rely heavily on department leaders to complete detailed budgets for their departments. The pharmacy director should consult with the CFO to understand the specific responsibilities for budget development.

The completed budget is subjected to an extensive review process. Approvals are obtained from senior leadership, the board of trustees, and any other governing entity (such as the corporate office, in the case of a health system). Once approved, the budget becomes the measuring stick against which monthly performance is compared.

In most hospitals, department leaders are responsible for analyzing and explaining performance variances with the budget. Action plans are often required for ongoing performance that is projected to vary significantly from the budget. This requires a thorough understanding of the departmental operations or responsibility reports and the general accounting processes influencing those reports.

The Monthly "Close"

The controller and staff "close" the general ledger at the end of every month. The ledger may be held open for a designated number of days in the following month to ensure that the accounts are reviewed, complete, and accurate. Some organizations strive to close the ledger within 5–10 days. Others allow additional time for account reconciliation. Once the general ledger is closed, the financial statements and departmental reports can be prepared and distributed for management to review.

The monthly close process can be a stressful time for the controller and staff. There is often a very short window to close the ledger and to consider numerous accounts and issues. Department leaders can assist the close process by ensuring that invoices are processed promptly, and that critical information about trends and operational changes is communicated to the controller in a timely manner.

Basics of Accounting

This section will provide a general overview of the basics of accounting, including the basic accounting methods, the general ledger chart of accounts, and the types of accounts used.

Accounting Methods

There are three basic accounting methods used by health-care organizations: cash basis, accrual basis, and fund accounting.

Cash-basis accounting recognizes income and expense only when cash is received or disbursed. It is a simple method of accounting that ignores liabilities for purchases made but not yet received, and assets earned but not yet collected. Financial reports generated by cash-basis accounting can be grossly misleading and inaccurate. Cash-basis accounting is typically limited to individuals or small community organizations.

The accrual basis of accounting is used for most businesses. This method seeks to "accrue" revenues and expenses to the proper period in which they are earned. This is a large part of the monthly close process for the controller and staff. For the monthly financial statements to be accurate, the controller and staff must ensure that all transactions for the month are properly recorded, regardless of whether cash has been received or paid. Most of the examples and discussion in the remainder of this chapter focus on the accrual basis of accounting.

Fund accounting is typically used by governmental entities and academic medical centers. Fund accounting establishes specific funds for a variety of uses. Two examples include an equipment replacement fund and the general fund. The equipment replacement fund would be used to replace specific equipment in the future. The general fund serves as the operating fund for the entity. Many of the funds extend beyond the normal one-year cycle. This makes budgeting and maintenance of the funds a bit more complex.

General Ledger Chart of Accounts

The general ledger uses a set of accounts organized according to their type. The term *chart of accounts* simply refers to the listing of all available general ledger account numbers. The number of digits varies by hospital, but a typical number is six. The following table demonstrates a typical configuration for organizing the chart of accounts:

Account Range	General Account Category
1xx.xxx	Assets
2xx.xxx	Liabilities
3xx.xxx	Equity or Fund Balance
4xx.xxx	Revenues
5xx.xxx	Deductions from Revenues
6xx.xxx and 7xx.xxx, if needed	Expenses

General ledger accounts are further organized within the category listed above. For example, 100.000 may be used for the general cash account, whereas 120.000 may be used as a patient receivables account. Some hospitals maintain detailed general ledgers using a separate account for tracking specific details. Other hospitals organize the general ledger in a broader manner and use subsidiary ledgers to provide detail.

Each revenue-producing department is assigned a revenue center code beginning with the first digit of the revenue account range identified in the chart of accounts (in the example above, 4). For example, the emergency department may be assigned 460, and the pharmacy department may be assigned 480. Therefore, all revenues recorded in the general ledger for those departments will be reflected in the account series starting with 460 and 480, respectively. The last three digits are often assigned to the type of revenue (inpatient, outpatient, etc.), the payer (Medicare, Blue Cross, self pay, etc.), or a combination of both.

All departments are assigned a unique cost-center code for tracking expenses. For example, the emergency department may be assigned 660, and the pharmacy department may be assigned 680. The last three digits, referred to as the subaccount or subcode, are often standardized by type of expense. For example, 200 may be supplies, and 300 may be repairs and maintenance. The subaccount may be further refined to provide additional detail. For example, 210 may be chargeable supplies, 225 may be implant devices, and 266 may be minor office equipment.

Along with the general ledger chart of accounts, most controllers have a list of expense subaccounts and their definitions to be used by all departments. Department leaders should understand the organization of the chart of accounts and the appropriate use of the subaccounts because they are often responsible for coding purchase requisitions and invoices as well as performance results within their department.

Financial Reporting

Financial reporting for health-care organizations is regulated by a number of different entities. The American Institute of Certified Public Accountants publishes an Audit and Accounting Guide for Health Care Organizations that summarizes the reporting requirements. This section introduces the basic financial statements and their application to operational management.

The Balance Sheet

The first financial statement typically reported is the balance sheet. The balance sheet lists assets owned by the organization on the left side of the report, and the liabilities owed and the equity of the organization on the right side of the report. Equity, or fund balance, represents the difference between the assets and the liabilities. It is called "net assets" because it reflects the amount of ownership in the organization after payment of liabilities. The financial statement derives its name from the fact that the total of the left side of the report must "balance" or equal the total of the right. In other words, assets must equal liabilities and equity.

The balance sheet represents a given date in time. It is often referred to as a "snap-shot" of the entity's assets and liabilities as of that specific date. It is a valuable statement that assists management in understanding the overall health of the organization. Managing an effective organization is dependent on understanding how quickly accounts receivable can be converted to cash and how much cash is available to pay upcoming liabilities. For this reason, the balance sheet is mostly used by senior leadership and the board rather than by department leaders.

Table 1.2 is an example of a typical balance sheet. Quite often, the balance sheet compares both current year and prior year totals. Table 1.3 lists definitions for typical line items reported on the balance sheet.

The Income or Operating Statement

The income statement, also referred to as the operating statement or the statement of revenues and expenses, reports the financial performance of the organization for a designated period of time. The designated period may be the end of the month and the year-to-date period ended that month. The income statement details the revenues earned and the related expenses incurred in the operation of the organization.

The income statement is used by hospital leadership to manage the operation. The individual departmental reports are modeled after the income statement and reflect the revenues and expenses for the specific department. The income statement is generally presented with the prior year information and the current year budget. This assists management in analyzing trends.

Table 1.4 is an example of an income statement for a typical for-profit hospital. Table 1.5 is an example of a statement of revenues and expenses for a typical not-for-profit hospital. Table 1.6 is a listing of definitions for the typical line items reported on the income statement.

The following provides a brief overview of the concept of net revenue, reimbursement methodologies, and the excess of revenues over expenses or EBIDTA—earnings before interest, depreciation, taxes, and amortization.

Net Revenue

Hospital organizations typically do not collect 100 percent of the amounts charged for services. Because of negotiated discounts with insurance payers and mandated contractual adjustments from government payers, hospitals only collect a percentage of the amounts charged for services.

Hospitals charge specified rates for the services and supplies provided to patients. These charges include room and board, also referred to as "routine charges," and ancillary services, such as imaging, operating room charges, and lab. The charges result in "gross revenue" on the income statement.

The negotiated discounts and mandated contractual adjustments are recorded in accounts labeled as "Deductions from Revenue" on the income statement. Another important deduction from revenue is the write-off for charity care.

Gross revenue less the associated deductions equals net revenue. Net revenue is the amount of revenue earned and expected to be collected. In retail terms, net revenue most closely reflects "cash sales." Because net revenue is the real measure of the revenue earned by the hospital, the financial reporting guidelines for published financial statements

Table 1.2. Typical Balance Sheets
As of December 31, 2006 and 2005

	12/31/06	12/31/05
Assets		
Current Assets		
Cash and Cash Equivalents	103,930	203,851
Accounts Receivable:		
Patient Receivables	20,292,328	17,049,650
Less: Allowance for Deductions From Revenue	(6,277,112)	(5,328,811)
Less: Allowance for Bad Debt	(6,767,871)	(4,699,947)
Net Patient Receivables	7,247,345	7,020,892
Net Final Settlements—Governmental Programs	458,797	559,333
Net Accounts Receivable	7,706,142	7,580,225
Inventories	1,131,869	906,737
Prepaid Expenses	237,421	197,028
Other Receivables	210,041	69,794
Total Current Assets	9,389,403	8,957,635
Property, Plant & Equipment		
Land and Land Improvements	495,889	495,889
Buildings and Building Improvements	24,546,453	22,447,943
Equipment	14,179,321	12,863,605
Construction in Progress	78,509	1,641,170
Gross Property, Plant & Equipment	39,300,172	37,448,607
Less: Accumulated Depreciation	(20,350,104)	(18,800,937)
Net Property, Plant & Equipment	18,950,068	18,647,670
Other Assets		
Intangible Assets, Net	504,566	504,566
Investment in Subsidiaries	1,018,125	0
Total Other Assets	1,522,691	504,566
Total Assets	29,862,162	28,109,871

Table 1.2. Typical Balance Sheets
As of December 31, 2006 and 2005 (Continued)

	12/31/06	12/31/05
Liabilities And Equity		
Current Liabilities		
Accounts Payable	1,727,020	1,531,920
Accrued Expenses	2,257,618	1,804,463
Accrued Payroll	611,500	1,223,527
Total Current Liabilities	4,596,138	4,559,910
Long-Term Debt		
Notes Payable	4,500,000	5,650,000
Total Long-Term Debt	4,500,000	5,650,000
Other Liabilities		
Misc. Long-Term Obligations	82,610	12,365
Total Other Liabilities	82,610	12,365
Total Liabilities	9,178,748	10,222,275
Equity		
Capital In Excess of Par Value	514,395	514,395
Retained Earnings—Start of Year	18,138,801	15,420,606
Net Income—Current Year	2,030,218	1,952,595
Total Equity	20,683,414	17,887,596
Total Liabilities and Equity	29,862,162	28,109,871

Table 1.3. Balance Sheet Definitions

Assets

Cash and Cash Equivalents	This represents the cash on hand and short term cash investments as of the balance sheet date.
Accounts Receivable	
Patient Receivables	This represents the accounts receivable from patients or payers on behalf of patients (Medicare, Medicaid, Blue Cross, Cigna, etc.). For several payers, the receivable is reduced to the net amount expected to be collected and is shown on this line at the net amount. For other payers, the gross receivable is shown on this line and an allowance for deductions from revenue is accrued.
Allowance for Deductions From Revenue	This represents the difference between negotiated or regulated rates expected to be received and the gross charges in accounts receivable. An allowance is calculated and accrued for all payers whose accounts are not discounted and reported net in the line above. Often referred to as Allowance for Discounts and Contractual Adjustments.
Allowance for Bad Debt	This represents the estimated amount of bad debt included in patient receivables. Often referred to as Allowance for Uncollectible Accounts.
Net Patient Receivables	This represents the net amount expected to be collected from patients or payers on behalf of patients.
Net Final Settlements— Gov. Programs	This represents receivables (or payables) anticipated from filed Medicare and Medicaid cost reports. These amounts are not finalized until the cost report is final settled by the intermediary.
Inventories	This represents supplies on hand as of the balance sheet date. Supplies includes medical and surgical supplies, lab, and diagnostic imaging.
Prepaid Expenses	This represents invoices paid which benefit future periods and are therefore expensed over those future periods.
Other Receivables	This represents miscellaneous receivables not from patients and patient services.
Current Assets	This represents assets which are highly liquid. Generally, current assets are assets that are expected to be converted to cash in less than one year.
Property, Plant & Equipment	
Land and Land Improvements	This represents the historical cost of land and any improvements (such as sidewalks and landscaping). Depreciation is not calculated on land.
Buildings and Building Improvements	This represents the historical cost of the buildings and building improvements.
Equipment	This represents the historical cost of major moveable equipment (typically large, stationary equipment that is capable of being moved, such as lab analyzers, imaging equipment, and autos), fixed equipment (typically large equipment attached to the

Table 1.3. Balance Sheet Definitions (*Continued*)

	buildings, such as boilers, HVAC, and back-up electrical generators), and certain minor equipment (typically office furnishings and equipment greater than an established dollar threshold . . . amounts below that threshold are typically expensed to supplies).
Construction in Progress	This represents the costs of construction projects currently in progress that have not yet been placed in service.
Accumulated Depreciation	This represents the depreciation expense recorded over time associated with the property, plant & equipment assets noted above. Depreciation is not calculated on land and on construction in progress.
Net Property, Plant & Equipment	Often referred to as "net book value", this represents the depreciated cost of the property, plant & equipment assets.
Other Assets	
Investments	This represents the cost of long-term investments. Often, specific investment categories will be reported on the Balance Sheet.
Intangible Assets, Net	This represents specific intangible assets associated with the organization. Goodwill from a purchase of the facility is one example.

Liabilities

Accounts Payable	This represents invoices and check requests which have been approved and are awaiting payment. These invoices have been processed through the accounts payable system.
Accrued Expenses	This represents known expenses for the period which have not been processed through the accounts payable system. These expenses may be awaiting receipt of the final invoice, be in transit to the accounts payable department, etc.
Accrued Payroll	This represents an accrual for the end of period payroll expense (payroll earned by employees but not yet paid).
Current Liabilities	This represents those liabilities that are expected to be paid within one year.
Notes Payable	This represents long-term debt evidenced by a signed note.
Misc. Long-Term Obligations	This represents other long-term debt or commitments by the facility.

Equity

Capital in Excess of Par Value	This represents the initial capital recorded upon the purchase or startup of the organization (only applicable to a for-profit facility).
Retained Earnings	This represents the accumulated earnings (losses) of the organization since its inception.
Net Income—Current Year	This represents the current year's net income.

Note: The equity section for a typical not-for-profit Balance Sheet is called Fund Balance, and generally does not have additional categories similar to Capital in Excess of Par Value, etc. like those listed above.

Table 1.4. Typical Income Statements (For a For-Profit Hospital) For the Years Ended December 31, 2006 and 2005

	Actual 12/31/06	Budget YTD 12/31/06	Variance	Actual 12/31/05	Variance
Routine	22,401,329	21,260,601	1,140,728	20,589,364	1,811,965
Ancillary	100,643,253	96,342,124	4,301,129	87,273,058	13,370,195
Total Inpatient Revenue	123,044,582	117,602,725	5,441,857	107,862,422	15,182,160
Outpatient Revenue	73,052,290	73,467,933	(415,643)	62,946,349	10,105,941
Total Patient Revenue	**196,096,872**	**191,070,658**	**5,026,214**	**170,808,771**	**25,288,101**
Other Revenue	1,035,102	1,054,363	(19,261)	1,127,139	(92,037)
Gross Revenue	**197,131,974**	**192,125,021**	**5,006,953**	**171,935,910**	**25,196,064**
Provision for Charity Care	8,589,652	7,985,650	604,002	7,015,685	1,573,967
Other Revenue Deductions	131,251,287	127,236,628	4,014,659	109,783,362	21,467,925
Total Deductions from Revenue	139,840,939	135,222,278	4,618,661	116,799,047	23,041,892
Net Revenue	**57,291,035**	**56,902,743**	**388,292**	**55,136,863**	**2,154,172**
Salaries & Benefits	26,246,788	24,394,341	1,852,447	23,793,777	2,453,011
Contract Labor	220,302	230,652	(10,350)	235,492	(15,190)
Supplies	8,023,455	8,521,581	(498,126)	8,416,809	(393,354)
Professional Fees	3,025,032	3,050,608	(25,576)	3,015,879	9,153
Contract Services	4,105,601	3,652,013	453,588	3,501,605	603,996
Repairs and Maintenance	3,250,602	3,106,405	144,197	3,095,659	154,943
Rents and Utilities	1,252,465	1,249,463	3,002	1,235,652	16,813
Bad Debts	2,869,715	2,659,546	210,169	2,354,628	515,087
Other Operating Expenses	519,272	428,285	90,987	415,982	103,290
Total Operating Expenses	**49,513,232**	**47,292,894**	**2,220,338**	**46,065,483**	**3,447,749**

	Actual 12/31/06	Budget YTD 12/31/06	Variance	Actual 12/31/05	Variance
EBIDTA	7,777,803	9,609,849	(1,832,046)	9,071,380	(1,293,577)
Capital Costs					
Depreciation & Amortization	2,610,976	2,147,640	463,336	2,622,198	(11,222)
Total Capital Costs	2,610,976	2,147,640	463,336	2,622,198	(11,222)
Pretax Income	5,166,827	7,462,209	(2,295,382)	6,449,182	(1,282,355)
Income Taxes	2,066,731	2,984,884	(918,153)	2,579,673	(512,942)
Net Income	3,100,096	4,477,325	(1,377,229)	3,869,509	(769,413)

Table 1.5. Typical Statement of Revenues and Expenses (For a Not-For-Profit Hospital) For the Years Ended December 31, 2006 and 2005

	Actual 12/31/06	Budget YTD 12/31/06	Variance	Actual 12/31/05	Variance
Routine	22,401,329	21,260,601	1,140,728	20,589,364	1,811,965
Ancillary	100,643,253	96,342,124	4,301,129	87,273,058	13,370,195
Total Inpatient Revenue	123,044,582	117,602,725	5,441,857	107,862,422	15,182,160
Outpatient Revenue	73,052,290	73,467,933	(415,643)	62,946,349	10,105,941
Total Patient Revenue	**196,096,872**	**191,070,658**	**5,026,214**	**170,808,771**	**25,288,101**
Other Revenue	1,035,102	1,054,363	(19,261)	1,127,139	(92,037)
Total Revenue from Operations	**197,131,974**	**192,125,021**	**5,006,953**	**171,935,910**	**25,196,064**
Provision for Charity Care	8,589,652	7,985,650	604,002	7,015,685	1,573,967
Other Revenue Deductions	131,251,287	127,236,628	4,014,659	109,783,362	21,467,925
Total Deductions from Revenue	139,840,939	135,222,278	4,618,661	116,799,047	23,041,892
Net Patient Service Revenue	**57,291,035**	**56,902,743**	**388,292**	**55,136,863**	**2,154,172**
Professional Care of Patients	20,246,788	18,494,341	1,752,447	17,993,777	2,253,011
Dietary Services	2,220,302	2,230,652	(10,350)	2,235,492	(15,190)
General Services	8,023,455	8,521,581	(498,126)	8,416,809	(393,354)
Fiscal and Administrative Services	4,025,032	4,050,608	(25,576)	4,015,879	9,153
Employee Health and Welfare	4,105,601	3,652,013	453,588	3,501,605	603,996
Medical Malpractice Costs	3,250,602	3,106,405	144,197	3,095,659	154,943
Depreciation	2,610,065	2,596,856	13,209	2,578,965	31,100
Interest	3,519,272	4,328,285	(809,013)	3,415,982	103,290
Provision for Bad Debts	2,869,715	2,659,546	210,169	2,354,682	515,033
Total Operating Expenses	**50,870,832**	**49,640,287**	**1,230,545**	**47,608,850**	**3,261,982**
Income from Operations	**6,420,203**	**7,262,456**	**(842,253)**	**7,528,013**	**(1,107,810)**

	Actual 12/31/06	Budget YTD 12/31/06	Variance	Actual 12/31/05	Variance
Nonoperating Gains (Losses)					
Interest Earnings	865,900	845,980	19,920	795,650	70,250
Unrestricted Donations	65,982	75,900	(9,918)	74,300	(8,318)
Rental Income	15,324	15,300	24	14,987	337
Gain (Loss) on Disposal of Assets	5,623	5,685	(62)	4,988	635
Development Expenses	(9,826)	(8,650)	(1,176)	(8,549)	(1,277)
Other Income (Expense)	10,987	9,850	1,137	9,652	1,335
Total Nonoperating Gains (Losses)	**953,990**	**944,065**	**9,925**	**891,028**	**62,962**
Excess of Revenues Over Expenses	**5,466,213**	**6,318,391**	**(852,178)**	**6,636,985**	**(1,170,772)**

Table 1.6. Definitions of Income Statement Items

Gross Revenue

Inpatient Routine	Patient service gross charges generated from room and board
Inpatient Ancillary	Gross charges for ancillary services provided to inpatients (such as lab, imaging, operating room, and pharmacy services).
Outpatient Ancillary	Gross charges for ancillary services provided to outpatients (such as lab, imaging, operating room, emergency room, and pharmacy services).
Other Revenue	Revenues generated from other sources such as gift shop sales, cafeteria sales, charges for release of health information, and capitation payments.

Deductions from Revenue

Provision for Charity Care	Discounts provided to indigent patients in accordance with established facility policies. Many policies provide a 100% discount (full write-off) for patients with incomes less than 100% of the published Federal Poverty Level (FPL). Typically, for patients with incomes of greater than 100% of the FPL but less than 200% of the FPL, a substantial discount is offered on a sliding scale. Some facilities extend the full 100% discount to patients with incomes up to 200% of the FPL.
Other Revenue Deductions	Represents the discounts negotiated with insurance and managed care payers, and the mandated contractual adjustments from governmental payers. Often, the financial statement includes more detailed line items such as Medicare Contractual Adjustments, Medicaid Contractual Adjustments, HMO/PPO Discounts, etc. In some cases, these details are disclosed in the notes to the financial statements.

Net Revenue

Represents the amount of gross revenue expected to be collected from the appropriate payers.

Operating Expenses

Salaries and Benefits	Represents the cost of payroll and related fringe benefits.
Contract Labor	Represents the cost of outsourced labor, such as temporary nursing labor.
Supplies	Represents the cost of medical, surgical, and office supplies used by the organization. Often includes the cost of minor equipment (such as office equipment and furnishings).
Professional Fees	Represents the cost of fees to professional medical staff for services rendered under contract. Examples may include emergency room services, medical directorships, clinical reading contracts, etc.
Contract Services	Represents the cost of services outsourced under contract to external organizations. Examples may include an outsourced pharmacy or lab, or a grounds keeping contract.
Repairs and Maintenance	Represents the cost of repairs and maintenance on equipment and buildings, including maintenance agreements.

Table 1.6. Definitions of Income Statement Items (*Continued*)

Rents and Utilities	Represents the cost of leases for equipment and buildings, and the cost of building utilities (such as gas, water, and electric).
Bad Debts	Represents the write-off of uncollectible accounts for patients who are unwilling to pay their balance. Hospitals are required to have a collection process and to ensure that every patient account follows that process to completion.
Other Operating Expenses	Represents a variety of miscellaneous operating expenses such as legal and professional fees, marketing, advertising, community support, etc.
EBIDTA	Represents Earnings Before Interest, Depreciation, Taxes, and Amortization
Capital Costs	
Depreciation & Amortization	Represents the cost of capitalized or fixed assets spread over the expected useful life of those assets.
Income Taxes	Represents an estimate of the income taxes due on the pretax income shown. Includes both federal and state taxes.

The expense descriptions listed above are grouped to reflect general categories or departments of expense on the Statement of Revenues and Expenses for Not-For-Profit Hospitals.

recommend that net revenue be the starting point on the income statement, and that gross revenue and the associated deductions only be disclosed in the notes of the financial statements.

Reimbursement Methodologies

The payment for services provided by hospitals is often referred to as "reimbursement." Over the years, hospitals have been reimbursed under a number of different methodologies. Each methodology shifts the risk of high-cost services to different stakeholders. Table 1.7 is a listing of the various payment methodologies and who bears the risk. These methodologies will be explored further in subsequent chapters. The pharmacy director should understand the different methodologies and the operational strategies that he or she should undertake based on their impact on net revenue.

Excess of Revenues over Expenses or EBIDTA

Net revenue less operating expenses equals earnings before interest, depreciation, taxes, and amortization (EBIDTA for for-profit reporting) or the excess of revenues over expenses (for not-for-profit reporting). This line item on the financial statement roughly equates to "cash income," but only to the extent that the depreciation expense is reported separately. It is an important measure of the success of the organization.

Table 1.7. Various Hospital Reimbursement Methodologies

Methodology	Description	Typically Used By	Risk for High Cost Services
Fee for Service	Patient is charged for services rendered and remits payment at 100% of charges	This methodology was used primarily before the advent of Medicare and health insurance as an employee benefit	The payer (which was typically the patient) held the risk for service utilization
Discounted Fee for Service	Patient is charged for services rendered at full rates, but the bill is discounted by some negotiated percentage	Indemnity insurance plans, uninsured discount programs, and other smaller payer sources	The payer continues to hold risk for service usage
Fixed Payment by Clinical Diagnosis	Hospital is reimbursed based upon a fixed or pre-determined payment amount for a specific medical diagnosis	Medicare and other governmental payers	Shifts more of the risk for service usage to the hospital. Typically, there is a provision to provide additional reimbursement for outlier/catastrophic cases
Per Diem Rates	Hospital is reimbursed a fixed, pre-negotiated amount per day for the care of the patient regardless of the services provided to the patient	Managed care and similar insurance payers	Shifts more risk to the hospital for service usage. Typically, the payer requires a daily review of the patient's case and approves the number of days allowed
Per Case Rates	Hospital is reimbursed a fixed, pre-negotiated amount per case for the care of the patient regardless of the diagnosis and the services provided	Managed care and similar insurance payers	Shifts most of the risk for service usage to the hospital. Typically, there is separate negotiated coverage for outlier/catastrophic cases
Capitation	Hospital is paid in advance a negotiated amount per insurance subscriber per month to provide for all of the medical services required by the designated subscribers during that month	Managed care and similar insurance payers	Shifts all of the risk for service usage to the hospital. This payment methodology is not very common in most markets in the United States. It is a common methodology in physician reimbursement

Table 1.8. Typical Key Operating Indicators
For the Years Ended December 31, 2006 and 2005

	Actual YTD 12/31/06	Budget YTD 12/31/06	Budget Variance	Actual YTD 12/31/05	Variance
Admissions	4,074	4,062	12	3,898	176
Adjusted Admissions	6,493	6,600	(107)	6,173	320
Patient Days	27,932	27,255	677	27,605	327
Adjusted Patient Days	44,515	44,281	234	43,715	800
Average Length of Stay (ALOS)	6.86	6.71	0.15	7.08	(0.22)
Average Daily Census (ADC)	76.53	74.67	1.86	75.63	0.90
Outpatient Visits	43,765	51,582	(7,817)	44,181	(416)
Deliveries	600	620	(20)	598	2
ER Visits	12,814	10,410	2,404	10,631	2,183
Inpatient Surgeries	1,690	2,027	(337)	1,722	(32)
Outpatient Surgeries	8,716	9,879	(1,163)	8,769	(53)
Total Case Mix Index	1.29	1.28	0.01	1.27	0.02
Medicare Case Mix Index	1.31	1.34	(0.03)	1.32	(0.01)
Performance Ratio	(1.7)	2.7	(4.4)	(0.2)	0.2
Labor Cost Per Man-hour	23.29	22.55	0.74	21.56	1.73
MHPAPD	20.67	20.07	0.60	20.68	(0.01)
MHPAA	141.73	134.64	7.09	146.45	(4.72)
FTEs—Employed	425	408	17	407	18
FTEs—Contract	16	18	(2)	26	(10)
Total Personnel % NR	45.80%	42.90%	2.90%	43.20%	2.60%
Overtime % Personnel	2.90%	2.90%	0.00%	3.30%	(0.40%)
Adjusted EPOB	3.62	3.51	0.11	3.62	0.00
Supply Expense % NR	14.00%	15.00%	(1.00%)	15.30%	(1.30%)
Net Days in AR—Net	53	54	(1)	51	2
Bad Debt/Charity % NR	11.50%	7.10%	4.40%	6.60%	4.90%
EBIDTA % of Net Revenue	13.60%	16.90%	(3.30%)	16.50%	(2.90%)
Per Adjusted Patient Day:					
Gross Revenue	4,428.42	4,338.75	89.67	3,933.09	495.33
Deductions from Revenue	3,141.42	3,053.72	87.70	2,671.81	469.61
Net Revenue	1,287.00	1,285.03	1.97	1,261.27	25.73
Operating Expenses	1,112.28	1,068.01	44.27	1,053.76	58.52
EBIDTA	174.72	217.02	(42.30)	207.51	(32.79)
Per Adjusted Admission:					
Gross Revenue	30,361.94	29,111.92	1,250.02	27,853.47	2,508.47
Deductions from Revenue	21,538.07	20,489.68	1,048.39	18,921.34	2,616.73
Net Revenue	8,823.87	8,622.24	201.63	8,932.12	(108.25)
Operating Expenses	7,625.95	7,166.10	459.85	7,462.57	163.38
EBIDTA	1,197.92	1,456.14	(258.22)	1,469.56	(271.64)

Table 1.9. Definitions for Key Operating Indicators

Volume Statistics

Admissions	Inpatient statistic representing incremental inpatients admitted to the facility overnight for services.
Patient Days	Inpatient statistic representing the total number of days patients are in-house and occupying a bed during the month.
Average Length of Stay (ALOS)	Inpatient statistic representing the average length of time each patient stays in-house. Calculated as **Patient Days/Admissions**.
Average Daily Census (ADC)	Inpatient statistic representing the average number of patients in-house during a defined time period. Calculated as **Patient Days/Number of Days in Period**.
Deliveries	Inpatient statistic representing the number of births in the period.
Outpatient Visits	Outpatient statistic representing the number of visits from patients on an outpatient basis. This is generally determined from the specific tests/procedures performed on the patient. Generally, this number is larger than outpatient registrations.
ER Visits	Outpatient statistic representing the number of patient visits to the ER.
Adjusted Admissions, Patient Days, & ADC	An overall statistic representing both inpatient and outpatient volumes in terms of admissions and patient days. Adjusted statistics seek to "convert" outpatient volumes to an IP statistic. Calculated as **Admissions/(Inpatient % of Total Revenue)** (substituting patient days or ADC for Admissions as necessary.) (or as **Admissions * the Adjustment Factor**) The adjustment factor is **Total Revenue/Total IP Revenue**. **This is a key statistic used in the comparison of facilities.**
Surgeries—Inpatient and Outpatient	A count of the total surgeries performed, separated between inpatient and outpatient. The statistic is further classified as C-Sections, pain cases, endoscopy cases, lithotripsy, and all other.

Intensity of Services

Total Case Mix Index (CMI)	A measure of the relative complexity of cases treated by the facility. The CMI is determined as a result of medical record coding on patients seen during the time period. Generally, the higher the number, the more complex the patient base.
Medicare Case Mix Index	Same as total case mix index but applied only to the Medicare population. For the Medicare DRG system, generally the higher the Medicare CMI, the higher the DRG reimbursement.

Table 1.9. Definitions for Key Operating Indicators (*Continued*)

Operational Statistics

Performance Ratio	A measure of the overall operational performance of the facility. The % change in NR - the % change in Operating Expenses × 100 should be positive. The actual calculated value is less meaningful than its sign. Calculated as **(% Change in net revenue between 2 periods - % Change in Expenses between the same 2 periods) × 100**
Labor Cost Per Man-hour	Employed (salaries and wages only) costs per man-hour.
Total Man-hours per Adjusted Admission or Adjusted Patient Day (MHAA or MHAPD)	A productivity statistic which compares total man-hours (both employed and contracted) to adjusted volumes (inclusive of both inpatient and outpatient).
FTEs	A measure of employees (both employed and contracted) stated in terms of "full-time equivalents" (part-time employees' hours are converted to full-time equivalents).
Total Personnel % of Net Revenue	A productivity statistic measuring total personnel costs (salaries, wages, contract labor, and benefits) as a % of net revenue.
Overtime % Personnel	The % overtime to total personnel time. Calculated as **OT Hours/Total Paid Hours.**
Supply Expense % Net Revenue Supply Expense per AA	Measurements of supply cost management comparing with net revenue and per adjusted admission.
Net Days in AR—Net	An AR management statistic representing the number of average net revenue days in net accounts receivable. The calculation is based on a three-month rolling average net revenue per day.
Percent of Net Revenue and per Adjusted Patient Day and per Adjusted Admission	Measurements of total financial results (gross revenue, net revenue, operating expenses, and EBIDTA).
Adjusted EPOB	Measures the *Employees Per Occupied Bed* as adjusted for outpatient volume. It is calculated as Total FTEs/Equivalent ADC.

Table 1.10. Payer Mix
For Periods Ended December 31, 2006 and 2005

	YTD 12/31/06	% to Total	YTD 12/31/05	% to Total
Inpatient	**Revenue**			
Medicare	80,640,727	65.5%	69,288,124	64.2%
Medicaid	10,844,996	8.8%	9,013,203	8.4%
Workers' Compensation	446,365	0.4%	2,334,866	2.2%
Commercial	9,274,010	7.5%	4,177,251	3.9%
Champus	204,527	0.2%	369,843	0.3%
HMO/PPO	12,369,215	10.1%	13,977,674	13.0%
Other	697,469	0.6%	428,993	0.4%
Blue Cross	6,406,675	5.2%	6,216,344	5.8%
Self Pay	2,157,665	1.8%	2,126,698	2.0%
Total	123,041,648	100.0%	107,932,996	100.0%
Outpatient	**Revenue**			
Medicare	25,564,673	35.5%	21,723,290	34.8%
Medicaid	3,434,542	4.8%	3,170,689	5.1%
Workers' Compensation	1,577,624	2.2%	1,338,974	2.1%
Commercial	2,632,861	3.7%	2,549,689	4.1%
Champus	670,903	0.9%	629,172	1.0%
HMO/PPO	25,571,206	35.5%	24,001,358	38.4%
Other	81,463	0.1%	2,542	0.0%
Blue Cross	10,867,280	15.1%	7,834,216	12.5%
Self Pay	1,651,484	2.3%	1,258,520	2.0%
Total	72,052,036	100.0%	62,508,450	100.0%
Total	**Revenue**			
Medicare	106,205,400	54.4%	91,011,414	53.4%
Medicaid	14,279,538	7.3%	12,183,892	7.1%
Workers' Compensation	2,023,989	1.0%	3,673,840	2.2%
Commercial	11,906,871	6.1%	6,726,940	3.9%
Champus	875,430	0.4%	999,015	0.6%
HMO/PPO	37,940,421	19.4%	37,979,032	22.3%
Other	778,931	0.4%	431,535	0.3%
Blue Cross	17,273,955	8.9%	14,050,560	8.2%
Self Pay	3,809,149	2.0%	3,385,218	2.0%
Total	195,093,684	100.0%	170,441,445	100.0%

Table 1.10. Payer Mix
For Periods Ended December 31, 2006 and 2005 (*Continued*)

YTD 12/31/06	% to Total	YTD 12/31/05	% to Total	YTD 12/31/06	% to Total	YTD 12/31/05	% to Total
Admissions				**Patient Days**			
2,776	68.1%	2,575	66.1%	19,426	69.5%	18,297	66.3%
391	9.6%	294	7.5%	2,357	8.4%	1,958	7.1%
19	0.5%	32	0.8%	106	0.4%	1,007	3.6%
148	3.6%	137	3.5%	2,358	8.4%	1,255	4.5%
13	0.3%	12	0.3%	(2)	0.0%	76	0.3%
416	10.2%	500	12.8%	2,052	7.3%	2,833	10.3%
17	0.4%	24	0.6%	174	0.6%	116	0.4%
212	5.2%	232	6.0%	1,057	3.8%	1,589	5.8%
82	2.0%	92	2.4%	404	1.4%	474	1.7%
4,074	100.0%	3,898	100.0%	27,932	100.0%	27,605	100.0%
Registrations				**Visits**			
16,827	34.2%	15,934	33.7%	20,670	32.1%	20,333	32.5%
3,801	7.7%	3,139	6.6%	4,183	6.5%	3,609	5.8%
2,233	4.5%	1,244	2.6%	3,488	5.4%	2,174	3.5%
2,000	4.1%	1,782	3.8%	5,278	8.2%	2,162	3.5%
222	0.5%	232	0.5%	238	0.4%	258	0.4%
15,541	31.6%	16,960	35.8%	17,410	27.0%	19,342	31.0%
20	0.0%	5	0.0%	20	0.0%	5	0.0%
5,883	12.0%	5,166	10.9%	7,226	11.2%	6,436	10.3%
2,623	5.3%	2,861	6.0%	5,963	9.2%	8,152	13.0%
49,150	100.0%	47,323	100.0%	64,476	100.0%	62,471	100.0%

Statement of Owner's Equity or Fund Balance

Another standard financial statement is the statement of owner's equity or fund balance. This statement provides a detailed account of the equity balance at the beginning and the end of the reporting period. The net income or loss (excess of revenues over expenses, in the case of a not-for-profit organization) is often the most significant transaction on this financial statement. Net income increases equity on the balance sheet, whereas net losses decrease equity. The statement of owner's equity or fund balance is reviewed by senior leadership and the board. Most organizations do not use this financial statement at the departmental level.

Statement of Cash Flows

The final financial statement is the statement of cash flows. This statement identifies the sources and uses of cash in the organization. The statement of cash flows must tie to the cash balance reported on the balance sheet. Although this statement is useful for senior leadership and the board, it is not typically used by the department leaders.

Statistical Analysis and Key Operating Indicators

Hospitals are driven by statistical analysis. Nearly every clinical department maintains statistical indicators that reflect the quality, efficiency, or effectiveness of the services they provide. Hospital finance is no exception. Table 1.8 is an example of a typical key operating indicators report that measures a facility's financial performance. Table 1.9 is a listing of the definitions, including calculations, for many of the key indicators.

Key financial indicators allow benchmarking comparisons with other facilities of different patient and service mixes. Many of these indicators are available for a specific department, thus allowing for detailed comparisons between departmental operations both inside and outside the organization.

One additional statistical report that is often reviewed by management is the payer mix of the hospital. Payer mix can be based on admissions or cases, patient days, or revenues. Table 1.10 is a typical payer mix report.

Conclusion

Understanding the relationships between accounts and the financial implications of operational decisions is an essential role of the department leader. Managing yearly trends, keeping current operations in line with budget expectations, and understanding future opportunities require clinical department leaders to be savvy financial professionals as well. The remainder of this book will explore many of these basic financial concepts in-depth, providing a greater understanding of the crucial role the pharmacy director plays in hospital finance.

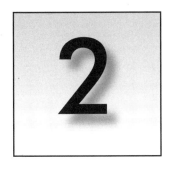

A Review of Hospital Financial Management and Cost Accounting

Roy J. Ward, Jr.

Introduction

Chapter 1 provided an overview of the health-care industry and introduced the key components of the accounting process. In this chapter, we build upon this foundation by examining the hospital's financial model (focused on the income statement) and reviewing financial tools that will help manage the pharmacy department and contribute to the hospital's overall financial success.

The current state of the financial model for health care in the United States is a topic of much discussion. The issues are many and complex, with almost everyone agreeing that health care is expensive, perhaps too expensive. Federal and state governments express concern over rising health-care costs consuming a growing percentage of their budgets; business leaders cite health-care costs as a major issue in the prices they charge for their products and services; the uninsured and underinsured contend that they are forced to pay higher prices than everyone else.

None of this is new. One of the first things that President Clinton tried to establish in the early 1990s was a national health insurance plan, in part to control rising costs. There were calls for a national health insurance program during the 1970s. So how did we get into this situation? A historical review of the hospital financial model will provide some insight.

Financial Model—The Hospital Profit Box

The hospital financial model, the hospital profit box, focuses on the income statement. Profits are the economic engine that drives all businesses, including hospitals. Businesses that cannot generate and sustain annual profitability will eventually cease to exist.

We start our analysis of the hospital profit box in the early 1960s. Figure 2.1 presents a picture of how the hospital profit box looked at that time. The entire box represents the hospital's gross revenue, with the shaded area representing the expenses, or hospital costs. The unshaded area represents the hospital's potential profit and bad debts. Bad debts are shown in this manner because they vary greatly by facility, and their fluctuation has a dollar-for-dollar inverse impact on profits. Figure 2.1 can also serve as a financial model for many non-health-care businesses today.

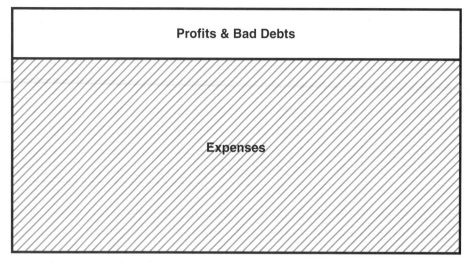

Figure 2.1. The Hospital Profit Box – **BEFORE** the introduction of cost-based payers

In the mid-1960s, the Medicare and Medicaid programs were enacted as part of President Lyndon Johnson's Great Society programs. The goal of the programs was to provide access to and pay for medical care for the aged and disabled (Medicare) and the poor and indigent (Medicaid). Both programs cover physician, home health, and other medical services, but we will limit our review to the hospital services.

Both Medicare and Medicaid were designed to pay hospitals for the cost of services provided, rather than what the hospitals charged for the services. This introduced a new phenomenon into the hospital profit box: the cost-based payer (see Figure 2.2).

Cost-based Payers	Charge-based Payers
Contractual Adjustments	Profits & Bad Debts
Expenses	

Figure 2.2. The Hospital Profit Box – Reflecting the introduction of cost-based payers

In Figure 2.2, the entire box still represents the hospital's gross revenue, and the lightly shaded area still represents the hospital's expenses. The new area of the hospital profit box is the darker shaded area, which is called contractual adjustments. Notice that the potential profit area has been significantly reduced.

In addition to creating a two-tiered system of payers (charge-based and cost-based), the introduction of the Medicare and Medicaid programs created the need for hospitals to file annual cost reports with the government to determine the ultimate amount the Medicare and Medicaid programs would pay. This requirement also created a whole new industry for consultants. The two-tiered structure also created the opportunity for strategic pricing and overhead cost shifting.

Industry-Driven Evolution of the Hospital Profit Box

Figure 2.3 reflects the impact of strategic pricing efforts, with the areas identified with the vertical lines (llllll) reflecting the gross revenue amounts shifted from the cost-based payers to the charge-based payers.

Although the entire box still represents the hospital's total gross revenue and the shaded area still represent expenses and contractual adjustments, the top line of the box (as adjusted for the strategic pricing effort) can also be considered as the average price charged per admission to the two classes of payers. The charge-based payers receive a higher average charge per admission

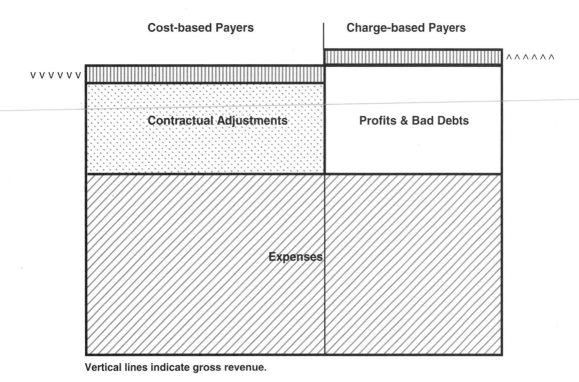

Figure 2.3. The Hospital Profit Box – Reflecting the introduction of cost-based payers and the impact of strategic pricing

than the hospital-wide average, and the cost-based payers receive a lower average charge. Total gross revenue (and total gross revenue per admission) remains the same. The potential profit area now includes the area of vertical lines on the charge-based payer side of the box.

Later in the chapter, we will discuss a report called the procedure analysis. Strategic pricing efforts use the same database that produces the procedure analysis report, but analyzes each procedure code by payer source (charge-based or cost-based). The goal of strategic pricing is to place as much of the price increase as is possible on procedures with high usage by charge-based payers, and as little as possible on procedures with a high usage by cost-based payers. (Business leaders refer to the practice of strategic pricing as cost-shifting, which should not be confused with the shifting of overhead cost to cost-based payers, which is our next step.)

Figure 2.4 adds the impact of overhead cost shifting to the hospital profit box and is represented by the areas identified by horizontal lines (=====). The Medicare and Medicaid cost-reporting process requires overhead (expenses in departments that do not generate revenue, such as maintenance, administration, or human resources) to be allocated to revenue-generating departments, such as the pharmacy. Both programs specify statistical methods for overhead allocations but also allow alternative methods to be used—provided that they are approved by the program prior to being used.

For example, departmental square footage is the specified statistic for the allocation of the housekeeping department. The basic assumption is that housekeeping is responsible for cleaning all areas of the hospital equally. However, the cleaning of the surgical suites is

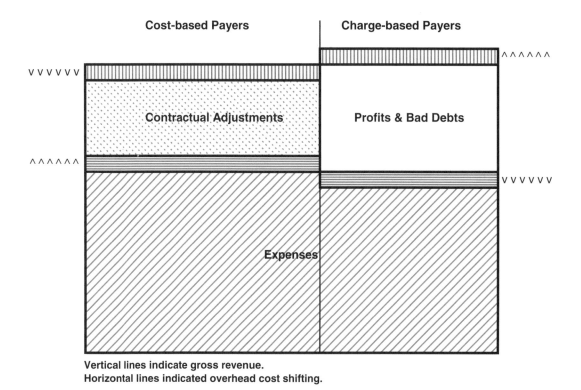

Figure 2.4. The Hospital Profit Box – Reflecting the introduction of cost-based payers and the impacts of strategic pricing and overhead cost shifting

often accomplished by staff directly assigned to the operating room department (cost center), which reduces the cleaning effort required by the housekeeping department. Because the operating room square footage is not cleaned by housekeeping equally to all other square footage, the recommended statistic allocates too much cost to the operating room. This is especially concerning, as the operating room generally has a large amount of square footage and a lower than average usage by cost-based payers.

The approved alternative statistic for allocating housekeeping costs is hours spent cleaning each department. This statistic is determined by performing quarterly time studies of at least one-week duration, preferably two weeks. Because the operating room has a relatively high usage by charge-based payers, properly reflecting the overhead allocation to that area results in a lower cost per admission for the charge-based payers, and a higher cost per admission for the cost-based payers. The potential profit area of the hospital profit box has now been expanded to include the areas of cost shifting and strategic pricing on the charge-based payer side of the box.

Although there were adjustments (eliminations) to what costs Medicare and Medicaid would cover, Figure 2.4 remained virtually unchanged as the model for hospital finances from the late 1960s to the early 1980s.

Government-Driven Evolution of the Hospital Profit Box

The Tax Equity and Fiscal Responsibility Act of 1982 (TEFRA) changed the Medicare program from a cost-based payer to a fixed-price payer for inpatient acute care admissions, leaving outpatient, physical rehabilitation, transplant, and behavioral health services as cost-based payers. TEFRA (or "Take Everything Favorably Reimbursed Away," as it was disparagingly referred to within the hospital industry) resulted in the implementation of the Medicare Prospective Payment System (MPPS), which bundles inpatient admissions into diagnosis-related groups (DRGs), and introduced the fixed-price payer into the Hospital Profit Box (see Fig. 2.5).

Under this system, hospitals in the same geographical area are all paid the same base rate for each admission. This base rate is then multiplied by the program-determined cost weight for the DRG to determine the actual payment by Medicare to the hospital. There are provisions within the system to provide additional payments for very expensive cases, called "outliers."

The impact of the fixed-price payer on the hospital profit box is evident in two areas. When compared to Figure 2.4, the potential profit area in Figure 2.5 has been reduced; the strategic pricing area in the charge-based section of the box is now much higher.

The MPPS went into effect with hospital business years that began on or after October 1, 1983. At that time, the "managed care" movement within the health-care industry was still in its infancy in many parts of the country, and many of the payment contracts were based on a percentage discount from gross charges.

The introduction of the fixed-price payer minimized the potential profit that could be achieved through the overhead cost-shifting process and required even more aggressive strategic pricing efforts to achieve the historical potential profit portion of the hospital profit box.

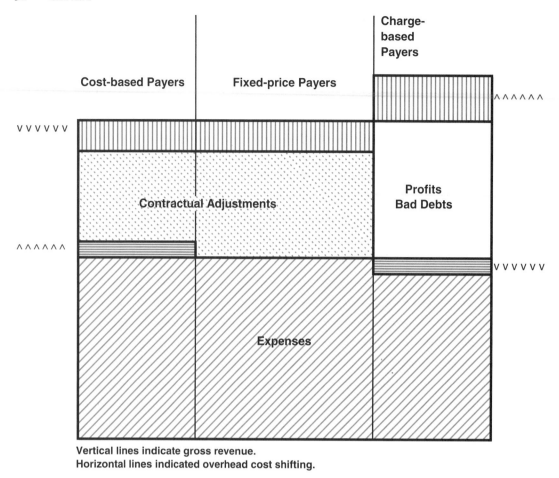

Vertical lines indicate gross revenue.
Horizontal lines indicated overhead cost shifting.

Figure 2.5. The Hospital Profit Box – Reflecting the introduction of cost-based payers, the impacts of strategic pricing and overhead cost shifting, and the introduction of fixed-price payers

Insurer-Driven Evolution of the Hospital Profit Box

As the managed care movement grew and matured, the health insurers gained strength in the negotiation process and were able to effect more favorable (to them) payment methodologies than a percentage discount from billed charges. Insurers moved out of the charge-based portion of the Hospital Profit Box and into the fixed-price payer section (see Fig. 2.6).

As was experienced with the transition from Figure 2.4 to Figure 2.5, the same two areas of the hospital profit box are affected in the transition from Figure 2.5 to Figure 2.6. The potential profit area has been compressed, and the strategic pricing impact on the charge-based payers is even more dramatic.

Perhaps the most favored payment methodology of health insurers is the fixed-price per patient day, referred to as a "per diem rate." The per diem rate methodology gave the

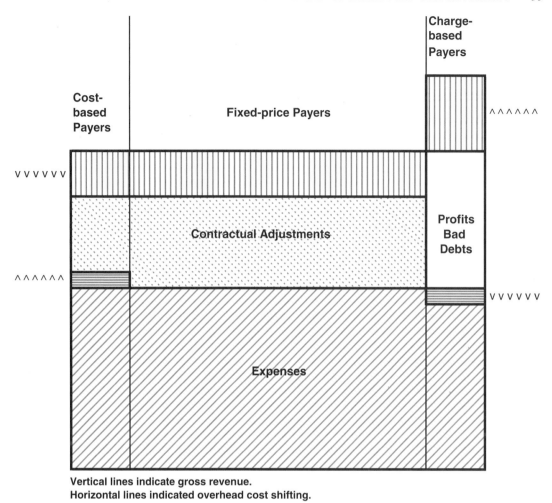

Vertical lines indicate gross revenue.
Horizontal lines indicated overhead cost shifting.

Figure 2.6. The Hospital Profit Box – Reflecting the introduction of cost-based payers, the impacts of strategic pricing and overhead cost shifting, and the introduction of fixed-price payers, and the dramatic increase in charges to charge-based payers

insurers a negotiated cap on the cost increases they would experience but also presented them the opportunity to reduce their cost (and the hospital's net revenue) by reducing the number of days a patient would stay in the hospital through utilization review and case management efforts. Although a per diem rate determined from historical payment data might appear to be favorable to the hospital, the reduction in length of stay could result in a significant decline in the hospital's net revenue.

To counter these efforts by insurers, hospital financial managers began negotiating rates on certain cases, such as obstetric, orthopedic, and cardiac surgery. This approach assured an adequate payment level despite any efforts to reduce length of stay, but introduced the risk of inadequate payment for long stay cases. Hospital financial managers can minimize this risk through the negotiation of provisions called "stop loss," in which additional payments are generated from the insurer when an individual admission reaches a certain charge level. (This is similar to the outlier payments under the MPPS, mentioned above). These additional payments can take any form (per diem, case rate, percentage of charges), with percentage of charges being preferred by the hospital financial manager.

Another potential area for generating incremental hospital net revenues and profits from the managed care insurers lies in the area of the pharmacy—high-cost (per dose) medications. The pharmacy director can be instrumental in a number of ways: advising the hospital's chief financial officer (CFO) concerning what drugs currently fall into the high-cost category; helping to determine what the high-cost threshold should be; and keeping the list of high-cost drugs as current as possible—especially as new medications are added to the hospital's approved drug formulary.

The Hospital Profit Box—Current State

Figure 2.6 represents the current state of the hospital financial model, with fixed-price payers being the largest category—a category that is growing. The ability to negotiate a payment level from managed care insurers that will cover the costs of patient care and provide a profit is critical to the facility's financial success. (This payment level is not depicted on Fig. 2.6). Keep in mind that the payment rate from Medicare and Medicaid (in states where they are fixed-price payers) are set by the government—with no negotiation.

With the growth of fixed-price payers and the public scrutiny over hospital charges—including calls for pricing transparency and the growing bad debt/uninsured problem—the potential profit area of the hospital profit box is clearly under attack. There are three ways to increase it: provide more service (making the entire hospital profit box larger), negotiate skillfully with managed care insurers, and reduce expenses.

Although expense control has always been a focus of hospital financial managers, the evolution of the hospital profit box has elevated its importance to unprecedented heights. Aggressive expense control can be a significant factor in determining the hospital's financial success. The pharmacy director, perhaps more than any other department manager, is positioned to play a major role in the hospital's expense control efforts.

The Pharmacy Director and the Hospital Profit Box

Like most department managers, the pharmacy director is expected to manage personnel costs, primarily through productivity management. This is especially important because the average hourly rate for the entire pharmacy department often exceeds the hospital-wide average hourly rate. It may even be the highest departmental hourly rate in the entire facility. We will discuss personnel management later in this chapter.

The pharmacy director is uniquely positioned to assist the CFO in exercising expense control over supply cost, which is usually the second largest line item on the hospital's income statement. It is not unusual for supplies to represent 20–30 percent of total expenses, consuming as much as 10–25 percent of the hospital's net revenue. Drugs are a major component of the hospital's supply expense. Depending on the services the hospital provides, drugs can range from 15–45 percent of the facility's total supply expense. For example, an active outpatient infusion program or an open heart surgery program can push the drug cost percentage to the higher end of the range. Conversely, a hospital with a very active orthopedic implant program could find its drug cost percentage at the lower end of the range.

The pharmacy director can help the CFO reduce the total drug expense by playing an active role in operational efficiencies and in appropriate medication management. Both of these areas can be managed with a well-designed clinical program that includes converting intravenous medication administration to oral administration (when feasible from a drug bioavailability standpoint), using generic medications when possible and appropriate, and suggesting less costly therapeutic substitutions.

Intravenous to oral therapy programs have long-established cost savings and cost avoidance to hospital pharmacy departments. Studies have also shown patients have few complications and shorter hospital stays when converted to an oral therapy earlier in their hospital visit. To be successful with the programs, the pharmacy director should work with the medical staff to develop automatic pharmacy-initiated conversion based on established patient criteria.

The use of generic drugs is standard practice within hospital pharmacy; however, two elements that ensure cost savings include having policies and procedures for automatic substitutions and converting early to the generic equivalent when a brand-name drug goes off patent. One major wholesaler recently estimated that a generic introduction to the market produced an 18–85 percent price reduction, depending on the number of entrants.

Therapeutic substitutions also play an important role in cost reductions. The more streamlined or closed the hospital formulary is, the greater control over expenses the facility will have.

A relatively new area in which the pharmacy director can help reduce supply cost is by being active in programs that replenish or rebate medications given to the medically indigent. Because the indigent patient population is growing, pharmacy departments need to look for ways to offset the cost of pharmaceuticals used to treat these individuals. This can be done through various means, such as disproportionate share hospital (DSH) program pricing, individual patient-assistance programs, or bulk pharmaceutical replacement from the manufacturer.

Disproportionate share hospital program pricing, or 340(b) Drug Pricing Program, provides discounts on the cost of certain pharmaceuticals. Typically, to qualify for 340(b) pricing, a hospital must provide care to a certain percentage (>11.75%) of low-income individuals.

Most major pharmaceutical companies sponsor patient-assistance programs, which provide opportunities for individuals with no insurance or prescription coverage to gain low-cost or free pharmaceuticals. These programs can be difficult for the indigent population to access, and the pharmacy department can help the hospital by identifying eligible patients and by assisting in enrolling the patients.

Bulk pharmaceutical replacement is another avenue that hospital pharmacies should consider. Again, these programs are typically sponsored by the pharmaceutical companies and have guidelines the facility must meet, similar to the 340(b) program.

Thus far, we have gone to great lengths to convince you that the major contribution the pharmacy director can make to the hospital's financial success is through aggressive expense control and expense management. Although gross revenue and net revenue remain very important to the hospital's profitability, the pharmacy director's actions can have only a modest impact on them in today's economic environment. Entrepreneurial efforts and business plans in pharmacy are discussed in later chapters. The focus on program development where profitability is a factor is also discussed. The pharmacy director should focus his or her primary efforts on the cost-side management of providing excellent patient care.

In the rest of this chapter, we will discuss some tools that will assist the pharmacy director in meeting this goal.

Financial Management Responsibilities

Managing the finances of an organization as complex and diverse as a hospital is a huge undertaking. Although the CFO sets the tone and leads the effort, the individual department managers accomplish much of the work.

Accounting reports that are furnished by the CFO to help individual department managers manage their departments fall into two categories: responsibility accounting and cost accounting. Important management reports in the area of responsibility accounting include the following:

1. Department Operations Report
2. Procedure Analysis Report
3. Accounts Payable Reports
4. Departmental Payroll Register Reports
5. Department Productivity Reports

The first three are usually prepared on a monthly cycle, with the payroll register matching the hospital's pay cycle (biweekly, semimonthly). The most effective productivity reports are those that are prepared daily. All of these reports are part of the hospital's overall general ledger accounting system.

Cost accounting reports are usually generated from a separate system that uses the hospital's general ledger accounting system data in conjunction with data from the hospital's patient billing system to generate specific-purpose reports, such as service line profitability. These reports will be discussed later in this chapter.

Responsibility Accounting

The basic goal of responsibility accounting is to show the department manager his or her responsibility in the financial picture. A basic principle of responsibility accounting is to present *only* those items that the manager is, or should be, directly responsible for in his or her department, and nothing else. Some hospital financial managers disagree and present additional items on their responsibility-accounting reports.

Department Operation Report (DOR)

The most common responsibility-accounting report is the monthly DOR, which serves as a summary of volumes, revenue, and expenses (including staffing information) for the department. Information on this report is usually supported by other, more detailed reports.

DOR Volume

The DOR should start with a volume indicator. For the pharmacy, this would likely be doses, units, prescriptions, or a calculation of pharmacy-adjusted patient days. If doses, units, or prescriptions are the selected volume indicator, the source of the data will be the procedure analysis report. The procedure analysis report depicts the current price, current month and year-to-date volumes, and gross charges (revenue) for each procedure code in the pharmacy, and includes departmental totals of volumes and revenue. The volumes and revenue amounts should be separated by inpatient and outpatient (includes emergency department and ambulatory surgery) service types.

If the pharmacy-adjusted patient days is the selected volume indicator, the procedure analysis report remains a key component of the volume indicator. The total pharmacy department revenue (inpatient and outpatient) is divided by the pharmacy inpatient revenue to generate a multiplier, or "adjustment factor." This adjustment factor is then multiplied by the hospital's total patient days for the month to generate pharmacy-adjusted patient days. The formulas for computing pharmacy-adjusted patient days are reflected in Table 2.1, below.

DOR Revenue

The departmental revenue information should be reported immediately below the volume information on the DOR. As discussed in the volume section above, the procedure analysis report is the source for the gross revenue information presented on the DOR. The gross revenue should be presented in its inpatient and outpatient components. The totals on the DOR should agree with the procedure analysis, giving the pharmacy director a clear picture of how the department's gross revenue is generated.

Some CFOs may choose to reflect revenue deductions (contractual adjustments, charity, etc.) on the DOR, feeling that the presentation of departmental net revenue is important information. Because the pharmacy director is not responsible for what the hospital is actually paid for its services (Hospital Profit Box discussion), some CFOs do not feel that it is appropriate to include revenue deductions on the DOR. Furthermore, such presentation requires allocations that are more suited to the cost accounting system than to the responsibility-accounting system.

DOR Expenses

Now, let's turn our attention to the departmental expenses portion of the DOR. In preparing responsibility-accounting reports, expenses are classified into two major categories: *direct* expenses and *indirect* expenses. Direct expenses are those expenses that can be clearly

---

Table 2.1. The computation of pharmacy-adjusted patient days

$$\text{Adjustment Factor} = \frac{\text{Inpatient Revenue} + \text{Outpatient Revenue}}{\text{Inpatient Revenue}}$$

$$\text{Pharmacy-Adjusted Patient Days} = \text{Adjustment Factor} \times \text{Hospital Patient Days}$$

identified as having been incurred in the operation of a department of the hospital. Indirect expenses, such as employee benefits, or depreciation, are similar in nature to revenue deductions in that they require an allocation to be made. Because the pharmacy director is not responsible for the cost of employee benefits offered by the hospital, Finance leadership in some hospitals does not reflect these items on the DOR.

Personnel costs usually represent the largest area of expense on the DOR, and consist of salaries and wages, contract labor (temporary agency staffing), and employee benefits, if they are allocated to departments. (Some CFOs may show the FICA tax and Social Security on the DOR without allocating other employee benefits, such as health insurance, pension, etc.) The source for the salaries and wages line item is the departmental payroll register report. This report should provide the pharmacy director with the name of each employee and the hours (by type—regular, overtime, sick, vacation, etc.) and expenses charged to the pharmacy department during each pay period.

Bear in mind that the DOR is a monthly report, and the payroll register covers only one pay period, which is usually a biweekly, or 14-day, period. In order to properly match expenses to revenue, the CFO must estimate the amount of salary and wage expense incurred between the end of the last pay period of the month and the end of the month. This estimate is called an "accrual" and is appropriately recorded as a direct expense to each department of the hospital. (A similar estimate is made for hours paid.) This accrual is reversed at the beginning of the next month and replaced by a new end-of-month accrual. The pharmacy director must keep in mind that the number of days of salaries and wages expense on the DOR will match the number of days of departmental revenue, whether it be 28, 29, 30, or 31.

Contract labor is used primarily to fill temporary staffing vacancies, or shortages, but can also represent a more permanent situation, such as an outsourced department. We will limit our discussion to the temporary staffing scenario. These expenses are paid through the hospital's accounts payable system and will be reflected on reports from that system. Although the name of the report may vary by hospital, we will call it the accounts payable accounting report.

The accounts payable accounting report is most likely produced on a monthly basis. This report should be sorted by general ledger account number, which facilitates research, and distributed to department managers. Within each general ledger account number, the report should list the following information across the page:

1. Vendor Name
2. Purchase Order Number (if applicable)
3. Invoice Number
4. Invoice Date
5. Date Paid
6. Amount Paid

Each account number should have a grand total. This report will provide the pharmacy director with the information necessary to ensure that the amount of contract labor reflected on the DOR is appropriate.

If employee benefits are reflected on the DOR, they should appear immediately after salaries and wages and contract labor, which facilitates a summary of personnel costs for the department. These amounts would be allocated to the department, perhaps as a percentage of salaries and wages, and it is unlikely that there is a formal report to support the amounts reflected on the DOR.

Supplies, as we discussed in the pharmacy director's role of the Hospital Profit Box section, represent the largest area of non-personnel expenses in the hospital. In addition to the cost of drugs, supply line items on the DOR could include office supplies, minor equipment (items below the hospital's capital threshold), uniforms, and so forth. The pharmacy director should work closely with the CFO to ensure that a sufficient number of general ledger accounts are allotted to separately report major drug categories, such as intravenous solutions, blood products, chemotherapy, thrombolytics, and so forth on the DOR. Table 2.2 represents an example of general ledger accounts that can be used. Multiple accounts are advantageous in that they allow the pharmacy director to clearly identify and trend drug expenses.

The major supporting document for supply expenses will be the accounts payable accounting report (introduced and described above in the Contract Labor section). However, because not all invoices applicable to a particular reporting period (month) are paid prior to the end of the month, the CFO must accrue these unpaid invoices and show them as current expenses on the hospital's accounting records, including the DOR. A formal report to support this accrual is part of the hospital's general ledger system, although it is may not be distributed to department managers because of its size.

Table 2.2. Example of detail drug accounts for the hospital general ledger

Sub_Account	Description
xx1	IV Fluids
xx2	Blood Products
xx3	Glycoprotein lib/llla
xx4	Drugs and Pharmaceuticals
xx5	Dietary Products
xx6	Pharmacy Supplies
xx7	General Anesthetics
xx8	Anti-Infectives
xx9	Cardiovascular
x10	Ionic Contrast Media
x11	Nonionic Contrast Media
x12	Biotech
x13	Biologicals
x14	Antineoplastics
x15	Thrombolytics
x16	Antithrombotics

This report will contain much of the same information as the accounts payable accounting report, with the date received replacing the date paid. The name of the report may vary by hospital but will probably be called "Unpaid Invoice Accrual," "Outstanding Payments Due," or something similar. Accounting rules require that any item received by the end of the month must be reflected as a liability (and expense) on the hospital's accounting records, because the act of receiving the item establishes a liability to pay for it.

Another source of supply expense occurs when items are requisitioned from the hospital's general storeroom. These items were initially acquired in bulk and kept in inventory until needed. To obtain these routine supplies (pens, paper, staples, Band-Aids, etc.), the department manager, or representative, is normally required to complete a requisition form.

A formal accounting system report is generated each month to charge each department with the items requisitioned from the storeroom. We will call this report the "Storeroom Issues Report," and it will be similar to the accounts payable accounting report. Information contained on this report should include the following:

1. Requisition Number
2. Requisition Date
3. Item Description
4. Quantity Ordered/Furnished
5. Unit Cost
6. Total Cost
7. Grand Total Cost

Additional expense line items that the pharmacy director should expect to see on their DOR would include (but not be limited to) the following:

1. Repairs and Maintenance—includes service contracts on departmental equipment
2. Leases and Rentals—includes the monthly cost of equipment used in operating the pharmacy but not owned by the hospital, such as drug dispensing machines
3. Travel/Professional Development—includes the costs of educational seminars attended by pharmacy staff (registration fees, travel, meals, lodging, etc.)
4. Consultant Fees—possibly used to prepare for JCAHO surveys
5. Licenses—state and federal licenses and permits required to operate the pharmacy.

Details on what individual items comprise these expenses on the DOR can be found in the accounts payable accounting report and the unpaid invoice accrual report.

After all expense line items are listed on the DOR, total departmental expenses will then be reported, possibly followed by a "contribution margin" line. The term contribution margin, as used here, is the amount by which total departmental revenue exceeds total departmental expenses. We will use the contribution margin again when we discuss cost accounting later in this chapter.

DOR Staffing/Productivity Data

The DOR should also contain information on staffing levels for the pharmacy. Total man-hours for the period will be reflected on a fully accrued basis (refer to the discussion of salaries and wages and the payroll register report). The man-hours should be detailed by employed hours, contract hours, and total hours.

On some DORs, you may also see FTEs reported. An FTE is a full-time equivalent employee, which is computed by dividing the number of man-hours for the period by the number of man-hours a full-time employee would be paid for that period. For a 28-day month, use 160 hours; for a 30-day month, use 171 hours; for a 31-day month, use 177 hours. (These amounts were derived by taking the product of 40 hours per week for 52 weeks, or 2,080 hours, dividing it by 365 days in a year to get 5.6986 hours per calendar day, then multiplying that by the number of days in the month.)

The departmental average hourly rate should also be reported on the DOR. Total reported salaries and wages expense is divided by total employed man-hours to produce the average hourly rate. This rate should be monitored for changes over time, as changes in staffing mix (professional vs. non-professional), overtime levels, turnover, and routine pay raises will cause the average hourly rate to fluctuate. The pharmacy director will be expected to know the cause of any significant changes in the average hourly rate.

A measure of productivity, such as man-hours per statistic, is often reported on the DOR. This computation of total reported man-hours (employed and contract) divided by total reported volume provides an elementary level of productivity tracking. Many hospitals have separate productivity monitoring systems, which focus on daily reporting of man-hours and volumes. These systems facilitate active management of departmental staffing levels, which is not possible under the monthly timeframe of the DOR. However, in the absence of such productivity systems, tracking productivity on the monthly DOR is better than not tracking it at all.

DOR Reporting Periods

So far, our discussion of the DOR has focused on what items should appear on the report, where they came from, and what documentation exists to support the amounts shown on the report. The time periods reported on the DOR will be the current month and the fiscal year-to-date information.

For each period reported, the current period information should be compared to the budgeted information (with computed variances for each line item noted) and to the actual information for the same period from the previous year (with computed variances for each line item noted). The pharmacy director's ability to analyze and understand these variances will determine his or her ability to manage the department in a fiscally responsible manner.

Subsequent chapters will detail the development of the budget information used on the DOR and discuss the productivity process.

Cost Accounting Systems

To supplement the financial management efforts supported by the responsibility-accounting system, many hospitals use a cost accounting system, also called a decision-support system. These systems use information from the hospital's general ledger system applied to individual patient accounts from the hospital's billing system to perform detailed data analysis on issues affecting more than a single department of the hospital.

Although these systems are called cost accounting systems, they differ from what accountants and MBA students study as cost accounting, which is primarily what manufacturing companies use as cost accounting systems. These systems deal with actual expenses to produce an item, measured against a standard cost (expected or budgeted).

The cost accounting systems used in hospitals today would be more accurately described as cost-allocation systems, as they allocate the hospital's total cost to the patient database and make no comparisons to budget, or a standard cost. Nonetheless, they are an important tool in managing the hospital's finances.

Before the advent of personal computers in the early 1980s, many hospitals relied on the cost-allocation process used to prepare the Medicare Cost Report to generate information about the cost of providing specific services to patients. The value of the information provided by this method was limited by time. First, it was a manual process, which took many hours to prepare. Second, the data used to prepare the cost information were from the prior accounting period, rendering it out of date. Finally, the cost information only represented a department-wide cost-to-charge ratio, which was not of sufficient detail to generate accurate costing information at the individual procedure code level. Because of the power and speed of the personal computer, more timely and sophisticated analysis became possible.

In reviewing cost accounting systems, we must first change our definitions of how expenses are classified. Under the responsibility-accounting process, we classified expenses as either direct or indirect. In the cost accounting process, we will classify expenses as fixed and variable.

Fixed expenses are defined as those expenses that do not fluctuate as volumes in the hospital change. An example of a fixed expense would be the monthly lease payment for office space or equipment. In the cost accounting process, many other expenses are considered to be fixed, including core staffing levels in some revenue-producing departments, and such overhead departments as administration, human resources, and fiscal services.

Variable expenses are defined as those expenses that *do* fluctuate as volumes in the hospital change. Pharmacy drug cost is an example of a variable expense—the more patients that the hospital has, generally, the higher the total drug cost is, and vice versa. Clearly, other factors, such as type of patients (cardiac, chemotherapy, etc.), also contribute to fluctuations in drug cost, but volume is generally the primary driver.

The proper determination of the fixed and variable costs associated with each item for which the hospital generates a patient charge is the foundation for any successful cost accounting system. To accomplish this, an accountant, or system specialist, will conduct detailed "costing" meetings with each department manager. For example, the amount of time to prepare an IV admixture must be assigned to the drugs administered in this manner, making them more expensive in pharmacist time than a drug administered orally or by injection. (This example demonstrates why the cost accounting system is more accurate than the use of a department-wide cost-to-charge ratio.)

At the conclusion of the costing meeting, it will become apparent that some costs considered to be direct under the responsibility-accounting process can fall into the fixed category under the cost accounting process, whereas other direct costs will fall into the variable cost category. Likewise, costs considered to be indirect under the responsibility-accounting process will also be classified into both the fixed and variable categories.

Once the costing process is complete, the cost accounting system is ready to be tailored for the hospital's use. Master files containing the hospital's identification numbers for its medical staff, its departments, its service line definitions, and so on must be established. Upon completion of this effort, the cost accounting system is ready to accept input, so it can be used to generate reports.

There are two major sources of data input to the cost accounting system: patient bills and accounting system general ledger information. These data sources are loaded into the cost accounting system, typically on a monthly basis, after the books have been closed for the previous month. They are maintained in the system's database perpetually, enabling multiperiod, multiyear reporting.

Cost Accounting Reports

As stated at the beginning of the chapter, profit is the economic engine that drives all businesses. Using the cost accounting system, we can now analyze the profitability of the individual service lines the hospital provides. This analysis is most easily done separately for the inpatient and outpatient (including emergency and outpatient surgery) environments.

On an inpatient basis, the diagnosis-related group (DRG) is typically used to assign cases to the hospital's service lines. The service lines can be as specific, or general, as the CFO desires. For example, orthopedic surgery can be separated out from general orthopedics, and major joint surgeries can be separated out from other orthopedic surgeries. Cardiac implants (pacemakers and automatic implantable cardioverter defibrillators, known as AICDs) can be separated out from cardiac surgeries and medical cardiology cases, and so on.

In the outpatient arena, the service line assignment is more difficult, as there is no DRG assignment to parallel the inpatient environment. Generally, the emergency department cases are assigned to their own service line. Outpatient surgery cases are typically assigned a service line based on the type of invasive procedure performed (ear, nose, and throat, cosmetic, neurosurgery, urology, orthopedic, cardiac catheterization, etc.). The remaining outpatient cases are assigned to a service line based on the department rendering the service, such as infusion, imaging, radiation oncology, cardiac testing, and so forth.

Service line profitability can be judged at various levels. Two of the more common levels are earnings before interest, depreciation, taxes, and amortization (EBIDTA) and net income (usually before income taxes for tax-paying hospitals). Regardless of the level of profitability selected for analysis and presentation, the following items should be reflected on the service line profitability report:

Patient Volumes (Discharges, Patient Days, Outpatient Cases)
Profitability Components:

+ Gross Revenue
− Revenue Deductions
= Net Revenue
− Variable Cost
= Contribution Margin
− Fixed Cost
= Profit (EBIDTA, Net Income)

Contribution margin is an important measure of service line profitability, as it presents the amount of earnings a service line generates and contributes toward the hospital's fixed costs and profits. Contribution margin is perhaps the most important measure financial managers study when considering which service lines to emphasize for volume growth. Contribution margin is effective because it measures profitability before fixed costs are assigned, and fixed costs, by definition, do not change as volumes fluctuate (increase). Stated differently, the contribution margin is the measure of incremental profits that can be generated by volume changes in the service line.

Having highlighted the importance of the contribution margin in evaluating service line profitability, we must remember that the hospital-wide fixed costs must eventually be covered to generate an overall profit. Businesses that fail to generate a contribution margin in excess of their fixed cost eventually fail.

The cost accounting system can be used for other purposes besides service line profitability. Any data element on the patient bill (all hospitals must generate a uniform bill, presently the UB-04) can be used to extract data from the cost accounting database. Because the patient zip code is on the UB-04, the system can be used to determine from which geographic areas the hospital's patients are drawn. Additional demographic data gathering can be gathered on age, sex, employer, primary insurer, and so on.

Pharmacy Director Use of the Cost Accounting System

The pharmacy director should be one of the most active users of the cost accounting system. Certain service lines, such as oncology, cardiology, and outpatient infusion, make extensive use of high-cost drugs. Their profitability should be carefully monitored and decisive action taken if their profitability should slip.

The cost accounting system provides the ability to drill down into the details of the service line's profitability and to determine what is driving the overall results. The process is similar to peeling an onion—going layer by layer.

Using the oncology service line as an example, drilling down into a DRG might reveal that DRG 409—chemotherapy—has a low-contribution margin when compared to the rest of the service line. Drilling down by physician might reveal length of stay issues in which the patients of one physician have an average length of stay that significantly exceeds the patients of the other physicians in DRG 409. If so, the cause of the higher length of stay should be determined. Drilling down into the DRG by physician might also reveal that the patients of one physician have a higher drug cost than the patients of the other physicians treating patients in DRG 409. Drilling down into the drug cost of these patients might reveal a preference for a high-cost drug that has a less costly substitute. Other causes may be determined by additional drill-down queries.

As you can see, the cost accounting system can be an effective tool in the pharmacy director's efforts to identify areas to reduce expenses and to develop implementation plans to bring the identified cost reductions to fruition.

Summary

Hospital financial management has evolved over the past forty years to the point in which expense control and management are arguably the most important topics. This chapter has traced that evolution. The review of responsibility accounting and reports and the review of cost accounting and reports have presented some tools that the pharmacy director can use in the control of expenses within the department and the hospital.

Subsequent chapters will examine other aspects of financial management, including budgeting, benchmarking, and productivity analysis.

References

The source of the hospital profit box is not known. It was first seen by this author in a presentation in the early 1970s. I have used it and "evolved" it throughout my 38 years in hospital financial management.

The remaining concepts presented in this chapter are my own thoughts, which have been formed over my 38-year career in health care—nearly 26 years of which was spent within the HCA system. This chapter has been submitted to HCA for their approval.

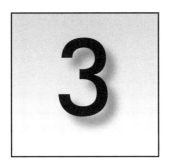

The Health Care Budget Process

Andrew L. Wilson

Introduction

Financial management and cost control are crucial activities for pharmacists in leadership roles in health system practice. The high cost of pharmaceuticals, growing salaries for pharmacists, changing and growing hospital services, and the continuing need for safe, effective pharmacy services and medication delivery require thoughtful, cost-conscious management to deliver success. Increasing scrutiny and regulation and the growth of support systems and technology to manage the safety, efficiency, and effectiveness of the medication use process, including automation and information systems, add to the span of financial management and cost-control responsibilities of pharmacists.

Financial Planning: The Annual Budget

The annual budget is an important part of the pharmacy manager's financial responsibility. A budget is a plan for future expenses and revenue, typically over a 12-month period. A budget does not represent the actual amount of money available to be spent but is a plan based on history and an understanding of the future. The pharmacy budget is designed to be a thoughtful, data-driven forecast of future expenses and revenue, and a yardstick for measuring financial performance over the course of the financial year.

Professional Practice Standards

ASHP practice standards and guidelines refer to the budget and financial leadership responsibilities of pharmacists and identify key roles and responsibilities related to financial management of a pharmacy service[1,2]:

- Budget management: The pharmacy should have a budget consistent with the organization's financial management process that supports the scope of and demand for pharmaceutical services.

- Workload and productivity management: Oversight of workload and financial performance should be managed in accordance with the organization's requirements.

- Analysis and control methods: Management should provide for (1) determination and analysis of pharmaceutical service costs, (2) analysis of budgetary variances, (3) capital equipment acquisition, (4) patient revenue projections, and (5) justification of personnel commensurate with workload productivity.

- Processes should enable the analysis of pharmaceutical services by unit of service and other parameters appropriate to the organization (e.g., organization-wide costs by medication therapy, clinical service, specific disease management categories, and patient health plan enrollment). The director should have an integral part in the organization's financial management process.

- Drug expenditures. Specific policies and procedures for managing drug expenditures should address such methods as competitive bidding, group purchasing, utilization review programs, inventory management, and cost-effective patient services.

- Revenue, reimbursement, and compensation. The director should be knowledgeable about revenues for pharmaceutical services, including reimbursement for the provision of drug products and related supplies and compensation for pharmacists' cognitive services.

ASHP policies and practice standards are the underpinnings of professional leadership expectations for pharmacy leaders in meeting the goals of their health system.

The Budget Process

To ensure the effective use of resources and to meet the organization's mission, the health system develops an annual plan. Nearly every health system must select and prioritize activities for the coming year from numerous and varied challenges and opportunities. Organizational, structural, and financial constraints challenge the health system's leadership to select a course and to identify the means to steer the health system through the year. Because a health system is a complex, highly regulated, and often financially constrained organization, the CEO, CFO, and board of trustees work from a strategic plan to develop goals for services, activity levels, expenditures, and revenues for the upcoming budget, and, in some instances, for longer periods. Planning and budgeting that requires building facilities, acquiring technology, developing business relationships or joint ventures, or extended implementation periods often are budgeted up to five years in advance.

Planning and forecasting activities are typically initiated 6–9 months before the fiscal year begins. Forecasts for admissions, service activity, growth, expansion, or other program changes are developed based on past activity, an understanding of the local and regional market, and with a systematic approach to engaging partners, including medical leadership and key governmental and community partners. The health system's board and finance committee are key stakeholders, and health system leadership must work diligently to secure their support and concurrence. When bonds or other debt obligations must be issued to complete a project, external regulatory authorities, banks, and other lenders must also be comfortable that the health system has a sound financial base and the wherewithal to sustain both its mission and its bottom line. Following development by leadership and approval by the finance committee or board, the health system's budget plan is shared with managers and leaders in the health system who work to prepare the annual budget. The budget planning process involves key senior leaders in the health system and may engage the pharmacy director when drug therapy intensive services or activities are considered.

The pharmacy budget process is a 12-month activity. Maintaining accurate and current accounts and keeping a dashboard or other continuing monitoring system to understand the pharmacy's current state and likely direction is a vital part of the knowledge and understanding necessary for effective budgeting. When the director of pharmacy receives the forecasts, he or she can begin the formal process of developing the pharmacy budget. Each health system's budget process varies slightly, and the expected inputs, reviews, and sequence of deadlines may be unique. However, in all cases the CFO or health system budget office provides a budget manual or other instructions, including a calendar and deadlines, budgeting format, and an indication of required approvals and reviews. Budget instructions may also specify the method or target for forecasting supply (drug) and labor cost inflation and other price increases to be used in budget development.

Portions of the budget represent fixed costs that will not vary with activity, such as leases or office supplies, whereas others are variable costs that will grow or shrink based on admissions or patient days, such as drug costs and human resources, requiring the manager to carefully review forecasts for admissions, patient days, and other volume indicators.

Capital Budget

The budget cycle typically begins with the development of a capital budget. The capital budget is typically comprised of items that cost more than a fixed threshold (e.g., an expense >$5,000) and have a useful life greater than a specified number of years (e.g., five years). Capital budget thresholds are set by the health system's board but are generally in this range. Capital expense budgets are typically set several years in advance because many capital expenses can be forecast. The need to replace equipment, to renovate or build facilities, or to incur expenses for a new program lends itself to forward planning, and the high costs mean that funds must be set aside. Accounting methods can report capital expenses spread across several years. Pharmacy examples of capital expenses might include installing new IV admixture hoods, remodeling a pharmacy, or building a new pharmacy satellite.

Capital budget needs and requests are typically greater than a health system can afford, so a process to prioritize the needs and capital requests is generally undertaken by the CFO. This process is typically a focused review of each proposed capital expense, assessing the level of need (Is the item required by a new regulation or standard? Is the current equipment broken, nonfunctioning, or insufficient to current or projected needs? Is the equipment or renovation necessary to support a new patient care program?) and the direct and related costs (Will additional staff need to be hired? Will facilities need to be renovated? What resources are needed to implement and make the equipment or resource operational?).

A review of the return on investment (ROI) is also used to prioritize or assess the financial wisdom of the capital expense. ROI is a structured calculation of the operating cost and revenue changes that the health system will incur with the new capital expense. (Will fewer employees be needed because of increased productivity? Will additional patient volume be generated because of increased capacity or throughput? Will more revenue be collected?) ROI calculations are often stated in the number of months or years that a capital purchase takes to pay back its purchase cost. Shorter payback periods are generally more favorable, and capital expenses that do not result in payback of their costs may not be easily approved and

Table 3.1. Pharmacy Volume Budget

LOCATION	Jan	Feb	Mar	Apr	May	Jun
Inpatient Pharmacy	452,593	408,794	451,133	437,993	455,513	436,533
Inpatient Pharmacy Total	**452,593**	**408,794**	**451,133**	**437,993**	**455,513**	**436,533**
Orders/Day	*14,599.77*	*13,186.89*	*15,037.77*	*14,128.81*	*15,183.77*	*14,081.72*
Outpatient Pharmacy #1	8,500	7,677	8,473	8,226	8,555	8,198
Outpatient Pharmacy #2	2,260	2,041	2,253	2,187	2,275	2,180
Outpatient Pharmacies Total	**463,353**	**418,512**	**461,858**	**448,406**	**466,342**	**446,911**
Rx/Day	*19,580*	*17,686*	*20,168*	*18,949*	*20,364*	*18,886*
Home Infusion Pharmacy	712	643	710	689	717	687
Rx/Day	*22.97*	*20.75*	*23.66*	*22.23*	*23.89*	*22.15*
GRAND TOTAL:	**916,658**	**827,949**	**913,701**	**887,088**	**922,572**	**884,131**

budgeted, unless they are required to meet a legal or accreditation standard. Although there are a variety of objective methods to determine the patient care, regulatory, and financial wisdom of a given capital expenditure, the conflicting or equivocal results from the structured review often mean that subjective elements are a component of the health system's capital budget decision process. A capital expense supporting a marketing opportunity for a new patient care service may take precedence over a more mundane internal purchase of similar financial and patient care impact because of the opportunity for public visibility or the ability to build relationships with key physicians or other constituencies.

The Operating Budget

The operating budget is a forecast of the daily expenses required to operate the pharmacy, including labor, drugs, supplies, and other support below the capital expense threshold. Development of the health system operating budget generally takes advantage of the fact that most expenses are similar in size and scope to prior years. In many organizations, the pharmacy director is presented with a preliminary budget based on the activity and expenses of the prior fiscal year. In some health systems the preliminary budget may be adjusted for forecast volume and service changes. In all cases, the pharmacy director must review the proposed expenses and revenues against the activity and finances of the prior one to two fiscal years and to base changes on institutional and industry trends, news, and other information. The budget review and approval process typically uses this method to ensure continuity and prevent errors.

Volume Budget

The volume budget is prepared by the CFO and budget office support team and supplies the number of admissions, patient days, CMI, outpatient visits, emergency department visits, and other activities. Key physicians, nursing leadership, and others review these

Table 3.1. Pharmacy Volume Budget (*Continued*)

Jul	Aug	Sep	Oct	Nov	Dec	TOTAL	Monthly Average
408,794	452,009	421,933	467,193	405,874	454,053	5,252,415	*437,701*
408,794	**452,009**	**421,933**	**467,193**	**405,874**	**454,053**	**5,252,415**	***437,701***
13,186.89	*16,143.18*	*13,610.76*	*15,573.09*	*13,092.70*	*15,135.01*		*14,413.37*
7,677	8,489	7,924	8,774	7,623	8,527	98,644	*8,220*
2,041	2,257	2,107	2,333	2,027	2,267	26,228	*2,186*
418,512	**462,755**	**431,965**	**478,300**	**415,523**	**464,848**	**5,377,286**	***448,107***
17,686	*21,650*	*18,254*	*20,886*	*17,559*	*20,298*		*19,330.41*
643	711	664	735	639	714	8,263	*689*
20.75	*25.40*	*21.41*	*24.50*	*20.60*	*23.81*		*22.67*
827,949	**915,475**	**854,562**	**946,228**	**822,035**	**919,615**	**10,637,964**	***886,497***

estimates to ensure that they reflect the historical perspective described earlier and take the external environment, competitors, and other changes into consideration. The pharmacy director should examine historical relationships between these volume statistics and pharmacy activity to develop a pharmacy volume budget. When possible, pharmacy volume statistics should be tied to a patient care program, site of care. Table 3.1 is an example of a pharmacy volume budget based on the CFO's base statistics.

Pharmacy work volumes consist of work units and paid hours. Pharmacy workload volume for inpatient services is reported as adjusted discharges or patient days. Outpatient pharmacy workload is reported as prescriptions filled and may include patient counseling or other direct patient care activities in some settings. Health system pharmacy volume projections may be based on patient counts, such as admissions or discharges, prescriptions filled, orders processed, doses dispensed, or combinations of these components. Typical indicators for pharmacy volume are adjusted using case mix index (CMI) or another indicator of acuity to recognize the additional cost and resources required to care for sicker patients. Pharmacy volume should also be adjusted to reflect the significant amount of effort and cost required to support outpatient surgery, the emergency department, outpatient infusion services, and other areas not reflected in patient day and admission counts.

Expense Budget

An expense is a payment made by the health system to others for value received. Pharmacy expenses can be divided into three categories: supplies, human resources, and other expenses. Direct expenses in each category are those expenses that are incurred by the pharmacy to deliver services and products. Supplies are the largest category of direct expense—predominately pharmaceuticals. Other categories of supplies managed by pharmacy include blood products, intravenous fluids, syringes and needles, administration sets, and other non-patient care supplies, such as packaging materials, paper, labels, and other office supplies. Human resources are often the second largest category of direct expense. Human resource expenses consist of the salary and benefit costs for pharmacists, pharmacy technicians, pharmacy managers, and others.

Other direct expenses incurred by the pharmacy include:

- Leases for hardware and software to manage medication delivery, including automated medication cabinets, dispensing robots, pharmacy computer systems, and intravenous pumps
- Services, including hood certification, service agreements for technology and equipment, and maintenance and repairs for pharmacy facilities
- Professional education and development expenses, including meetings, travel, and competency programs
- Licenses, taxes, and other fees associated with accreditation, including pharmacy residency program accreditation

Direct expenses can also be classified as fixed or variable. Fixed expenses are defined as costs that do not vary significantly in the short-term with the volume of activity. Property and equipment are examples. Variable expenses are costs that vary in the short-term with the level of activity. Purchase costs for drugs are an example; costs rise and fall as the number of patients and prescriptions change. Pharmacy activity volume may be expressed based on the number of patient days, prescriptions or orders processed, or on the number of doses dispensed. Most health system budgets base variable costs for pharmacy supply and labor on a combination of inpatient days, emergency department visits, and clinic or other ambulatory volumes. This calculated figure is often referred to as an adjusted patient day or an adjusted patient discharge.

Indirect expenses are payments for services that support the pharmacy but are not directly paid by the pharmacy. These include housekeeping, heat and air-conditioning, electricity, health system administration, health system purchasing, information systems support, human resources, finance, and others. The cost of these indirect services may also be referred to as overhead. In the modern health system, the magnitude of these costs is substantial. Because the costs are beyond the control of the pharmacy manager, they are not generally part of regular financial reports. However, indirect costs may be considered when business plans and profitability of a service or program are reviewed, including pharmacy services.

Human Resource Expense Budget

Human resource expenses include the salaries for all professional, technical, and support staff and their benefits, including insurance, workers' compensation, disability, and so on. The pharmacy manager takes the number of approved positions in each job class (pharmacist, pharmacy technician, secretary, etc.) and multiplies them by the number of paid hours and the hourly rate for the year to arrive at the salary cost. Benefits are added as a percent of the final salary figure. The cost of benefits is typically stated as a percentage of the annual salary. Benefit costs can run as high as 25–30 percent. Benefit percentage for budget calculation is typically provided by the CFO in the budget manual or budget instructions.

A spreadsheet, detailing the hours worked, salary, and other calculations for each incumbent employee (with vacant positions listed), ensures a correct calculation. Projected raises and salary increases for the coming year should be included in this calculation. New positions added to the pharmacy service should also be added to this calculation during the budget review and approval process as they are approved. The internal systems that support the health system's time and attendance and payroll functions take the pharmacy human resource budget and translate it into biweekly or monthly budget allocations, accounting for holidays, sick, vacation, and other non-worked time and for expected vacancy rates, proposed pay increases, and other known or forecasted events. To the extent possible, the pharmacy director's estimates should reflect this level of detail as well.

When new positions are tied to a new pharmacy program or service, they may be approved separately, contingent on the approval of the service itself during the budget process. Budgeting for these and other new positions should reflect start dates, new service activities, and likely hire dates. Changes in salary across the year for merit and other raises or for anticipated increases to meet hiring market conditions should also be done in a way that marks their occurrence during the budget year. Again, the internal systems that support the health system's time and attendance and payroll functions will translate the approved positions into biweekly or monthly budget allocations.

Supply Expense Budget

The overwhelming majority of pharmacy supply expense is drugs, and the size and scope of drug expense have material impact on the health system's overall budget. A thoughtful, well-supported supply budget for drugs is critical for the pharmacy's success and has a material impact on the health system's budget. Forecasting drug and other supply expense is a combination of four factors: (1) price inflation, (2) drug usage, (3) drug mix, and (4) a blend of usage and mix representing expensive, innovative medications. The authors of a continuing series of articles examining trends in drug cost recommend a nine-step process to ensure success in forecasting this expense:

Step 1: Collect data. Historical purchase data can be gathered from distributor data systems and usage data from health system and pharmacy information systems. Group purchasing organizations provide reports on anticipated contract price changes and an annual forecast that serves as a resource for predictions of new drug approvals, adoption of recently approved drugs, generic drug introductions, and overall trends.

Step 2: Review financial history. Evaluate the pharmacy's performance against the budget for the most recent full fiscal year and for the current fiscal year (annualizing current fiscal year-to-date data). Compare actual fiscal year data to identify local inflationary trends by drug and by disease, diagnosis, or service. Identify areas of exceptional variance for more detailed assessment. Review the performance of current cost-containment efforts.

Step 3: Build a high-priority drug budget. A relatively small number of drugs (50–60 products) typically represents 80–90 percent of total drug purchases and usage in most health systems. Create a drug product-specific budget for these drugs based on historical usage, and project changes in volume of use.

Step 4: Build a new product budget. Consider new drugs expected to be approved during the period covered by the budget. Work with prescribers to identify which new drugs will be used, how they will be used, and how often.

Step 5: Build a nonformulary drug budget. Budget commonly used nonformulary products separately for financial monitoring purposes.

Step 6: Build a low-priority drug budget. The low-priority drug budget represents a small portion of the total drug budget and can be safely budgeted as a lump sum. This component of the budget should be predicted on a volume-specific basis, taking into consideration any anticipated change in overall patient volume. Other medical supplies and general supplies can also be forecast using this method.

Step 7: Establish a drug cost-containment plan. Include drug-use evaluation results, indicating inappropriate prescribing, drug classes with multiple competing agents, and reports of successful cost-containment efforts published by other health systems. For each cost-containment target identified, produce a targeted prediction that includes the scope of the plan, what the intervention will entail (e.g., guideline implementation, formulary change), the timing of intervention implementation, and an estimate of the costs for a successful plan.

Step 8: Finalize and present the total drug budget. The total drug budget is the sum of expected expenditures on the high-priority list, new products, nonformulary agents, and low-priority products, minus the total cost impact expected from the cost-containment plan. In many cases, the initial estimate of expenditures will be higher than health system leadership is comfortable with. Using this budgeting model, requests for additional cuts can be met in a variety of ways.

Step 9: Vigilance. Budgets established using the eight steps above provide a level of detail and a robust baseline for comparison with actual performance and variance reporting.[3]

The director of pharmacy, and key members of the pharmacy staff, including clinical pharmacists and business and purchasing managers, should collaborate with the pharmacy and therapeutics committee and other stakeholders to develop the most thoughtful and accurate forecasts for this part of the budget. Because of the high cost of drug therapy, health system administration and boards rely on pharmacists to contribute to the understanding of the impact of medication costs and to develop a plan for this expense. Pharmacy leadership must articulate a plan for clinical pharmacists and other pharmacy staff to have an impact on the balance of cost and benefit and patient care outcome and to communicate the resulting savings, cost avoidance, and leverage for the drugs purchased.

Other Fixed Expense Budget

Other expenses generally vary only in response to inflation and price changes. Table 3.2 shows a full range of expenditures budgeted on this basis, including general supplies, purchased services, and telephone. Where data exist to budget these expenses and accounts fully and correctly (for example in the case of a lease or contract in which terms and costs are specified or in which prior year activity is a good guide), these figures should be used to develop and support the final budget. The health system budget office or the purchasing department generally supplies supporting documentation and guidance regarding price changes and inflation-specific accounts, services, or supply categories.

Revenue Budget

Revenue is defined as money received for products or services provided to customers. Pharmacy revenues consist primarily of patient charges. Patient charges may arise from doses administered in an inpatient setting or from prescriptions dispensed in an outpatient setting. Pharmacies may also generate revenue by providing professional services, including consultation, management of research studies, providing education and other support services, and for medication therapy management.

Inpatient pharmacy revenues appear on patients' hospital bills as charges. A total of all charges posted by the pharmacy to all bills for an accounting period (e.g., a month) are reported as the pharmacy's gross revenue. Few, if any, payers actually pay full charge for pharmacy items. However, the development of a revenue budget remains an important component of the budget process. Charges offer an opportunity to track the operations of the pharmacy and serve as a proxy for net revenue after discounts and allowances.

Outpatient (retail) pharmacy revenue is often posted in a similar fashion as prescriptions are filled. The pharmacy contracts with a third party—insurance provider, state Medicaid program, or pharmacy benefits manager (PBM)—to fill prescriptions at a fixed rate based on medication costs and service fees. Rate structures are often based on a percentage of a benchmark drug cost and a filling fee. Outpatient prescription payments are handled electronically at the time of dispensing; generally referred to as adjudication at the point of service.

The pharmacy may also bill and receive payment for professional services, including management oversight of nursing homes, prescription plans, and medication therapy management (MTM). Budgeting for these fees and revenues can be accomplished in a similar fashion by estimating work volumes and fees received in detail over the course of the budget year.

Pharmacy revenue can be forecast from workload volume and from supply expense. Because a detailed volume budget has been developed for the pharmacy, the charges associated with this volume can be forecast. However, because most pharmacy charges are driven by the cost of service, including drug cost, it is important to account for the influence of changes in case mix and new services, the impact of price changes in specific drugs, and the overall effect of increased drug supply cost. In addition, revenue changes set by the health system's CFO are often set as an overall increase in the department's gross revenue. The pharmacy manager must develop a detailed plan that meets the overall revenue target using the expense budget as a foundation. Benchmarking performance across the fiscal year and adjusting services and targets requires an in-depth, detailed plan and an understanding of current activity.

Budgeting for a New Program

New pharmacy programs that involve operating expense must also be considered carefully and planned in detail. New drug and supply expense, additional personnel, and other expenses merit careful consideration. The budget for a new pharmacy program should be considered a smaller version of the budget process identified above. A spreadsheet identifying the costs by category as described above and as outlined in Tables 3.1 and 3.2

Table 3.2. Pharmacy Operating Budget

INPATIENT PHARMACY	JAN	FEB	MAR	APR	MAY
PATIENT SERVICES REVENUE					
INPATIENT SERVICES					
ANCILLARY SERVICES	7,880,727	8,485,475	8,822,211	8,714,977	7,949,128
TOTAL INPATIENT REVENUE	7,880,727	8,485,475	8,822,211	8,714,977	7,949,128
OUTPATIENT SERVICES					
SPECIAL MEDICAL SERVICES	1,183,946	1,274,799	1,325,387	1,309,278	1,194,222
EMERGENCY SERVICES	102,952	110,852	115,251	113,850	103,845
TOTAL OUTPATIENT REVENUE	1,286,898	1,385,651	1,440,638	1,423,128	1,298,067
PATIENT SERVICES REVENUE	9,167,625	9,871,126	10,262,849	10,138,105	9,247,195
DEDUCTION FOR CONTRACTUAL	(5,075,959)	(5,653,838)	(5,900,828)	(5,803,603)	(5,292,160)
TOTAL CONTRACTUAL ADJUSTMENT	(5,075,959)	(5,653,838)	(5,900,828)	(5,803,603)	(5,292,160)
NET PATIENT REVENUE	4,091,666	4,217,288	4,362,021	4,334,502	3,955,035
SALES-NP DRUG SALES	15,711	16,916	17,588	17,374	15,847
TOTAL OTHER OPERATING REVENUE	15,711	16,916	17,588	17,374	15,847
TOTAL REVENUE	4,107,377	4,234,204	4,379,609	4,351,876	3,970,882
SALARY-MGMT & SUPERVISION	32,243	32,485	32,485	31,216	32,703
SALARY-TECHNICIAN	359,852	360,198	361,293	344,871	364,614
SALARY-SUPPORT STAFF	9,957	10,043	10,043	9,586	10,043
SALARY-OTHER	2,057	2,057	2,057	1,964	2,057
TOTAL SALARIES	404,109	404,783	405,878	387,637	409,417
WAGES-TECHNICIAN	32,930	33,180	33,391	32,068	33,695
WAGES-AIDES & ORDERLIES	4,651	4,664	4,664	4,452	4,669
TOTAL WAGES	37,581	37,844	38,055	36,520	38,364
OVERTIME-TECHNICIAN	9,805	9,818	9,845	9,845	9,880
OVERTIME-SUPPORT STAFF	367	370	370	370	370
TOTAL SALARIES OVERTIME	10,172	10,188	10,215	10,215	10,250
OVERTIME-SUPPORT STAFF	171	172	172	172	172
TOTAL WAGE OVERTIME	171	172	172	172	172
SHIFT-DIFFERENTIAL TECHNICIAN	9,146	9,146	9,146	9,146	9,146
TOTAL SHIFT DIFFERENTIAL	9,146	9,146	9,146	9,146	9,146
ON CALL-TECHNICIAN	262	262	262	262	262
TOTAL ON CALL	262	262	262	262	262
VACANCY REDUCTION-SALARY	(6,428)	(6,439)	(6,458)	(6,163)	(6,545)
TOTAL OTHER PERSONNEL	(6,428)	(6,439)	(6,458)	(6,163)	(6,545)

Table 3.2. Pharmacy Operating Budget (*Continued*)

JUN	JUL	AUG	SEP	OCT	NOV	DEC	TOTAL
8,363,443	7,568,410	8,069,571	7,671,084	7,646,254	7,621,188	8,239,793	97,032,261
8,363,443	7,568,410	8,069,571	7,671,084	7,646,254	7,621,188	8,239,793	97,032,261
1,256,466	1,137,025	1,212,317	1,152,451	1,148,720	1,144,955	1,237,889	14,577,455
109,258	98,872	105,419	100,213	99,889	99,561	107,643	1,267,605
1,365,724	1,235,897	1,317,736	1,252,664	1,248,609	1,244,516	1,345,532	15,845,060
9,729,167	8,804,307	9,387,307	8,923,748	8,894,863	8,865,704	9,585,325	112,877,321
(5,449,855)	(4,905,266)	(5,130,224)	(4,890,408)	(4,876,444)	(4,935,855)	(5,233,475)	(63,147,915)
(5,449,855)	(4,905,266)	(5,130,224)	(4,890,408)	(4,876,444)	(4,935,855)	(5,233,475)	(63,147,915)
4,279,312	3,899,041	4,257,083	4,033,340	4,018,419	3,929,849	4,351,850	49,729,406
16,673	15,088	16,087	15,293	15,243	15,193	16,426	193,439
16,673	15,088	16,087	15,293	15,243	15,193	16,426	193,439
4,295,985	3,914,129	4,273,170	4,048,633	4,033,662	3,945,042	4,368,276	49,922,845
34,388	31,700	30,191	34,720	31,700	33,210	33,210	390,251
382,704	350,186	333,908	384,153	351,847	369,005	371,322	4,333,953
10,650	9,723	9,261	10,724	9,791	10,257	10,257	120,335
2,151	1,964	1,870	2,151	1,964	2,057	2,119	24,468
429,893	393,573	375,230	431,748	395,302	414,529	416,908	4,869,007
35,227	32,163	30,638	35,234	32,212	33,781	33,880	398,399
4,881	4,457	4,245	4,887	4,462	4,725	4,791	55,548
40,108	36,620	34,883	40,121	36,674	38,506	38,671	453,947
9,900	9,923	9,941	9,947	9,991	10,007	10,072	118,974
376	376	376	378	378	378	382	4,491
10,276	10,299	10,317	10,325	10,369	10,385	10,454	123,465
172	172	172	172	172	174	176	2,069
172	172	172	172	172	174	176	2,069
9,146	9,146	9,146	9,146	9,146	9,146	9,146	109,752
9,146	9,146	9,146	9,146	9,146	9,146	9,146	109,752
262	262	262	262	262	262	262	3,144
262	262	262	262	262	262	262	3,144
(6,860)	(6,278)	(5,989)	(6,895)	(6,322)	(6,634)	(6,675)	(77,686)
(6,860)	(6,278)	(5,989)	(6,895)	(6,322)	(6,634)	(6,675)	(77,686)

Table 3.2. Pharmacy Operating Budget (*Continued*)

INPATIENT PHARMACY	JAN	FEB	MAR	APR	MAY
FICA	33,692	36,278	37,718	37,259	33,985
GROUP HEALTH INSURANCE	40,517	43,626	45,355	44,806	40,869
RETIREMENT BENEFITS	26,957	29,026	30,178	29,810	27,191
WORKER'S COMP INSURANCE	2,323	2,501	2,602	2,569	2,343
GROUP LIFE INSURANCE	1,789	1,927	2,004	1,979	1,805
DISABILITY INSURANCE	1,464	1,577	1,640	1,619	1,477
TOTAL EMPLOYEE BENEFITS	106,742	114,935	119,497	118,042	107,670
TOTAL PERSONNEL EXPENSE	561,755	570,891	576,767	555,831	568,736
DRUGS	1,723,980	1,573,726	1,647,390	1,636,774	1,456,395
INTRAVENOUS SUPPLIES	30,092	32,401	33,689	33,278	30,353
BLOOD & BLOOD PRODUCTS	163,614	458,717	465,707	450,639	447,582
REAGENT & CHEMICALS	9,066	9,761	10,150	10,025	9,144
GENERAL MED/SURG SUPPLY	12,549	13,512	14,049	13,878	12,658
TOTAL SPECIAL SUPPLIES	1,939,301	2,088,117	2,170,985	2,144,594	1,956,132
OFFICE SUPPLIES	489	527	548	541	493
OFFICE EQUIPMENT	57	61	64	63	57
COMMUNICATION EQUIPMENT	148	159	165	163	149
COMPUTER SUPPLIES	42	45	47	47	43
TOTAL GENERAL SUPPLIES	736	792	824	814	742
REPAIR OF MEDICAL EQUIP	229	247	258	254	231
REPAIR NON-MEDICAL EQUIP	92	99	103	102	93
FREIGHT	8	8	8	8	8
PRINTING	4,632	4,987	5,184	5,122	4,672
PHARMACY SCHOOL SERVICE CONTRACT	41,539	41,539	41,539	41,539	41,539
GENERAL SERVICES	28	30	32	31	29
TOTAL PURCHASED SERVICES	46,528	46,910	47,124	47,056	46,572
TELEPHONE	489	527	547	541	493
TOTAL OTHER EXPENSES	489	527	547	541	493
TOTAL NON-PERSONNEL EXPENSES	1,987,054	2,136,346	2,219,480	2,193,005	2,003,939
TOTAL OPERATING EXPENSES	2,548,809	2,707,237	2,796,247	2,748,836	2,572,675
TOTAL EXPENSES	2,548,809	2,707,237	2,796,247	2,748,836	2,572,675
NET EXCESS	1,558,568	1,526,967	1,583,362	1,603,040	1,398,207

Table 3.2. Pharmacy Operating Budget (*Continued*)

JUN	JUL	AUG	SEP	OCT	NOV	DEC	TOTAL
35,756	32,357	34,500	32,796	32,690	32,583	35,227	414,841
42,999	38,912	41,488	39,439	39,312	39,183	42,363	498,869
28,608	25,889	27,603	26,240	26,154	26,069	28,185	331,910
2,465	2,231	2,379	2,261	2,254	2,247	2,429	28,604
1,899	1,718	1,832	1,742	1,736	1,730	1,871	22,032
1,554	1,406	1,499	1,425	1,421	1,416	1,531	18,029
113,281	102,513	109,301	103,903	103,567	103,228	111,606	1,314,285
596,278	546,307	533,322	588,782	549,170	569,596	580,548	6,797,983
1,534,187	1,385,952	1,508,429	1,382,728	1,402,981	1,384,655	1,519,980	18,157,177
31,935	28,900	30,813	29,292	29,197	29,101	31,463	370,514
469,026	426,834	424,396	454,651	428,451	440,773	453,616	5,084,006
9,621	8,706	9,283	8,825	8,796	8,767	9,479	111,623
13,318	12,052	12,850	12,215	12,176	12,136	13,121	154,514
2,058,087	1,862,444	1,985,771	1,887,711	1,881,601	1,875,432	2,027,659	23,877,834
519	470	501	476	475	473	511	6,023
60	55	58	55	55	55	59	699
157	142	151	144	143	143	154	1,818
45	41	43	41	41	41	44	520
781	708	753	716	714	712	768	9,060
244	220	235	223	223	222	240	2,826
98	89	95	90	90	89	97	1,137
8	7	8	7	7	7	9	93
4,915	4,448	4,743	4,508	4,494	4,479	4,843	57,027
41,539	41,539	41,539	41,539	41,539	41,539	41,542	498,471
30	27	29	28	27	27	30	348
46,834	46,330	46,649	46,395	46,380	46,363	46,761	559,902
519	470	501	476	475	473	511	6,022
519	470	501	476	475	473	511	6,022
2,106,221	1,909,952	2,033,674	1,935,298	1,929,170	1,922,980	2,075,699	24,452,818
2,702,499	2,456,259	2,566,996	2,524,080	2,478,340	2,492,576	2,656,247	31,250,801
2,702,499	2,456,259	2,566,996	2,524,080	2,478,340	2,492,576	2,656,247	31,250,801
1,593,486	1,457,870	1,706,174	1,524,553	1,555,322	1,452,466	1,712,029	18,672,044

should be prepared. A narrative supporting the new program, including objectives, program description, advantages, competition, required resources, program outcomes, and a bottom line, should be developed. If a capital expense such as renovation or purchase of equipment is required, this should be done in concert with the capital budget process described earlier. Many organizations also consider indirect costs for new programs, although these costs are generally not a significant part of the annual budget process for the pharmacy.

The first step in proposing a budget for a new pharmacy program or service should be a review of the existing pharmacy operations, workload, and budget to ensure that current resources are leveraged effectively. Some health systems engage a separate budget review process for new programs and require specific reports, forms, and presentations beyond the formal annual operating budget process.

Budget Negotiation, Review, and Approval

After all of the health system departments have developed their respective budgets, they are returned to the budget office for a roll up, in which the individual department budgets are aggregated and the first version of a working health system budget is created. Because the budget development process takes place somewhat independently at the department level, the resulting budget draft may need substantial work. The CFO works to balance the budget, to identify errors and problematic assumptions, and to develop a workable plan.

The health system's administration, led by the CEO and CFO, and advised by the board and medical leadership, set priorities for funding programs and may ask departments to reduce or otherwise modify their budget requests. In some cases, a department may be asked to explain or justify its projections and to rework the budget plan to meet a projection more agreeable to administration. In the case of pharmacy, projected growth in service volumes, addition, and usage of new, expensive drugs on the formulary or the basis for drug price inflation may be the focus of this review.

Pharmacy budgets are evaluated against prior fiscal year experience to ensure that they are realistic and reasonable. The integrity of the development process and the level of support for key assumptions, such as pharmacy volumes, drug price increases, and new drug adoption are also a factor in considering how the pharmacy budget is accepted. The record of accomplishment of the pharmacy and pharmacy manager in meeting prior budgets often has significant influence on the outcome of the current budget review. A thoughtful, well-developed budget supported by data has the greatest chance of success and provides the health system with the best forecast of the future.

In the negotiation process, budget requests may be deferred to future years, sent back to be re-scoped and reworked, or denied outright. Budget development is both a rational and a political process; negotiations center on the organization's highest priorities and on the quality of preparation and presentation made by the respective department leaders. Preparation is critical to ensure the best response from leadership and the highest utility outcome for pharmacy and for the health system.

Monitoring the Budget

Volume, expense, and revenue data are collected in real time by the health system's data financial management systems. Monthly activity and financial reports are provided to pharmacy managers. These reports should be reviewed and action taken to ensure that the pharmacy department meets targets set during the budget process. Alternatively, if changes occur, such as declining prescription volume, deferral of a new program or service, or a delay in the introduction of a new drug, and the pharmacy will not meet the budget target as a result, regular review will ensure that action is taken to resolve the problem or to appropriately alter the budget to reflect the new reality.

Budget Variance Analysis

Budget performance should be reviewed monthly. The monthly operating statements show expenses incurred each month and are compared to the budget for the current month and for the fiscal year-to-date. A budget variance is a difference between the budgeted amount and the actual amount spent for a period. Variances are generally evaluated monthly, and an assessment is made of the monthly variance and the variance from the start of the fiscal year-to-date. Variances can be described as positive (expenses lower than forecast; revenues higher than forecast) or negative (expenses higher than forecast; revenues lower than forecast). Variances can be absolute: the total actual amount is higher irrespective of volume, or volume-adjusted, or the variance in cost cannot be explained solely by changes in activity volume.

Some variation in expense and revenue is expected. Pharmacy leaders are expected to have a continuing, current understanding of the nature and source of budget variance. Their understanding should include their clinical therapeutics and pharmacy service operations knowledge, combined with an understanding of the business principles and practices. The regular discipline of monthly analysis provides an opportunity to understand the pharmacy's contribution to the health system. Budget variance analysis is covered in detail in chapter 8.

Conclusion

Thoughtful financial management is critical to the success of the organization's pharmaceutical care plan. Development of an organized budget based on data, monitoring of variance, and the assessment and management of costs and revenues supports the modern pharmacy department.

Pharmacists are charged with maintaining a medication use system that provides the highest quality of care and serves the medical and pharmaceutical needs of the patient to its fullest. However, in a health system in which resources are finite, the pharmacy leader must monitor, allocate, and actively manage financial, pharmaceutical, and professional resources to achieve success.

References

1. American Society of Health-System Pharmacists. ASHP guidelines: minimum standard for pharmaceutical services in ambulatory care. *Am J Health-Syst Pharm.* 1999; 56:1744–53.

2. American Society of Health-System Pharmacists. ASHP guidelines: minimum standard for pharmacies in hospitals. *Am J Health-Syst Pharm.* 1995; 52: 2711–7.

3. Hoffman JM, Shah ND, Vermeulen LC et al. Projecting future drug expenditures—2005. *Am J Health-Syst Pharm.* 2008; 65: 234–53.

Forecasting Pharmaceutical Expenditures

Lee C. Vermeulen
James M. Hoffman
Nilay D. Shah

Introduction

One of the most challenging aspects of financial management in health system pharmacy is the forecasting of future medication expenditures. Drugs are the largest component of every health system pharmacy department's operating budget, so accurate financial planning for drug purchases is crucial to the department's overall financial management efforts. Further, with continuing growth in drug expenditures, drug expense represents a meaningful component of the entire hospitals operating budget. As a result, pharmacy leadership performance in this arena will attract scrutiny from the institution's senior leadership. Developing an accurate prediction of future spending on drugs requires a manager to have a clear understanding of the phenomena that will influence future pharmaceutical expenditure trends. It also requires retaining accurate information about patterns in past medication spending to form the basis for future planning.

Figure 4.1 illustrates a conceptual model that outlines the relationships between the drivers of drug expenditures and the actions that pharmacy leaders must take to manage medication technology and expenditures. As described in detail below, a number of medication cost drivers exist, and the pharmacy leader must respond with multiple planning approaches that are supported by data analysis. Further, a successful plan requires constant vigilance and assessment of medication use and expenditures. While this chapter focuses on financial planning, Figure 4.1 illustrates that strategic and tactical planning is also need for successful drug expenditure management.

The drivers of medication expenditure patterns are complex, including higher order and external factors that are often uncontrollable by any individual. For example, demographic changes in the United States population (i.e., the "graying" of the population), which have increased the US chronic disease burden and resulted in increased medication use, is an example of a higher order phenomenon that is well beyond the control of a pharmacy leader. On a more practical level, Food and Drug Administration (FDA) approval of a new, innovative, and expensive medication is an example of an external phenomenon that is largely uncontrollable, but to some extent pharmacy leaders can proactive plan for these cost drivers.

Other factors within the health system often related to organizational decisions regarding the scope and nature of care provided, may be somewhat controllable by a pharmacy

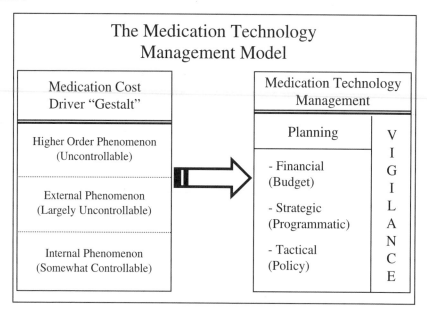

Figure 4.1. Medication Management Technology Model

manager (internal phenomenon as listed in Figure 4.1). For example, an organizational decision to open a new dialysis center which will add several high-cost products to the pharmacy drug budget may be influenced by information provided by a pharmacy leader, but the decision will ultimately rest elsewhere. In these situations, pharmacy leaders must be proactive and assertive to provide relevant information to health system leaders. Some internal phenomena are more easily influenced by a pharmacy manager, provided they are recognized and understood. For example, a decision to replace an expensive brand-name drug with a newly approved generic drug is in the purview of the pharmacy leader (or with a Pharmacy and Therapeutics Committee with which the pharmacy leader should have substantial influence).

With an understanding of the drivers of medication expenditures, pharmacy leaders can reflect upon local trends in utilization and spending to develop robust and accurate forecasts. For nearly 2 decades, the *American Journal of Health-System Pharmacy* has published annual expenditure forecasts that can provide guidance to pharmacy leaders as they develop financial plans and budgets. Recent installments have also included budgeting guidance, proposing a step-wise approach to the creation of an expenditure forecast.[1,2,3] This chapter details that approach, providing guidance to the pharmacy leader striving to forecast and manage medication expenditures. Table 4.1 summarizes the steps of the recommended approach to forecasting drug expenditures.

Step 1: Obtain and Analyze Data

Forecasting the future starts with a clear understanding of the past and present. The lack of valid, reliable data necessary for guiding financial decisions is one of the most challenging aspects of financial management in health systems. Financial data must be obtained, validated, and understood at the beginning of the forecasting process. Departmental financial statements,

Table 4.1. Summary of Steps to Forecast Drug Expenditures

Step	Action
1.	Obtain and Analyze Data
2.	Review Past Performance
3.	Build High Priority Medication Budget
4.	Build New Product Budget
5.	Build the Non Formulary Budget
6.	Build the Low-Priority Budget
7.	Establish a Cost Containment Plan
8.	Finalize Medication Budget
9.	Vigilance

including the previous completed fiscal year, the current fiscal year-to-date, and reports estimating expenditures through the end of the current fiscal year should be reviewed.

When analyzed at the drug product level, 60 to 80 drugs typically make up the majority (70–80%) of a hospital drug budget. Drug cost data analysis should therefore focus on the drugs that make up the majority of the drug budget. Table 4.2 provides an example of an approach to organize drug purchase data in an overall manner. This approach allows the pharmacy leader to understand the "big picture" view of the organizations top drug expenditures, and how the rankings of drug expenditures have changed over recent fiscal years, which will help focus and track expenditure management efforts on a global level.

A critical component of this step is obtaining data both from purchasing sources and from actual medication usage. Although many health systems monitor purchase data (acquired from wholesalers and distributors) as the source of financial reports, simply understanding that a certain quantity of a particular medication was acquired will not provide useful information regarding its eventual use (who prescribed the medication, in what dose, for what patient, with what diagnosis, etc.). In order to secure sufficient information to complete the next step in this process, data on actual usage must be obtained. This information is often available through medication use evaluation modules in pharmacy operations systems. Data may also be acquired through cost accounting systems and may need to be combined with data from admission/discharge and transfer systems.

While many health systems monitor purchase data (drugs actually acquired from wholesalers, distributors, or inventory systems) as the source of financial reports, only understanding that a certain quantity of a particular medication was acquired will not provide useful information regarding its eventual use (who prescribed the medication, in what dose, for what patient, with what diagnosis, etc.). In order to secure sufficient information to complete the next step in this process, it is essential that data on actual utilization be obtained and analyzed. This information is often available through medication use evaluation modules in pharmacy operations systems or through an institution's data warehouse. Data may also be acquired through health system cost-accounting systems, and may need to be obtained

Table 4.2. Example Simple Table to Track Drug Expenditures using Drug Purchase Data

Rank current FY07 projected cost	Rank past FY cost	Drug (Include all formulations as one line)	Total expenditures immediate past FY	Total expenditures 2 FY previous	$ Change between 2 previous FY (%)	Current expenditures FY to date (annualized)	Change current FY (annualized) to previous FY (%)
1	2	Enoxaparin					
2	1	Epoetin					
3	3	Pegfilgrastim					
4	5	Infliximab					
5	6	Cefepime					
6	10	Eptifibitide					
7	7	Rituximab					
8	15	Pipercillin/Tazobactam					
9	13	Iohexol					
10	8	Ceftriaxone					
11	21	Irinotecan					
12	18	Sevoflurane					
13	20	Caspofungin					
14	22	Pneumococcal vaccine, diphtheria conjugate					
15							

Continue to table to include all drugs that compose majority of drug expenditures (typically 60–80 drugs)

FY is Fiscal Year.

and combined with data from admission/discharge and transfer systems. Drug use data are especially useful when use of specific high cost drugs are organized and examined by medical service or area of use.

See Table 4.3 for an example of one approach to organizing drug use and expenditure data for a high cost drug. Multiple similar tables for other high cost drugs should be organized and reviewed for a complete picture of drug use and expenditures. This strategy typically requires the effort of a skilled data analyst to set up and organize these data on recurring basis. As already noted, data analysis should focus on the top 60 to 80 drugs that make up the majority of drug expenditures. Organizing drug use and cost data will often be a long term project, and organizations should start with the top 20 to 30 drugs and add additional drugs over time. These reports should be produced and reviewed on a routine basis (e.g. monthly or quarterly), therefore making drug expenditure management an ongoing effort.

The validation of data drawn from purchasing records and usage sources should include a reconciliation of discrepancies. Purchasing records may indicate a higher level of medication expenditure than usage records if inventory levels are increasing, either intentionally (for example, if "buying long" to avoid problems associated with an impending shortage) or because of inefficient purchasing and inventory control practices. Such a discrepancy can also indicate pilferage.[4] If purchasing records indicate a lower level of expenditure than usage records, other explanations may be possible. In many institutions, maintaining medication pricing information is often a challenge. As prices change, discrepancies between purchase price and charge can appear. Health systems should expect their group-purchasing organizations to assist with this aspect of data acquisition in support of financial planning, particularly with expected price increases.

Other sources of information should be obtained in addition to data on drug spending and usage. One of the most underappreciated sources of information are the pharmacists and physicians of your own health system. Early in the process of developing an expenditure forecast, pharmacy leaders should interview key individuals within their health system. These health-care professionals will help identify where new programs will be developed in the coming year, where expansions in existing programs will occur, and how these changes may affect medication expenditures. Individuals should be asked to predict the emergence of new medications in their area of practice and to reflect on changes in existing medication usage that may take place.

Step 2: Review Past Performance

Once financial statements are validated, they should be evaluated for trends and patterns. Comparisons of actual expenditures to the budget should be made, as well as comparisons in actual usage between fiscal periods (one month in one fiscal year compared to the same month the previous fiscal year; one month in one fiscal year compared to the previous month in the same fiscal year; etc.). Any discrepancies or unexpected changes should be explored. Simply identifying and explaining causes of variances is not sufficient. The pharmacy leader must understand the implications of these changes and their relationship to future expenditure patterns. When discrepancies between purchasing and usage records are seen, the pharmacy leader must distinguish between price and usage changes as the cause.

Table 4.3. Example Table of Drug Use and Cost Organized by Medical Service*

Drug	Service	Metric	August	September	October	November	December	Total
epoetin alfa	Nephrology	Expenditure	$9,457.40	$5,116.84	$2,507.47	$6,213.68	$11,176.65	$34,472.03
		Patients	36	24	13	28	32	133
		Doses	102	56	28	57	83	326
	Transplant	Expenditure	$1,263.97	$859.41	$2,536.21	$4,013.97	$2,896.45	$11,570.02
		Patients	5	8	5	14	13	45
		Doses	10	12	19	43	35	119
	Critical Care	Expenditure		$2,831.01	$2,102.71	$2,872.32	$1,771.06	$9,577.10
		Patients		8	5	7	6	26
		Doses		7	11	9	9	36
	Oncology	Expenditure	$2,558.80	$809.69	$2,086.86	$849.30	$2,245.02	$8,549.67
		Patients	6	5	6	4	4	25
		Doses	33	12	15	6	16	82
	Hematology	Expenditure	$809.11	$2,022.15	$1,617.72	$2,426.58	$808.86	$7,684.42
		Patients	2	5	3	5	2	17
		Doses	2	5	4	6	2	19
	All Others	Expenditure	$414.63	$1,819.94	$970.63	$1,253.73	$2,649.02	$7,107.96
		Patients	3	3	1	2	4	13
		Doses	6	24	12	18	35	95

*Data fictional.

For example, if purchases of a particular medication over a one month period of time total $100,000, yet it appears only $50,000 of that medication was utilized (administered to patients), several explanations are possible. It is possible that the standing inventory of the pharmacy has been increased by $50,000 (which may be an inventory management problem, or a deliberate decision to add inventory in response to an impending product shortage). It is possible that a large quantity of medication was prepared and wasted (an unfortunate occurrence with many high-cost injectable medications). It is possible that the price of the medication changed dramatically and was not updated in one of the two systems (either in the purchasing file or the utilization file). Of greater concern, the explanation may be that $50,000 worth of the medication was pilfered (inventory shrinkage). Identifying the cause of the variance, and responding accordingly, is a critical step in this process.

As variances are identified and understood, implications for the financial plan must be considered. Will a trend in higher cost or higher usage continue, plateau, or moderate in the future? Understanding the cause of the trend will help to make that determination and to plan a financial management response.

An increase in spending on a particular agent may be tracked back to the start of a new clinical program. Based on discussions with the physicians leading that program, the pharmacy leader may learn that the program is expected to grow (suggesting the need for increased involvement of clinical pharmacists to ensure efficient medication use), or that the new program has reached its intended capacity (suggesting that an observed upward trend may reach its peak and not grow further).

When variances are found that are attributed to price increases, a cost-containment strategy involving a change in a preferred formulary drug or the implementation of a new therapeutic interchange may be considered as a tactical response. When a variance is attributed to usage changes, the development of a clinical practice guideline or formulary restriction may be considered. As part of this step in the process, observed trends should lead to a general understanding of future expenditure patterns and should provide the starting point for the development of cost-containment plans.

Step 3: Build High-Priority Medication Budget

As a pharmacy leader begins to understand past performance and future expenditure trends, a list of high-priority medications should emerge. In most organizations, a list of 60 to 80 drug products represents as much as 80 percent of total annual expenditures. The list of drug products should be constructed at the level of "molecular entity," not as a drug product line item. For example, acetaminophen should not appear in this list as acetaminophen tablets as one item and acetaminophen liquid as another. Expenditures for all dosage forms of acetaminophen should be combined into a single number and included once. The drug list should be rank-ordered by descending total expenditures, and the agents representing approximately 80 percent of total cumulative spending should be considered the high-priority agents. As the financial forecast is developed, most of the pharmacy leader's time should be devoted to understanding and managing these medications.

For each high-priority medication, past purchasing and usage trends should be identified. Although the rank order of the high-priority product list should be conducted at the molecular-entity level, as purchasing trends are evaluated, each individual line item (e.g., at the NDC level) should be considered. Past pricing trends, the potential for brand-to-generic shifts, and other future price-related changes should be the focus of that evaluation. Each high-priority medication should also be evaluated using usage data, quantifying usage by prescriber and at the patient level (evaluating who prescribed the medication, for which patients, diagnoses, conditions, etc.). For each individual high-priority medication, a specific prediction of expenditures should be made, considering both expected price and usage changes. These product-specific "budgets" are then combined to complete the high-priority drug budget.

A pharmacy leader must also consider adding products that may not make the list based on recent purchase trends to the high-priority list. For example, newly approved medications that are expensive may not have yet diffused into routine practice, but, if expenditures can be expected to rise substantially over the following year, these medications should be included, with a product-specific profile for each. In some institutions, inexpensive products that are controversial (targets of cost containment or quality improvement) should also be included, because the product-specific profile can serve as a tracking mechanism to monitor the impact of the intervention.

For example, meperidine is an inexpensive medication that is associated with many costly adverse effects. While the total expenditure on this agent may not place it in the high-priority category, having it included will allow managers to monitor utilization at the prescriber and patient levels, tracking the impact of efforts to reduce use.

After a profile for each medication in the high-priority list is developed, the high-priority budget can be calculated by summing over all products in that list. Approximately 80 percent of total medication expenditures for the following fiscal year will then be budgeted.

Step 4: Build New Product Budget

Construct a separate expenditure forecast for new medications expected to be approved during the subsequent fiscal year. Budgeting for new agents on a product-specific basis can be far more accurate than simply adding an arbitrary amount of money in the budget that is intended to pay for any unknown new agents that arrive the subsequent year. This process allows pharmacy leaders not only to plan for the financial impact of the new agent but also to consider programmatic changes that may be necessary to accommodate the new medication. For example, the emergence of new, high-cost biological agents administered in the clinic setting may suggest the need to increase clinical pharmacist staffing in a hospital's ambulatory infusion center to manage both distribution and clinical interventions.

A pharmacy leader should draw information regarding new medications in the drug-development pipeline from several sources, including group-purchasing organizations, the annual expenditure forecast published in *AJHP*, and interviews with physicians and pharmacists. As each new medication is identified, expected price and volume of use must be predicted. Price estimates are particularly challenging to develop. Some estimates can be drawn from the cost of existing therapies in the same therapeutic class or from the price of other agents used to treat the condition for which the new agent will be used. Yet even the best pricing estimate will have considerable uncertainty, and conservative (high) estimates are often made.

More accurate usage estimates can be developed. By understanding the expected indications for the medication in development, it is possible to use data resources available within most

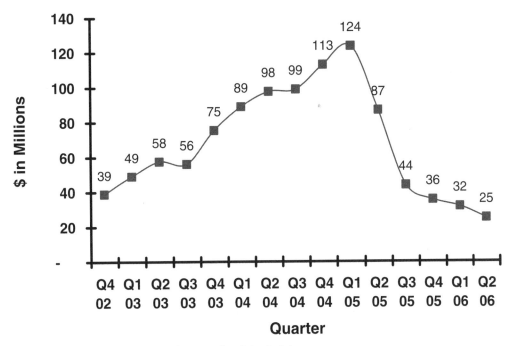

Figure 4.2. Quarterly Expenditures for Nesiritide

institutions to determine the number of patients who may be treated with that new agent. Those estimates can be based on the number of patients receiving particular medications that the new medication is expected to replace or add on to or based on the number of patients with a particular diagnosis. For example, if, based on input from infectious diseases physicians, a pharmacy leader discovers an antibiotic for gram-positive infections is being developed, it

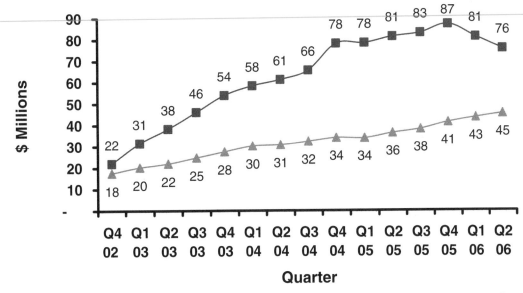

Figure 4.3. Quarterly Expenditures for Caspofungin (Squares) and Voriconazole (Triangles)

is possible to calculate the proportion of patients currently receiving other antibiotics with gram-positive activity who may be candidates for the new agent once it is approved.

As the forecast for new medications is developed, the expected approval time for each agent should be noted. An agent expected to be approved near the end of an upcoming fiscal year will have less impact than one that is expected to arrive early in that year. The impact of diffusion patterns should also be considered. As any innovation is brought to the market, it will diffuse into routine practice over time. As shown in Figures 4.2 and 4.3, rates of diffusion vary from product to product.[5] The pharmacy leader must factor in that expected rate of diffusion as the expenditure forecast for new agents is developed.

Step 5: Build the Nonformulary Budget

Insofar as the medication formulary of any health system reflects the standard of care for medication use within that system, the use of nonformulary agents represents both potentially inappropriate prescribing and a possible cost-containment opportunity. However, few organizations track nonformulary medication use in ways that facilitate the identification of those potential quality- and cost-improvement initiatives. These opportunities are emphasized by including expenditures for nonformulary medications as a separate component of the overall medication budget. For high-cost nonformulary agents and for those agents identified as potential targets for quality- or cost-improvement intervention, product-specific profiles (as described in step 3) should be developed. For the remaining portion of the nonformulary budget, a budget can be constructed by calculating a volume-adjusted estimate of expenditures that includes a fixed-price inflation factor, as described in detail in the next step.

Step 6: Build the Low-Priority Budget

After considering high-priority medications, new agents expected to arrive on the market, and nonformulary agents, a large number of medications will remain unbudgeted. The total cost of these products, as a proportion of the entire medication budget, however, will be small. It is appropriate to compute a "residual" budget for these drugs using a simple forecasting method.

The influence of patient volume in this calculation must be considered. Although many group-purchasing organizations provide annual estimates of overall forecasted price increase, simply applying that estimate to total purchases to produce a future expenditure estimate is not appropriate. Patient volume must also be considered using the following method. First, compute total expenditures for remaining unbudgeted agents in the current fiscal year (annualize year-to-date expenditures if that entire fiscal year has not yet been completed). Then divide that total by the number of discharges during that same period of time (again, annualized if necessary). Next, apply the price inflation factor to the expenditure per discharge figure, and, finally, project the next fiscal year expenditure total using the estimate of total discharges expected during that next fiscal year. This volume-adjusted approach is far more accurate, appropriate, and simple.

A note on the annualization procedures used in this step is necessary. Because months contain varying numbers of days, annualizing by dividing year-to-date expenditures by the number of months completed and multiplying by 12 introduces errors. For example, if a health system has a July-to-June fiscal year (starting July 1 and ending June 30 of the following year), there will be 181 days in the first half of their fiscal year and 184 days in the second half. Although the difference of 3 days may seem trivial, it represents nearly a 1 percent difference, or over $80,000 in a $10 million drug budget (enough to fund a substantial portion of a pharmacist's salary and fringe). As net margins continue to shrink in health systems, even small variances become significant. Annualization should be calculated using the number of fiscal days completed and remaining.

The pharmacy leader must also recognize that hospital admission patterns are not necessarily stable from month to month in any given year. Some hospitals experience higher volume in some months, and that pattern is often stable and predictable. An evaluation of monthly volume over 10 to 15 years can provide a valid adjuster that should be applied to data being annualized. For example, if volume is shown to consistently increase by 3 percent in the second half of a given fiscal year as compared to the first half of that fiscal year, the estimated volume should be adjusted as it is annualized.

The total low-priority budget should be calculated and added to the high-priority budget, the new medication budget, and the nonformulary medication budget to create the initial estimate of the total medication budget. This initial snapshot of expected expenditures should be compared to any spending target set by the organization and will guide the size of the cost-containment objective for the coming year.

Step 7: Establish a Cost-Containment Plan

Throughout the budgeting process, the pharmacy leader should maintain a list of ideas for possible quality-improvement and cost-containment initiatives. During the data gathering and analysis steps, while interviewing physicians and other thought leaders, document areas in which targeted interventions may improve quality and reduce cost. Although most initiatives may come from the high-priority budgeted items (because their cost is high, the potential for savings is also high), do not overlook less costly agents that may also be targeted for savings.

As cost-containment initiatives are identified, carefully document both the estimated savings (which should be taken out of the budget) and the tactical approach expected to achieve that reduction. In some cases it may be necessary to increase labor expense to achieve medication cost reduction. Tying requests for new positions to cost reduction is important, but, if new positions are denied, managers must also eliminate expected drug expenditure savings that will the not be achievable without that added manpower.

In considering cost containment, recognize that actual cost reduction (spending less in one year than the previous year) is seldom possible. Instead, most cost-containment opportunities succeed only in moderating the trend in increasing expenditures. For example, consider a cost-containment initiative that is successful in moderating the rate of increase for a particular medication from 30 percent per year (e.g., an increase from $200,000 in year 1 to $260,000 in year 2) to 10 percent per year (from $260,000 in year 2 to an estimated $286,000 in year 3). The initiative should be credited with a savings of 20 percent, or $52,000, in year 3. This savings is estimated based on the projected spending of $338,000 in year 3 if growth seen from year 1 to year 2 (30 percent) continues.

Moderating the growth trend, producing "cost avoidance," is arguably as relevant as actual cost reduction.

Furthermore, some cost-containment efforts must be continually conducted to achieve ongoing savings. Initiatives such as antibiotic stewardship programs that streamline anti-infective use produce savings that are only successful as long as manpower is devoted to the task. Should those human resources be redirected to focus on other interventions, growth in anti-infective use can be expected to rise to the level seen before the program was initiated. Therefore, it is appropriate to consider ongoing cost-containment efforts as part of the overall cost-containment plan from year to year, and the savings they produce should be counted as a part of the overall savings.

Step 8: Finalize Medication Budget

The final medication budget then becomes the sum of the high-priority, new medication, nonformulary, and low-priority budget components, minus the savings identified in the cost-containment plan. When the final budget is completed, document areas in which estimates included some degree of uncertainty. Given the finite amount of time and effort devoted to the budgeting process, some estimates will be necessary. By carefully documenting the areas in the budget in which potentially inaccurate estimates are made, it is possible to revisit the budget, to refine those estimates, and to reduce expenditure forecasts. For example, if the estimated expenditure growth for a particular high-priority medication is based on a conservative (and probably higher than actual) estimate of expected patient volume, that uncertainty should be documented on that particular medication profile in the high-priority budget. If hospital administration later returns to the pharmacy budget with a request for further reduction, the pharmacy leader can reconsider the budget for that particular high-priority medication and possibly reduce the estimated expenditure by calculating the expected volume growth more accurately.

As described in the nonformulary and low-priority medication steps above, developing volume-adjusted spending forecasts is also critical. If a medication budget increases from one period to the next, only a few potential categories of explanation exist. Medication prices may have increased. The use of higher-cost medications in situations where lower-cost medications were previously used may have increased (potentially suggesting inefficiency). Patient acuity may have increased, resulting in the need for more medications and more costly medications (not necessarily suggesting inefficiency). Finally, the total number of patients may have increased, resulting in more medication use (and again, not necessarily suggesting inefficient medication use). Appropriate budgeting and financial monitoring should focus on separating cost increases that are due to inefficient medication use from those that are appropriate and likely unavoidable. In the hospital setting, one important method for separating costs is to monitor expenditure trends as a function of medication expenditures per some unit of inpatient volume. Although some hospitals use patient days as a volume-adjusting denominator, hospital discharges should be used instead.

The logic behind this particular recommendation is important to understand. In most hospitals, cost-containment initiatives have focused attention on interventions that reduce length of stay as a means to reduce total cost. Although reducing an average length of stay does increase capacity (important for hospitals with limited capacity that must turn away potentially profitable admissions), the actual cost reduction will not be consistent from department to department. Recognize that drug expenditures (like some other resources consumed during an admission) do not occur in a linear fashion over the course of a hospital admission. Drug expenditures are often higher earlier in an admission (when high-cost medications are given) than later. Patients admitted to treat an infection of unknown pathogen may receive multiple high-cost, broad-spectrum antibiotics during the first 48 hours of admission. Once cultures and susceptibility results are known, therapy is often streamlined, and the total cost per day of antibiotic is lower. Similarly, in patients undergoing cardiac surgery, high-cost anesthetics and perioperative medications will be used early in the admission, but relatively low-cost agents will be used later in the admission. Shortened lengths of stay may reduce some costs, but because high-cost medications are used early in the admission, they will not be affected by eliminating the last day or two from any given admission.

If financial performance in medication expenditures is monitored on the basis of cost per patient day, as length of stay reduction initiatives succeed, performance will appear to worsen (medication expenditures will not change substantially, but the denominator will decrease, making that metric increase). A more appropriate measure of performance, recognizing the pattern of resource consumption over the course of an inpatient admission, should therefore be medication cost per discharge.

Step 9: Vigilance

After a medication budget is prepared using the first eight steps in this process, ongoing performance must be tracked. Fortunately, once these steps are followed, a great deal of information is available to make that monitoring process easier and more meaningful. Because each medication in the high-priority budget has its own profile that identifies price, volume, and details regarding an actual usage pattern (along with other information gathered from interviews, etc.), as each medication is purchased and used, the cause variances between estimated and actual can be identified more easily. Price increases, changes in total usage, changes in usage by prescriber, patient type, and so on can all be readily identified (and as necessary, intervened upon).

Financial performance in medication expenditure can be tracked in terms of variance from budget in purchases and usage (as described in steps 1 and 2), and volume-adjusted expenditures (as described in step 8), in total expenditures as well as by sub-budget (high-priority, new medications, nonformulary, and low-priority). Within each of the sub-budgets, variations in expenditures for individual medications can also be tracked in detail. Monitoring financial performance routinely throughout the year will make annual budget development easier.

Discussion

The development of expenditure forecasts and medication budgets is a complicated and often frustrating task. Institutions with insufficient data resources, limiting the first two steps in the nine-step process discussed here, are particularly concerning. Many institutions collect and store data but either do not maintain those data in a format accessible to managers or do not make that data available to managers. In some instances, it may be as simple as asking for data, whereas in other cases it may be necessary to explain why the data are needed, how they will be used, and what improvements in the financial management of medications are possible if the data are provided. Once data are obtained, pharmacy leaders must either develop the ability to manipulate the data (using data management tools such as spreadsheet and database software) or employ a data analyst to support that function. The latter approach is particularly beneficial, because having a dedicated staff resource can not only focus on annual forecast and budget preparation but can also conduct ongoing monitoring and complete a wide range of nonfinancial database activities (supporting medication use evaluation, formulary decision-making, etc.).

Obviously, the complexity of each organization should dictate the degree to which these steps are adopted. Small, less complex organizations may be successful by simply focusing on their high-priority budget and maintaining a modest ongoing vigilance process. Other larger, more complex organizations may need a more exhaustive (and exhausting) process. Although the focus of this nine-step process has been on inpatient medication expenditures, parallel processes can be used to forecast and budget outpatient, clinic-administered medication, and other expenditures. In each case, separate data streams will be needed, and accounting nuances should be considered. For example, although inpatient admissions are generally thought of as discrete encounters (one admission unrelated to another, even for the same patient), in the case of clinic-administered medications, individual doses or patient encounters are less relevant than the number of patients receiving long-term therapy with a particular agent. The fundamental process of forecasting and budgeting, however, remains the same.

Forecasting medication expenditures remains one of the most challenging aspects of pharmacy management in health systems. Although the process described herein does not simplify forecasting, the stepwise strategy helps clarify the components that contribute to expenditures and charts a course for pharmacy leaders to follow toward successful financial performance.

References

1. Hoffman JM, Shah ND, Vermeulen LC et al. Projecting future drug expenditures. *Am J Health-Syst Pharm.* 2006; 63:123–138.

2. Hoffman JM, Shah ND, Vermeulen LC et al. Projecting future drug expenditures. *Am J Health-Syst Pharm.* 2005; 62:149–167.

3. ———. Projecting future drug expenditures. *Am J Health-Syst Pharm.* 2004; 61:145–158.

4. Young D. Hospitals take action after theft of expensive drugs. *Am J Health-Syst Pharm.* 2003; 60:514–529.

5. Hoffman JM, Shah ND, Vermeulen LC et al. Projecting future drug expenditures. *Am J Health-Syst Pharm.* 2007; 64:298–314.

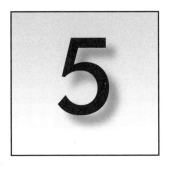

Understanding Drug Expense Using Administrative Data

Michael J. Oinonen

Introduction

Myriad sources of data exist to help pharmacy managers analyze their pharmaceutical usage and expense. These sources may include purchase invoices from wholesalers and distributors, medication use evaluations (MUEs), benchmarking projects, chart reviews, and surveys. To manage pharmaceutical resources successfully, managers must seek to identify these sources and learn how to transform these data into useful information to support decisions that ultimately will affect patient safety, quality of care, and the pharmacy budget. The focus of this chapter is to introduce the concept of using administrative datasets as one source of information to help clinically support the financial management of pharmaceutical resources. The fundamentals of setting up a dataset or applying statistical interpretation will not be covered; instead, this chapter will provide managers with an outline on how administrative data can lend powerful insight to the practice patterns of the institution and can monitor compliance with national or local evidence-based guidelines.

Background

Administrative data is generated anytime a patient has an encounter with a provider or facility and for which reimbursement for those services is sought. Although there are many sources of administrative data (enrollment into insurance plans, claims from hospitals, claims from providers, pharmacy claims, etc), this chapter will refer to data that are generated from acute care hospitalizations that contain demographic information on the patient, the diagnoses assigned, procedures performed, related clinical resources consumed, and any other elements typically associated with the encounter (admission/discharge dates, associated physicians, etc.). Information that is typically not administrative in nature, and therefore not usually part of these datasets, is patients' attributes, such as laboratory values, vital signs, and satisfaction or quality of life scores. The power of administrative data is that it allows individuals to associate drug usage and patient outcomes (length of stay, cost, morbidity and mortality, etc.) within specific, clinically defined populations.[1,2,3] This is complementary to the typical information gathered from purchase invoices, showing trends of what was purchased and when, to where and by whom the medications are being used.

This chapter narrows the scope to consider only the administrative datasets typically available at the institution and most pertinent to inpatient discharges. Hospitals vary in terms of how robust their administrative datasets are, as well as how user friendly they are in locating the information and generating queries. These databases are typically used by the hospital's quality or performance improvement departments but can also be found within the finance or billing offices. Many hospitals or health systems have a centralized data warehouse, or what is often called a clinical decision support system (CDSS), to analyze combined administrative, clinical, and financial data. Commercial software products and/or service companies exist that offer products to create and maintain these systems, but some institutions have homegrown systems in place.

Terminology

The Basics

Many pharmacists have had limited exposure to the elements found within administrative datasets. Their attention should be focused on the core elements of the administrative dataset; those essential pieces of information needed to conduct an analysis and that are also typically most readily available. Once the capabilities of the internal systems and data that are available have been investigated, a pharmacy manager might find that more information (lab values, patient satisfaction scores, etc) will make analysis much more robust. For ease of discussion, these core elements will be segregated into two groups, one called encounter level and the other the line item detail level (see Table 5.1). For most hospitals, the backbone of the encounter level is generated from the information supplied on the National Uniform Billing Committee's (NUBC) uniform billing form of 2004 (UB-04), also known as the CMS-1450 claim form. The NUBC membership includes participation from all major national provider and payer organizations and is responsible for developing a single billing form and standard dataset that can be used nationwide for submission of claims. Although 86 total elements are collected on the UB-04 form, the core elements considered here are defined in Table 5.1 and typically represent the patient level information that informs the insurer about the patient's encounter.

The line item detail level data is not on the UB-04 form, and is sourced from the pharmacy system, the electronic medical record, or the medication administration record and provides the transaction level detail on what the patient received (Table 5.1). For most institutions, these two groups of data are often combined and obtained from the CDSS.

Coding

The backbone of all administrative databases is the coding. The user of this data must be familiar with the coding system used to identify diseases and procedures and must understand the local coding practices within the health information management department when analyzing data. Most clinical information within administrative datasets employs the use of International Classification of Diseases, Ninth Revision (ICD-9) codes to document the diagnoses assigned and procedures performed for patients. This system, maintained by the World Health Organization (WHO), was designed for the classification of morbidity

Table 5.1. Essential administrative dataset elements

Encounter level elements (Usually sourced from the UB-04[1] form)	Description
Patient identification/Encounter ID/Medical Record Number	Unique identifier that allows for the tracking of this particular encounter separate from all others.
Demographics	Age, date of birth, gender, and race of the patient.
Principal diagnosis (coded with ICD-9-CM codes)[2]	The medical condition that is ultimately determined to have caused a patient's admission to the hospital. The principal diagnosis is used to assign every patient to a diagnosis related group. This diagnosis may differ from the admitting and major diagnoses.
Secondary diagnoses (coded with ICD-9-CM codes)[3]	Other diagnoses associated with the current stay that are: coexist at the time of admission, that develop subsequently, or that affect the treatment received and/or length of stay. Diagnoses that relate to an earlier episode which have no bearing on the current stay, are to be excluded.
Principal procedure (coded with ICD-9 CM codes) and date	The procedure (and date) performed for definitive treatment, rather than for diagnostic or exploratory purposes, or to resolve a complication. More than one procedure may meet this definition, but the one most related to the principal diagnosis should be listed on the claim.
Secondary procedures (coded with ICD-9-CM codes) and dates[3]	Other significant procedures or surgeries (and dates) that were performed on the patient.
Admission date and type	Formal acceptance by the hospital of a patient who is to receive services while receiving room, board, and continuous nursing services. Types include: emergent, urgent, elective, etc.
Discharge date and disposition	Formal release of the patient and termination of services. Patient can be discharged to home, another hospital or facility, leave against medical advice, or die.
Attending physician	The clinician who is primarily responsible for the care of the patient from the beginning of the hospital episode.
Operating physician	The clinician who performed the principal procedure.
Payer	Expected source of payment (government, commercial, self, charity, etc.).
Charges	Dollar charge for the service, usually summarized into industry standard revenue code groupings or cost centers (Lab, Blood, Imaging, Pharmacy & IV therapy, etc.). These usually reflect both the direct and indirect charges of providing the service/resource.
DRG[4]	Diagnostic-Related Grouping is assigned to each patient upon discharge and is primarily driven by the other encounter level information listed above.

Table 5.1. Essential administrative dataset elements (*Continued*)

Line item detail level elements (usually sourced from the charge master and detailed billing files)	Description
Patient identification/Encounter ID/Medical Record Number	To provide a link back to the encounter data.
Medication charge code	Unique alpha/numeric code internally used within the organization to represent a particular medication.
Medication description	Descriptions vary, but typically include the chemical name, form, and unit of measure (i.e., aspirin 325mg tab).
Quantity (Dose)	Quantity ordered. Should be interpreted with description, depending on how billing is structured.
Date of service	Generally the date the medication was administered to the patient.
Industry code	Typically a supporting code for the medication (National Drug Code most commonly used source for pharmaceuticals).
Revenue code	Corresponding UB-04[1] revenue or cost center code to which the charge code belongs. Used for grouping charges into similar buckets.
Charge/Cost	Dollar charge or cost of the transaction; depending on what is available.

1. UB-04 (Uniform Billing, 2004 version)
2. ICD-9-CM (International Classification of Diseases, Ninth Revision, Clinical Modification)
3. Generally speaking only the first position (primary) is most important. There is no particular order after the primary spot that indicates the degree of severity.
4. The DRG is not part of the UB-04 form but is determined primarily from the information obtained on the form, and can be considered part of the encounter level information.

and mortality information for statistical purposes, for the indexing of records, and for ease of data storage and retrieval. In the late 1970s the National Center for Health Statistics (NCHS) organized a committee, composed of other U.S. health-care associations, to modify the ICD-9 system to become more clinically relevant and precise than what was needed for simple groupings for analysis. As a result, providers in the United States use the ICD-9, Clinical Modification (ICD-9-CM) classification system, which is updated annually by NCHS and the Center for Medicare and Medicaid Services (CMS). The ICD-9-CM classification for diagnoses and injuries are grouped into 17 chapters that are typically arranged by body systems. These codes can be up to five digits in length, which provides for detailed descriptions (see Table 5.2). There are two supplementary classifications, the first includes V codes to represent factors influencing health status and contact with health services (V22 = normal pregnancy, which is not a disease but rather a condition that might have bearing on the admission). The other supplementary classification include E codes, used to represent the external causes of injury and poisoning

Table 5.2. ICD-9-CM Classification Codes for Diagnosis of Diastolic Heart Failure

428 Heart failure
    428.3 Diastolic heart failure
        428.30 Unspecified
        438.31 Acute
        428.32 Chronic
        428.33 Acute and chronic

ICD-9-CM (International Classification of Diseases, Ninth Revision, Clinical Modification) Effective October 1, 2006–September 30, 2007

(E854.0 = accidental poisoning by antidepressants). The ICD-9-CM surgical and diagnostic procedure codes are grouped into 16 chapters and are typically four digits in length. Table 5.3 includes a sample of procedure codes and their classification. Using the codes to identify a comprehensive clinical picture is, at times, more art than science. The information can sometimes tell a more complete story of a patient's clinical situation. For example, administrative data can tell us that a patient has physical symptoms (780.7 malaise and fatigue), a laboratory abnormality (275.41 hypocalcemia), or socioeconomic issues (payer = Medicaid or V61.0 family disruption) that might become useful in an analysis. As their experience with the data grows, pharmacy managers may need to become more creative in finding ways to leverage the codes.

Official coding guidelines exist and are typically coordinated between NCHS, CMS, the American Hospital Association, and the American Health Information Management Association. Adherence to these guidelines is required under the Health Insurance Portability and Accountability Act (HIPAA), and there are strict penalties in place for hospitals that are found to incorrectly "up code" a patient's condition or illness. Even with guidelines in

Table 5.3. ICD-9-CM Classification for Selected Operations on Vessels of the Heart

36 Operations on vessels of heart
    36.0 Removal of coronary artery obstruction and insertion of stent(s)
        36.03 Open chest coronary artery angiography
        36.04 Intracoronary artery thrombolytic infusion
        36.06 Insertion of non-drug-eluting coronary artery stent(s)
        36.07 Insertion of drug-eluting coronary artery stent(s)
        36.09 Other removal of coronary artery obstruction

ICD-9-CM (International Classification of Diseases, Ninth Revision, Clinical Modification) Effective October 1, 2006–September 30, 2007 place, coding is only as good as the physician documentation within the medical record. Coding is also left to interpretation, which can vary from place to place and person to person, all of which can lead to differences in coding patterns.[4,5,6,7] For example, unless the physician specifically documents "patient stool positive for Clostridium difficile toxin, started on metronidazole," the patient's record may not be coded with ICD-9-CM code 008.45 (intestinal infection due to Clostridium difficile). Conversely, a patient's record might be incorrectly coded if a physician's statement of "CDiff suspected on day 3" is interpreted as being infected, even if the diagnosis is not confirmed through laboratory testing.

The WHO revises the codes approximately every 10 years, and, although ICD-10 coding has been used in other countries since 1999, the implementation in the United States was delayed because of difficulties in coordinating the international and the appropriate national private and governmental committees, agencies, associations, and organizations. There is not yet an anticipated implementation date for the ICD-10-CM in the United States, but, once the final notice to implement has been published in the Federal Register, hospitals will have a two-year window to comply. A comprehensive overview of coding history and ICD-9-CM and ICD-10 structure can be found on the NCHS's Web site (www.cdc.gov/nchs). One final important element of the administrative dataset includes the patient's diagnosis related grouping (DRG), which is assigned upon discharge. Although not part of the UB-04 or line item detail level information, the DRG is an important patient assignment to know. In 1983, Congress mandated a prospective payment system for reimbursement of all Medicare inpatients. CMS bases their reimbursement for inpatient care on the DRG, because patients assigned to a given DRG are expected to have similar consumption of hospital resources. Reimbursement is complex and each hospital's rate will vary based on location and area wage indexes, but payments for each DRG are available from CMS (e.g., DRG 545= revision of hip or knee replacement, national average = $12,344 for 2006). A single DRG is assigned to each patient by a software program provided by CMS (Grouper version 24.0, effective through Sept 2007) and is based on ICD-9-CM diagnoses, procedures, age, sex, and the presence of complications or comorbidities that are presented for grouping. DRGs can also be segregated into medical versus surgical populations.

On October 1, 2007 CMS began paying inpatient Medicare claims based on version 25 DRGs, often referred to as the Medicare-Severity DRGs (MSDRGs). This represents a major shift in patient classification and reimbursement. Their intention was to align payments more closely with resource utilization. Most version 24 DRGs have now been broken-down into three categories based on the presence or absence of complications and comorbidities (CC).

Yet coding is always changing. Each year, ICD-9-CMs and DRGs are added, deleted, or modified based on clinical practice changes and technologic advances, so a pharmacy manager should conduct research before analysis. For example, effective for inpatient discharges after October 1, 2006, DRG 148 (major small and large bowel procedures with CC) was deleted, and in its place two new DRGs were created: 569 (major small and large bowel procedures with CC with major gastrointestinal diagnosis) and 570 (major small and large bowel procedures with CC without major gastrointestinal diagnosis). With the implementation of version 25 DRGs, these version 24 DRGs, 569 and 570 have been replaced with three categories; DRG 329, 330, and 331 (Major small and Large Bowel Procedures with

MCCs, with CCs, and without CCs, respectively). Collaborating with someone from the health information management department will be invaluable. Their knowledge of the coding system and their ability to explain the nuances between codes and how the hospital's discharge notes are interpreted by the coding staff will lend powerful insight to analysis of administrative databases.

Risk Adjustment

Studying patient outcomes, whether clinical or financial in nature, are often the primary reason administrative database analyses are conducted. Before drawing any conclusions about the impact interventions had on patients, the researcher must account for those patient characteristics that might have significant influence on the overall outcome of interest. The purpose of risk adjustment is to provide for meaningful comparisons across patient populations by accounting for these characteristics (e.g., age, sex, comorbidities, etc). By knowing these patient characteristics, a pharmacy manager can predict outcomes such as the patient's length of stay, total hospital costs, or the probability of mortality. Although the statistical methodologies used to calculate such predictions are beyond the scope of this chapter, the pharmacy manager should incorporate the concept of risk adjustment when discussing patient outcomes. Actually, the assignment of a DRG is one form of risk adjustment that helps predict total hospital charges or a patient's length of stay. It would be beneficial for the pharmacy manager to become more familiar with the various methodologies of risk adjustment as his or her experience with database analysis grows. Many texts are available on the subject and should become part of the pharmacy reference library.[8]

Putting It All Together

Managers can leverage this clinical administrative data to help answer questions concerning rising medication costs. Having an organized methodological approach to analysis will make conducting complex studies easier in the future.

Case Study

This is an evaluation of the use of recombinant human erythropoietin (EPO) within the inpatient population.

Background

Multiple areas in pharmacy are being scrutinized for opportunities to increase efficiency and decrease costs. In addition to labor expense, strategically managing pharmaceutical expense is often one of the largest challenges facing pharmacy managers and directors. Adopting a prospective approach to the monitoring of budget variances has been common practice at the institution. This is especially true with respect to medications that consistently contribute to a substantial portion of the total pharmacy expense. A report is presented that indicates purchases of EPO (separated from outpatient cost centers) have been steadily increasing over the last 12 months and have consistently made the top five list of most costly inpatient medications for the organization. Although a slight increased trend was predicted and budgeted

Table 5.4. Guidelines for the utilization of Epoetin Alfa (EPO)

FDA approved indications and unlabeled uses for the administration of Epoetin Alfa

Indications:

1. Treatment of anemia of chronic renal failure patients (CRF):
For the treatment of anemia associated with chronic renal failure, including patients on dialysis (end-stage renal disease [ESRD]) and patients not on dialysis. Epoetin alfa is indicated to elevate or maintain the RBC level (as manifested by the hematocrit or hemoglobin determinations) and to decrease the need for transfusions in these patients. Nondialysis patients with symptomatic anemia considered for therapy should have a hemoglobin less than 10 g/dL.

2. Treatment of anemia in zidovudine-treated HIV-infected patients:
For the treatment of anemia related to therapy with zidovudine (AZT) in HIV-infected patients. Epoetin alfa is indicated to elevate or maintain the red blood cell (RBC) level (as manifested by the hematocrit or hemoglobin determinations) and to decrease the need for transfusions in these patients. Epoetin alfa is not indicated for the treatment of anemia in HIV-infected patients because of other factors such as iron or folate deficiencies, hemolysis, or GI bleeding; manage these conditions appropriately.

3. Treatment of anemia in cancer patients on chemotherapy:
For the treatment of anemia in patients with nonmyeloid malignances where anemia is due to the effect of concomitantly administered chemotherapy. Epoetin alfa is indicated to decrease the need for transfusions in patients who will be receiving concomitant chemotherapy for a minimum of 2 months. Epoetin alfa is not indicated for the treatment of anemia in cancer patients due to other factors such as iron or folate deficiencies, hemolysis, or GI bleeding; manage these conditions appropriately.

4. Reduction of allogeneic blood transfusion in surgery patients:
For the treatment of anemic patients (hemoglobin greater than 10 to less than or equal to 13 g/dL) scheduled to undergo elective, noncardiac, nonvascular surgery to reduce the need for allogeneic blood transfusions. Epoetin alfa is indicated for patients at high risk for perioperative transfusions with significant, anticipated blood loss. Epoetin alfa is not indicated for anemic patients who are willing to donate autologous blood. The safety of the perioperative use of epoetin alfa has been studied only in patients who are receiving anticoagulant prophylaxis.

Unlabeled uses (Must get approval from pharmacy):
A. Use in critically ill patients to reduce the number of RBC transfusions
B. Anemia of prematurity in preterm infants
C. Anemia associated with myelodysplastic syndrome
D. Anemia associated with chronic inflammatory disorders (e.g. rheumatoid arthritis)
E. Prophylaxis of anemia associated with frequent blood donation
F. Treatment of anemia associated with ribavirin combination therapy in hepatitis C-infected patients
G. Treatment of anemia in cancer patients not receiving chemotherapy
H. Treatment of anemia associated with CRF in children not requiring dialysis
I. Treatment of anemia related to zidovudine therapy in HIV-infected children
J. Treatment of anemia in children with cancer on chemotherapy

for, a regular variance analysis indicated the increase was beyond an acceptable 10 percent threshold that was forecasted. Although there is not dedicated clinical pharmacy coverage on the renal service, no significant changes in patient volume or case mix in that area have been noted. Understanding the factors that lead to such trends is important to understand before attempting to manage these costs or to forecast future usage. The pharmacy manager is asked to evaluate the potential causes of this variance, judge the appropriateness of this usage, and identify any cost-saving opportunities associated with its use. Budgets need to be finalized and senior administrators would like a report to distribute at a meeting that is scheduled to occur in one week.

Initial Steps

Initial thoughts may include enlisting the help of a few students and residents to pull charts from a sample of the nearly 800 patients that received EPO last year, but it will take two to three days for the chart request to be processed. There is little time for such a manual process of review. The pharmacy manger identifies internal guidelines approved by the P&T committee two years ago, and notes that these guidelines follow the FDA-approved indications (see Table 5.4). A previous MUE conducted by a pharmacy student, based on a chart review of 30 medical records, found only a single patient who did not appear to follow the guidelines. The manager decides, given the time constraints, that an administrative database analysis is a logical next step, so she prepares to download the information that will be requested by the CDSS staff. Before collecting any data for research purposes, approval from the local institutional review board (IRB) may be necessary. Technically speaking, administrative data involves human subjects, and, although patients can be de-identified, issues of privacy and confidentiality are still of concern. In many cases, these types of analysis are considered quality improvement activities and IRB approval is waived, but it is the function of the IRB to determine whether patients are appropriately protected.

A successful approach to database analyses incorporates multiple data checks and validation exercises to establish confidence in the accuracy of the findings. This cannot be understated and should not be considered a one-time activity. Almost all database analyses require some modification because of data quality issues (i.e., missing or incomplete data points). It is therefore important to corroborate findings with other available information (trend report of EPO purchases) to ensure there are no glaring differences (see Figure 5.1). Limitations of the data should be understood, communicated, and minimized before making administrative decisions on drug use policy.

Step 1: Determining what to collect. If someone else is pulling the information, it might be beneficial to prepare a template or standard dataset layout of the essential elements most commonly requested. Standardizing requests will save time and avoid confusion on what exactly was requested. It also provides a structured format that facilitates analysis. Applying inclusion or exclusion criteria too restrictively may yield a dataset that is too narrow but not restricting criteria enough may require more manipulation in the end.

The pharmacy manager determines that the dataset should contain the following items: patient medical record number, basic demographics (age, sex, race), primary payer, admit and discharge date (plus calculated length of stay), admit status and source, discharge status,

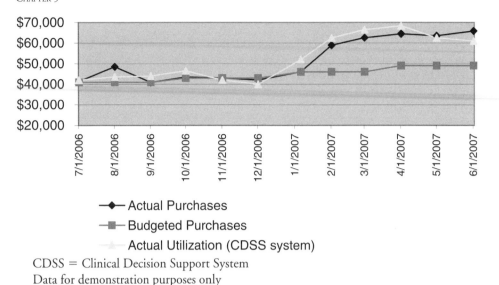

CDSS = Clinical Decision Support System
Data for demonstration purposes only

Figure 5.1. Budgeted and Actual Purchases versus Utilization of Epoetin Alfa; Inpatient only, July 2006–June 2007

all available ICD-9-CM diagnoses and procedures, DRG, attending physician ID and their specialty, EPO dose/date of administration/cost, and the total hospital cost for each patient. (Note the pharmacy manager should provide the charge codes or NDC codes for EPO, so it can be identified easily by the CDSS staff.)

Step 2: Translating EPO indications into ICD-9-CM codes. Appropriate usage of EPO could be determined in part by whether patients have met the criteria established by the P&T committee. This requires a creative look at each patient's coded profile for the presence of a clinical indication for EPO use. Grouping EPO usage into two general categories (potentially appropriate or inappropriate) is a manageable approach to this particular analysis. Appropriate use can generally be thought of as identifying patients with either an anemia that is kidney failure-related or chemotherapy-induced and not associated with iron deficiency. Although lab values would strengthen the inclusion or exclusion of these patients, they may not always be readily available. The key is to identify any diagnoses and/or procedures that support the conclusion that one of these conditions exist for a patient. If there are no clear-cut ICD-9-CM codes available (i.e., 285.21, anemia in end stage renal disease), surrogate measures might be a viable option (i.e., 39.95, patient underwent hemodialysis). The pharmacy manager must be cognizant of potential overestimations of appropriate use. The impact of these false positives can be minimized by combining codes that strengthen the argument. For example, simple inclusion of patients with a malignant neoplasm (140.XX–199.XX) does not necessarily indicate there is concomitantly administered chemotherapy or that anemia is even present. However, identifying the same patients receiving blood transfusions may (or may not) be acceptable inclusion criteria in this case. Therefore, being comfortable with the level of sophistication for specific code combinations provided

Table 5.5. Selected ICD-9-CM Codes For Identifying Potentially Appropriate Epoetin Alfa (EPO) Utilization

ICD-9-CM Code	Description	Comments
Diagnosis		
585.X	Various stages of chronic kidney disease	Code 585.6 indicates patient is in end stage renal disease (ESRD)
586	Renal failure, unspecified	May include acute as well as chronic renal failure
584.X	Acute renal failure (if worthy)	Often combined with 585.X codes to identify the stage of kidney disease
403.XX	Various forms of hypertensive kidney disease	
V45.1	Renal dialysis status	Indicates patient had previous kidney disease
V56.0	Encounter for extracorporeal dialysis	
V56.8	Encounter for peritoneal dialysis	
V58.11	Encounter for antineoplastic chemotherapy	Patient is or was on chemotherapy in the past
285.21	Anemia in chronic kidney disease	Does not include anemia from iron defficiencies, which are separate ICD-9-CM codes
285.29	Anemia in other chronic disease	
140.XX – 199.XX	Various malignant neoplasm	Does not necessary indicate patient is on active chemotherapy, but does mean there is a malignant neoplasm present
042	Human immunodeficiency virus infection	
Procedure		
39.95	Hemodialysis	Indication of kidney disease
54.98	Peritoneal dialysis	
99.25	Injection of cancer chemotherapy substance	Does not indicate which chemotherapy agent was given, but rather that the patient was treated during this stay
35.XX – 39.XX	Operations on the cardiovascular system	Use in combination with "elective" admission status to determine if the patient underwent a cardiovascular-related surgery

ICD-9-CM (International Classification of Diseases, Ninth Revision, Clinical Modification) Effective October 1, 2006–September 30, 2007

will ultimately be a decision that must be made for each analysis individually. It is certainly acceptable to have methodological changes after initial cuts of the data reveal gross over- or underestimations. Consulting with one of the hospital's coders can serve as confirmation of the reliability of any surrogate measures representing the medical necessity of EPO (Table 5.4). The outcome of this activity is a list of ICD-9-CM codes (see Table 5.5) and a modification to the pharmacy manager's

Table 5.6. Inpatient Utilization of Epoetin Alfa (EPO); July 2006 – June 2007

Patient demographics and selected outcomes

Total patients (n = 794)

		Mean	Median	Range (min-max)
Gender (% pts)	Patient Age (years)	68	62	25 – 82
Male (55%)				
Female (45%)	Length of Stay (Days)	5.2	4	1 – 29
Race (% pts)	EPO Total Cost/Patient	$795	$630	$102 – $10,254
White (42%)				
Black (36%)	EPO Dosing			
Other (22%)	Number of Doses/Patient Stay		2	1 – 15
	Renal Patient Individual Dose		10000 IU	2,000 – 32,000 IU
Payer (% pts)	Oncology Patient Individual Dose		40000 IU	4,000 – 60,000 IU
Medicare (65%)	Pts receiving multiple doses (81%)			
Commercial (24%)	Pts receiving single doses (19%)			
Other (11%)				

Summarized utilization of selected ICD-9-CM codes (see table 5.5)

Pts with any indication/code	79%
Pts without any apparent indication/code	21%
total	100%
Pts with renal condition codes (excludes anemia, HIV, neoplasm, and chemo inject codes)	59%
Pts with oncology condition codes	20%
Pts with HIV codes	0%
Pts with other conditions	21%
total	100%
Pts with elective surgical DRGs (excluding cardiac/vascular surgery)	65%

ICD-9-CM (International Classification of Diseases, Ninth Revision, Clinical Modification)
Data for demonstration purposes only.

original request to the CDSS staff, who now asks for the addition of zidovudine usage and lab values for each patient. Lab values will take longer to pull, so it will not be available until after the meeting.

Step 3: Aggregating the data. Having basic counts and a demographic breakdown of the population of interest can be informative (Table 5.6). When the final grouping of patients into their respective categories occurs, patterns may begin to emerge. The CDSS staff also provided the pharmacy manager with a medical or surgical designation for each patient and the clinical service (product lines) to which the patient belongs, allowing for easier grouping of DRGs. Assuming the manager is comfortable with the 79 percent of patients coded with a potential indication of

Service	Number of Patients receiving EPO	EPO Cost
Orthopedics	102	$55,740
Critical Care	23	$24,112
General Medicine	22	$16,345
Gastroenterology	10	$7,386
All Others	9	$3,217
Total	166	$106,800

ICD-9-CM (International Classification of Diseases, Ninth Revision, Clinical Modification)

Data for demonstration purposes only

Figure 5.2. Service lines with no apparent approved indications (lack of ICD-9-CM codes) for Epoetin Alfa (EPO)

appropriate EPO use, further attention should focus on the 21 percent of patients who did not make the first pass. Figure 5.2 provides the additional characteristics of those 21 percent of patients not meeting any of the inclusion criteria. A large portion of those patients fall into the critical care and orthopedic areas (see Figure 5.2). A quick trend analysis, by service or product line, might also highlight the increased usage of EPO by patients in one particular point of time (Figure 5.3), which may (or may not) have been as apparent if only analyzed by physician (Table 5.7).

Step 4: Interview and confirm suspicions. Although guidelines are in place to help guide appropriate EPO usage, they are not enforced at the institution. Orders for EPO are not routinely questioned; neither is there adequate clinical pharmacy coverage for those areas. Based on the analysis, it would appear that one of the main drivers of this increase in usage is the orthopedic service area, with an increased

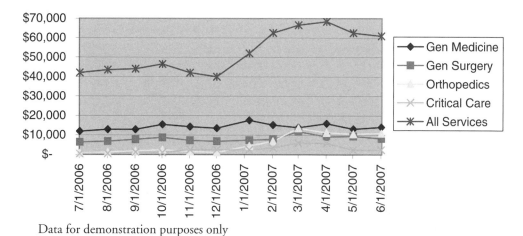

Data for demonstration purposes only

Figure 5.3. Trend of Epoetin Alfa Utilization, by Selected Services (July 2006–June 2007)

Table 5.7. Top 10 Physicians and Services Utilizing ($) Epoetin Alfa (EPO)

Top Physicians (represents ~62% of total EPO pts)

Physician ID	EPO Pts	Service	Total EPO Cost
234	102	General Medicine	$ 60,503
543	84	General Medicine	$ 49,825
654	77	General Surgery	$ 49,707
567	30	General Surgery	$ 38,055
876	22	Medical Oncology	$ 32,060
789	18	Medical Oncology	$ 31,988
98	55	Orthopedics	$ 31,080
765	15	Critical Care	$ 30,789
654	38	General Medicine	$ 29,010
345	48	Orthopedics	$ 28,804

Top Services (represents ~85% total EPO cost)

Service	EPO Pts	Total EPO Cost
General Medicine	230	$170,880
General Surgery	115	$ 98,012
Medical Oncology	89	$ 97,900
Orthopedics	112	$ 66,744
Cardiology	44	$ 39,600
Critical Care	32	$ 37,722
Urology	18	$ 13,899
Gastroenterology	15	$ 11,080
Cardiothoracic Surgery	6	$ 4,580
Neurology	6	$ 4,520

Data for demonstration purposes only

trend occurring around the first of the year. Although this group of patients does not represent the majority of EPO cases, it is surprising to see nearly 90 percent of the patients received EPO while undergoing knee or hip replacement/revision surgery toward the end of this period. In fact, further analysis shows that about half of those patients are receiving two doses prior to discharge. Of the four primary orthopedic surgeons with a substantial volume of cases over the period, two appear to be the primary drivers of usage. After reviewing the data with a supervisor, an appointment with the chair of orthopedics was in order to discuss the findings. The pharmacy manager's suspicions were confirmed: two new surgeons were brought to the hospital around the first of year to build up the presence of the orthopedic service offering in the community. Even without the lab data, the chair acknowledged that the majority of patients coming in were not anemic; it was simply the practice of these two physicians to "bulk" up the patients prior to discharge, in the belief that they had a better recovery in those first weeks post-surgery. What was not known, until this analysis, was the overall impact this practice was having on the pharmacy budget.

Step 5: *Determine if comparative data are needed.* It may become necessary to provide additional evidence to convince clinicians that this local assessment of practice varies across peer groups or is not commonly done. Although the opportunity in this particular case study might be apparent, using comparative benchmark data will offer insights as to the degree the practice may vary or where improvement is possible. This support may come in the form of literature reviews for evidence-based practices, informal surveys of peer organizations through Listservs or online communities, national patient registries, or from the mining of larger comparative databases maintained by various associations and consortiums. Because the UB-04 data is readily accessible, organizations such as the University HealthSystem Consortium (UHC) maintain national databases to allow participants to gain access to administrative data for performance improvement activities, ultimately allowing users to gain insight to the usage of specific resources in well-defined clinical populations and across custom compare groups. Similar limitations apply when interpreting these data, and the pharmacy manager must factor in certain influences that may explain possible variations in practice when such an analysis is done. For example, in this particular case study, the pharmacy manager might consider the following concerning the use of EPO in orthopedic patients:

- Could patients be receiving EPO after discharge (or before admission), which is not reflected in the data?

- Are the patients' beliefs or religious orientations driving the use of medications over blood products?

- Is the documentation and coding so poor in a particular hospital, that it lends itself to being a poor comparator?

- Are the hospital characteristics, patient complexity, or procedure volume similar to the hospital in which the pharmacy manager works?

- Has the analysis included all alternative yet similar medications within the therapeutic family?

These unknowns can be mitigated by addressing certain questions. Are the results similar when data is aggregated from a large group versus smaller custom groupings? Do the usage patterns appear consistent with approved indications, given the patient mix, when looking outside the orthopedic service line in other hospitals? If the hospital is a participant in a national database, are the results consistent with the internal CDSS source? Consider contacting the comparator hospital to confirm what their data appear to show. Remember, these data are meant to guide the pharmacy manager's decisions not to answer every question. Administrative database analysis, especially comparative usage, can provide quick confirmation that the direction a pharmacy manager has taken is on or off track. This may also be all that is needed to convince physicians that their practice patterns are not consistent with their colleagues.

Step 6: Final report preparation and recommendations. The final report to senior administrators or the P&T committee should be brief and to the point. Charts and graphs should be condensed as much as possible and able to stand on their own with little or no explanation needed on how to interpret them. A one- or two-page document should suffice with a brief background and methodology section, synopsis of the findings, limitations or uncertainties, and final recommendations. Double-check all counts and avoid the use of confrontational or punitive wording that will ultimately cause some readers to be distracted from the message. When appropriate, support recommendations with identified best practices or with a thorough review of the evidence published in the literature. Figure 5.4 provides a suggested layout for a final report.

The purpose of this case study was to provide some general direction on how pharmacy managers can quickly conduct an analysis using readily accessible information. Not all inclusion or exclusion criteria can be applied at all times, but these exercises can help with future action planning by determining the following:

- Whether the collection of more data is needed (e.g., number of transfusions a patient received)
- Whether a focused MUE across all services or just within the orthopedic service area should be conducted
- Whether clinical guidelines need to be updated or enforced
- Whether all orders for EPO need pharmacy approval
- Whether comparative benchmark data is needed to support recommendations

Limitations

An administrative database can provide powerful insight when used to its full potential. There are, however, inherent limitations that come with its use.

Coding

Most importantly is the issue of accurate and complete coding. Clinical interpretation of a patient's diagnosis, complication, or comorbidity relies on not only the physicians' documentation of its presence but on the interpretation of the person doing the coding. In addition, although thousands of ICD-9-CM codes are available, the lack of clear clinical definitions makes it difficult to ascertain precise differences among certain codes or the degree of severity. For example, a commonly used code for heart failure includes ICD-9-CM 428.9 (heart failure, unspecified). The anemia diagnosis codes (ICD-9-CM 280–285) do not specify hematocrit levels or how rapidly the condition developed. In fact, until the "present on admission" indicator is used on the UB-04 form, it is impossible to determine with 100 percent certainty if a condition developed in the hospital. Lack of other key pieces of clinical information would include knowledge of the patient's general physiologic status, such as blood pressure, oxygenation, renal function, allergies, or certain contraindications to medications that might exist but that are not necessarily coded for. Hospitals might limit the number of codes captured for diagnoses and procedures which may influence coding beyond what is needed for legitimate

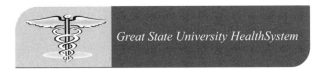

Medication Utilization: Epoetin Alfa(Epogen®/Procrit®)

Distributed July 12, 2007

If you have any comments regarding this report, please contact John Smith, Assistant Director of Pharmacy X4799 or the pharmacy dept at X2439.

Background

Epoetin Alfa currently is the only erythropoietin (EPO) agent on formulary at the medical center. EPO use represents a substantial pharmaceutical expense for the hospital and currently ranks 3rd, in terms of total pharmaceutical expenditures for the hospital. The Department of Pharmacy has observed a substantial increase in Epo costs over the past 12 months (see figure 1).

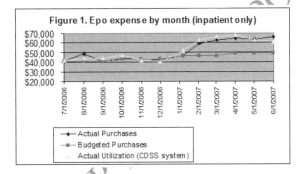

This increase can be partially explained by a small increase in the acquisition cost of Epo (5.5% increase in cost annually), but the majority can be attributed to an increase in utilization. P&T-approved guidelines do exist and can be referenced in the appendix of the current formulary binder.

Methods/Data Sources

Administrative data was collected and analyzed from three sources:
- Internal CDSS system, aka "gemini"
- Wholesaler XYZ, purchase report out of the pharmacy system
- Comparative benchmarking sourced from the University HealthSystem Consortium's (UHC) Clinical Data Products.

Data was collected from inpatients discharged between July 1, 2006 and June 30, 2007 that received at least one dose of Epo during their stay. Patients were placed into product lines (service lines) based on their DRG assignments and were further flagged as either potentially utilizing Epo appropriately or inappropriately based on the presence or absence of ICD-9-CM codes in their profiles. The included ICD-9 codes that were ultimately considered "potentially appropriate use of Epo" are listed in the table below. It was assumed that patients with malignant neoplasms and having encounters with chemotherapy substances were assumed to have anemia related to the chemotherapy itself.

Figure 5.4.

ICD-9-CM Code	Description
Diagnosis	
585.X	Various stages of Chronic kidney disease
586	Renal failure, unspecified
403.XX	Various forms of hypertensive kidney disease
V45.1	Renal dialysis status
V56.0	Encounter for extracorporeal dialysis
V56.8	Encounter for peritoneal dialysis
V58.11	Encounter for antineoplastic chemotherapy
285.21	Anemia in chronic kidney disease
285.29	Anemia in other chronic disease
140.XX -	Various Malignant Neoplasms
Procedure	
39.95	Hemodialysis
54.98	Peritoneal dialysis
99.25	Injection of cancer chemotherapy substance

A total of 10 patients were sampled for coding accuracy and determined to be within acceptable limits for purposes of identifying Epo utilization. All Epo cost data was gathered from the Gemini system, which is sourced directly from the internal pharmacy system. Comparative data gathered from UHC included hospitals that were determined to be of similar case mix, location, procedure volume, and bed size. In addition, key administrators and physicians were asked to select hospitals that they felt "comparable" to our hospital.

Key Findings

A total of 79% of the 794 Epo inpatients were considered to use Epo potentially appropriately (see table 1).

Table 1. Inpt use of Epo (July 06- June 07) Total patients (n= 794) Summarized utilization of selected ICD-9-CM codes (see table above)	
Pts with any indication/code	79%
Pts without any apparent indication/code	21%
total	100%
Pts with renal condition codes (excludes anemia, HIV, neoplasm, and chemo inject codes)	59%
Pts with oncology condition codes	20%
Pts with other conditions	21%
total	100%

Of the 21% of pts with potentially inappropriate use of Epo, the majority belonged to the orthopedic and critical care service lines. Table 2 shows the service lines, patient counts, and Epo cost for all of these patients.

Table 2. Service lines with no apparent indication (code) for Epo use	Number of Patients receiving Epo	Epo Cost
Orthopedics	102	$55,740
Critical Care	23	$24,112
General Medicine	22	$16,345
Gastroenterology	10	$7,386
All Others	9	$3,217
Total	166	$106,800

Figure 2 shows the trend of Epo costs by selected service lines. Other service lines were removed from this figure because they did not show any substantial variation across this time period. The chair of Orthopedics confirmed these results, indicating with the hire of new surgeons in Jan 2006, it was standard practice for them to use Epo routinely in their patients, regardless of their hemoglobin/anemia status upon admission.

Figure 5.4. *(Continued)*

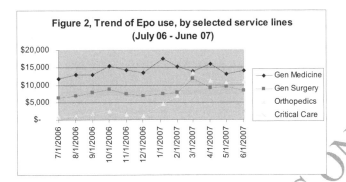

Figure 2, Trend of Epo use, by selected service lines (July 06 - June 07)

Utilization relative to peer organizations (UHC comparative data)

Table 3 displays the utilization information from 3 UHC hospitals considered to be good comparators to ours. The data clearly shows we use Epo in a greater percent of our orthopedic and critical care inpatients when compared to others.

Table 3. UHC comparison data on Epo use (July 06- June 07)	% inpts with potentially appropriate use	% of inpts with potentially inappropriate use	% orthopedic pts use	% critical care pt use
Great State Hospital (focus)	79%	21%	75%	15%
Specific Hospitals				
Hospital A	95%	5%	10%	5%
Hospital B	96%	4%	8%	7%
Hospital C	93%	7%	30%	1%
Average of 3 specific hospitals	**95%**	**5%**	**16%**	**4%**

Recommendations

The guidelines should be reviewed regularly as the environment changes, such as more research becoming available with respect to identifying optimal hemoglobin target levels, pricing or reimbursement changes that might occur, or when the institution experiences major shifts in the patient case mix. Currently, if the only change to occur was the enforcement of the current guidelines, our utilization would fall more in line with those practices from other institutions.

The orthopedic service line was identified as one of the largest contributors to the increased cost during this timeperiod. If the current volume of orthopedic procedures is maintained (increase of 15% each year), substantial increases in Epo will occur. There is little support in the literature that demonstrates Epo increases the quality of life or minimizes recovery times following orthopedic related procedures. It is therefore a joint recommendation from the pharmacy and surgery departments that this practice be further investigated under a small investigational trial over the next 6 months to determine if there are any positive patient outcomes related to the use of Epo in these patients. Further objectives of this study will include: identification of patients most likely to benefit from Epo therapy (i.e., patients especially deemed at risk for transfusion), optimal dosing regimen, and use of alternative blood-less therapies. Investigators will be in contact with the hospital's office of investigational drug services as a follow up to this report. During the study period, it is our recommendation to follow established guidelines until the results of the study are known. If desired, physicians can begin Epo therapy prior to admission on an outpatient basis for those patients undergoing elective procedures.

Figure 5.4. *(Continued)*

In addition, although the use of Epo in the critical care population is not as high as the orthopedic service line, the pharmacy dept will be conducting a focused drug utilization review (DUE) in this particular sub-group of Epo users to demonstrate the cost-effectiveness of this therapy. A final report on this DUE will be distributed within the next 30 days.

References for consideration

Correction of anemia with epoetin alfa in chronic kidney disease.
Singh AK, Szczech L, Tang KL, et al. *NEJM*. 2006:355:2085-98.
Synopsis of article: The use of a target hemoglobin level of 13.5 g per deciliter (compared to 11.3) was associated with increased risk and no incremental improvement in the quality of life in this open-label trial of 1432 chronic kidney disease patients.

Normalization of hemoglobin level in patients with chronic kidney disease and anemia.
Drueke TB, Locatelli F, Clyne N, et al. *NEJM*. 2006;355:2071-84.
Synopsis of article: In this 3 year study of 603 patients with chronic kidney disease, early complete correction of anemia does not reduce the risk of cardiovascular events.

An open-label, randomized study to compare the safety and efficacy of perioperative apoetin alfa with preoperative autologous blood donation in total joint arthroplasty.
Stowell CP, Chandler H, Jove M, et al. *Orthopedics*. 1999;Jan:22 (Suppl):s015-12.
Synopsis of article: In this study of 490 patients, compared with the autologous donor arm, mean Hb levels measured preoperatively, postoperatively on Day 1, and at discharge visits were significantly greater in the Epoetin alfa-treated arm (P < .0001).

Figure 5.4. *(Continued)*

reimbursement. For example, ICD-9-CM procedure code 99.02 (transfusion of autologous blood, collected before surgery) might have been helpful in the case study above but is rarely used in practice. Therefore it would be misleading to assume its absence from a patient's profile implied no pre-op donation was made.

Retrospective Nature

The timeliness of administrative data can also prove to be a limitation. These data provide only a retrospective look at usage. The retrospective nature may make it difficult to recall environmental influences that contributed to certain usage patterns (i.e., drug shortages or recalls).

Costs and Charges

Administrative data are claims for which the hospital seeks reimbursement. Therefore, on the transaction or even service line level, most systems are interested in applying the correct charge for the unit of service rather than tracking the cost. Depending on the institution's CDSS system, the cost of the transaction (medication ordered) may (or may not) be easily captured. The true acquisition cost often resides within the pharmacy's cost accounting system and may only be pulled the same time administrative data is pulled. This poses a problem when viewing historical usage with the only pricing (current) that might be available. Take the necessary time to determine how credits are applied and whether the figures represent direct and/or indirect cost related to the pharmaceutical transactions.

Given these inherent limitations, administrative database analyses offer certain advantages over randomized controlled trials, MUEs, or even chart reviews. Large sample sizes can be reviewed in a relatively short period with minimal cost. Other advantages include the ability to gain perspective on ordinary medical practice to the issues at hand, measure performance historically, and longitudinally track patients, if necessary.

Ensuring Success

The incorporation of administrative data in financial management activities is a valuable component in the process. Here are ways in which the pharmacy manager can ensure continued success with the use of this information.

Establishing a Data-Driven Culture

One of the most critical success factors is enabling the senior administration to see value in the information derived from the data. If a supervisor does not recognize or understand the benefits, the manager's efforts must be directed elsewhere, which may not be as productive. The manager must get as much face time with key decision makers to support the case and the value she brings as an informaticist. Pharmacy informatics, as an emerging subspecialty of informatics, can be thought of as the effective organization, analysis, management, and use of information in the delivery of pharmaceutical care. Traditionally, informatics' programs and departments have dealt heavily with the information technology aspect (computerized prescriber order entry, robotics, bar coding, etc.) of data transmission, storage, and retrieval of information. However, data analysis is another important component that needs just as much attention. Having a supervisor recognize the need for a pharmacy informaticist and incorporating these activities into a position information questionnaire (PIQ) will formally recognize the duties and responsibilities that go along with position. This may (or may not) be a separate function from staff that play a more traditional drug information role within the organization. In fact, there is continued growth in the offering of pharmacy residency training programs that specialize in the field of pharmacoinformatics.

Organizational Savvy

Knowing how to leverage other departments and staff will make the pharmacy department more efficient. Learning about other active projects within the organization, the gaps of information that others seek, or research interests of key individuals or other faculty might lend itself to assistance that will pay off. Networking with other departments or facilitating a regular user group meeting will allow the pharmacy manager to identify any potential synergies (or redundant work effort) among the various activities. Most people are interested in their individual or departmental performance as it compares to their peers. In addition to tracking budget variance or other operational performance metrics, producing monthly or quarterly reports for department chairs or individual physicians with the inclusion of pharmacy usage and expense will keep project goals and clinical data fresh in their minds. This must be approached with caution, because it could easily become a way to increase the manager's workload with more time being diverted to pet projects with little benefit to the organization. Becoming a standing agenda item on the P&T committee or presenting at grand rounds or seminar is another way to demonstrate the value of this information consistently. Providing historical or baseline performance information and future trends or monitoring the impact of post-policy implementation will help establish the pharmacy manager's role as a vital component of the decision making process. Once data have been turned into actionable information, a multidisciplinary approach to action planning is needed to maximize the return on investment. Physician buy-in is essential. The contacts should be the same individuals who will influence the rational use of medications and promote their usage in a fiscally responsible manner.

Personal and Professional Development

Continuous education is a lifelong process and is something that every pharmacist should practice. In addition to networking, the pharmacy manager should find an individual who analyzes this type of information on a regular basis, someone who might act in an advisory capacity. The manager should consider what he hopes to gain from the relationship in terms of both career and personal growth. Getting involved in professional organizations will offer more networking opportunities, seminars, or structured coursework as it relates to informatics. Outside of national and state pharmacy associations, organizations such as the American Health Information Management Association (AHIMA, www.ahima.org) and Healthcare Information and Management Systems Society (HIMSS, www.himss.org) are excellent resources for the health information manager. With the acknowledgment of the impact pharmacists have in this area, in the beginning of 2007, HIMSS established a Pharmacy Informatics Task Force for its members with a role in pharmacy informatics. Its purpose is to provide a professional forum for the advancement and adoption of information systems to reduce medication errors, improve patient safety, and bring measurable improvements to the medication-use cycle. This group has officially defined *pharmacy informatics* as "the scientific field that focuses on medication-related data and knowledge within the continuum of healthcare systems—including its acquisition, storage, analysis, use, and dissemination—in the delivery of optimal medication-related patient care and health outcomes."[9] The significant role that pharmacists play in medical informatics has also been reaffirmed in statements made by the American Society of Health-System Pharmacists.[10]

Honing Skills

The mining of administrative databases involves aggregating mounds of data into actionable information. Having a basic understanding of the proper use of simple descriptive statistics (mean, mode, median, etc.) is essential; however, once analyses become more complex in nature, an understanding of linear and logistic regression (especially for risk adjustment purposes), chi-squares, P values, sample sizes, and so forth become mandatory. A variety of software applications is available to make working with the data manageable. Having programming skills to create datasets or manipulate large volumes of data is no longer an absolute necessity. In fact, many applications that sit on top of data warehouses are becoming more user friendly, which minimizes the need for IT involvement. Most analysis, statistical application, and reporting can be accomplished with simple, off-the-shelf software products that are readily available (MS Excel, Access, PowerPoint, etc.). Whether pulling data or directing dedicated programmers, unlocking the full potential of the tools (aggregating, graphing, reporting, etc.) will help the pharmacy manager to budget time efficiently. Because each organization is structured differently and because of patient confidentiality concerns, the pharmacy manager must determine the most efficient way to access data. Once the data has been summarized into final charts, tables, and graphs, the written and oral presentation of the information becomes critical. Although presentation technique and style are beyond the scope of this chapter, there are many references available to help the pharmacy manager effectively persuade her audience through the thoughtful display of information.[11-14]

Continuous Quality Improvement (CQI) of the Data

CQI is a management philosophy that asserts that most things can be improved upon—a belief that should encompass the activities of coding patient information and the charge capture of the pharmaceuticals they consume. The more time that can be spent on cleaning pharmacy-related charge masters and billing practices, the better data will become. Too often, extensive analyses are performed only to find there are fundamental flaws in the quality (and quantity) of the inputs. Many companies and consultants are available to provide a comprehensive review of the institution's charge description master (CDM) from proper revenue or code assignment to strategic pricing and general maintenance of the CDM. These factors will directly affect reimbursement; however, when the CDM is used within the context of analysis, the researcher is faced with similar limitations of the data. Some potential issues to watch out for would include:

- The failure to establish charge codes for new medications in a timely manner. The finance department, which typically maintains the CDM, will often use a generic description of the charge until a new code is created weeks or even months after the medication's introduction into patient care.

- The lack of specific charge codes for nonformulary items. If a separate budget is maintained for nonformulary items, at some point the usage of those specific items should be tracked.

- General use of non-descriptive codes with little supporting information (i.e., lack of NDC codes). Referring to the EPO example above, if the pharmacy manager had to base his analysis on codes that came with descriptions of "EPO alfa 10,000–20,000 units" or "erythropoietin 1 unit," issues of quantity—or even whether it is the correct product—would come into question.

- Recycling of a charge code over time. This is especially damaging when the timeframe of the analysis spans a long period and the code's meaning has changed.
- A change in the billing unit increment, either over time or by the primary payer. One unit of use might represent 10,000 EPO units for one payer, whereas another requires submission in 1,000 EPO unit increments.

Proactively taking an interest in the accuracy, consistency, and timeliness of the data will diminish skeptical feedback and establish the pharmacy manager as the content expert. This will allow the manager to move beyond questioning data integrity and on to the more difficult challenges of the action planning and implementation phases.

Conclusion

As managers, we are inundated with enormous amounts of data on a day-to-day basis. Knowing how to analyze information effectively and efficiently from a variety of sources can be a daunting task. As pharmacists, we often have limited formal training in informatics, so each of us must identify these sources, understand their strengths and weaknesses, and learn how to use them in a complementary fashion. With advances in electronic capture, transmission, storage, and integration of computerized systems, administrative data is becoming more readily available to assess and manage the pharmacy budget.

References

1. Arnold LM, Crouch MA, Carroll NV et al. Outcomes associated with vasoactive therapy in patients with acute decompensated heart failure. *Pharmacotherapy.* 2006; 26(8): 1078–85.
2. Bonk ME, Krown H, Matuszewski KA et al. Potentially inappropriate medications in hospitalized senior patients. *AJHP.* 2006; 63:1161–5.
3. Hsing-Ting Y, Dylan ML, Lin J et al. Hospitals' compliance with prophylaxis guidelines for venous thromboembolism. *AJHP.* 2007; 64: 69–76.
4. Hsia DC, Krushat WM, Fagan AB et al. Accuracy of diagnostic coding for Medicare patients under the prospective-payment system. *NEJM.* 1988; 318(6): 352–5.
5. Hsia DC, Ahern CA, Ritchie BP et al. Medicare reimbursement accuracy under the prospective payment system, 1985 to 1988. *JAMA.* 1992; 268(7): 896–9.
6. Hsia DC. Diagnosis related group coding accuracy of the peer review organizations. *J AHIMA.* 1992; 63(9): 56–64.
7. Berthelsen CL. Evaluation of coding data quality of the HCUP National Inpatient Sample. *Top Health Inf Manage.* 2000; 21(2): 10–23.
8. Iezzoni LI, ed. Risk Adjustment for Measuring Health Care Outcomes. 3rd edition. Chicago: Health Administration Press; 2003.
9. Pharmacy Informatics. http://www.himss.org/ASP/topics_pharmacyInformatics.asp (Accessed February 15, 2007).
10. ASHP Statement on the pharmacist's role in informatics. *AJHP.* 2007; 64: 200–3.

11. Tufte E. The visual display of quantitative information. Cheshire, CT: Graphics Press; 2005.

12. Tufte E. Envisioning information. Cheshire, CT: Graphics Press; 1990.

13. Tufte E. Visual explanations: Images and quantities, evidence and narrative. Cheshire, CT: Graphics Press; 1997.

14. Tufte E. Beautiful evidence. Cheshire, CT: Graphics Press; 2006.

Financial Management of Human Resources

Andrew L. Wilson

Introduction

Human resources and related expenses represent the second-largest financial management responsibility of a health system pharmacy manager. Drugs and the specific services and activities that support their acquisition, distribution, and management rightly command significant attention when considering the impact of pharmacy services on the health system's finances. However, human resource costs and the management of expenses present unique challenges and are governed by significant organizational policies, regulations, and constraints, creating a different set of management challenges. Unlike drug costs, human resource costs are legitimately perceived to be more completely under the control of a pharmacy leader than drug costs. Effective, thoughtful, and precise management of human resources is a critical leadership activity for a hospital pharmacy manager. In an era when there are not sufficient pharmacists and pharmacy technicians to meet staffing needs and where growing medication use and increasingly complex care require greater numbers and more specialized pharmacy staff, a detailed plan for recruitment, retention, and use of pharmacy staff is necessary to meet organizational needs and to effectively articulate the financial and other resources required to support these efforts.

Aspects of the financial management of human resources are also covered in two other chapters: chapter 3, The Health-Care Budget Process, and chapter 12, Benchmarking and Productivity. The reader is referred to these chapters for a more extensive treatment of the role and impact of the finances of human resources in each of these areas.

Measuring Labor Volume and Cost

The key common unit of measure of labor is the full-time equivalent, or FTE. One FTE represents the number of hours budgeted or allocated for the efforts of one person paid for full-time employment, typically thought of as five 8-hour shifts each week over the 52 weeks of the year (e.g., 8 hours per day $\times$ 5 shifts per week $\times$ 52 weeks = 2,080 hours.) A half-time employee who is budgeted for 1,040 hours per year is valued at 0.5 FTE (e.g., 4 hours per day $\times$ 5 shifts per week $\times$ 52 weeks = 1,040 hours.) Likewise, creative scheduling, partial shifts, and additional hours paid or worked follow the same calculation for conversion to an FTE; a single hour is equivalent to 0.000481 FTE. FTE calculations are important in budgeting and staffing plans and can be performed for a single FTE as in the examples above or in aggregate

Table 6.1. Salary Budget Calculation

Position	Paid Hours Budgeted	Paid FTE	Salary per Hour	Annual Salary	Benefit Percent	Total Annual Salary and Benefit Cost
Pharmacy Director	2,080	1.0	$80.00	$166,400	30%	$216,320
Pharmacist 1	2,080	1.0	$47.00	$97,760	30%	$127,088
Pharmacist 2	2,080	1.0	$45.50	$94,640	30%	$123,032
Pharmacist 3	2,080	1.0	$51.00	$106,080	30%	$137,904
Pharmacist 4	1,040	0.5	$49.50	$51,480	30%	$66,924
Pharmacist 5	1,040	0.5	$48.75	$50,700	30%	$65,910
Clinical Pharmacy Specialist 1	2,080	1.0	$66.00	$137,280	30%	$178,464
Clinical Pharmacy Specialist 2	2,080	1.0	$72.00	$149,760	30%	$194,688
Technician 1	2,080	1.0	$21.00	$43,680	30%	$56,784
Technician 2	2,080	1.0	$19.50	$40,560	30%	$52,728
Technician 3	2,080	1.0	$18.75	$39,000	30%	$50,700
Technician 4	1,040	0.5	$19.00	$19,760	30%	$25,688
Technician 5	520	0.25	$19.25	$10,010	30%	$13,013
Technician 6	520	0.25	$19.50	$10,140	30%	$13,182
Technician 7	2,080	1.00	$19.50	$40,560	30%	$52,728
Technician 8	520	0.25	$20.00	$10,400	30%	$13,520
Technician 9	1,560	0.75	$19.00	$29,640	30%	$38,532
Secretary/Clerk	2,080	1.0	$15.00	$31,200	30%	$40,560
Total	24,960	12.00				$1,467,765

across all or part of a department's workforce to identify and quantify resource allocation and staffing. Table 6.1 shows an example calculation and aggregation of hours and positions into FTE. Additionally, the FTE calculation can be applied to budgeted and forecasted hours in a planning process, or to actual paid and worked hours when assessing resource use and productivity. This calculation can also be used across the entire hospital in building management reports. Salary and benefit costs, workload, and productivity can be expressed with FTE as the common denominator (e.g., salary cost per FTE, benefit cost per FTE, adjusted patient days per FTE, clinical interventions per FTE, doses dispensed per FTE, etc.).

The actual productive time available and work capacity of an FTE is calculated by deducting the non-worked benefit time, such as vacation, holiday, and sick time from the full paid 2,080 hours. In practice, this decrease is approximately 10 percent (e.g., 1.0 FTE = 2,080 paid hours – vacation @ 120 hours – holidays @ 64 hours – sick time used at 24 hours = 1,872 worked hours). This calculation may demonstrate greater available work time for employees with less benefit time or may show a greater discount in organizations where employees receive more benefit time. When used in local planning and assessment, the actual benefit time figures for each employee should be used, recognizing the impact of seniority and tenure to ensure correct assessment and calculation.

Developing a Staffing Plan

A thoughtfully developed, detailed staffing plan based on a thoughtfully considered practice model is the starting point for effective financial management of human resources.[1] The goal of a practice model and staffing plan is to create an optimal relationship between the available resources (hours of pharmacist and technician work time) to the coverage hours and activities of the pharmacy and to achieve the greatest utility and output while meeting the human needs of staff. The basis for a staffing plan includes the scope of services of the pharmacy, practice standards and regulatory requirements, the leverage provided by the skills and competencies of the pharmacy staff, the capabilities of automation and technology, and an understanding and acknowledgement of the support needs at practice interfaces with physicians, nurses, and others who work in the medication use process.

The plan and its implementation is typically constrained by the organization's financial resources and may also be circumscribed by productivity benchmarks and targets and tied to historical trends and manpower utilization. Significantly, the unique and summative impacts of a variety of factors make the development of a local staffing plan a necessity. The factors that influence an institution's pharmacy staffing plan are numerous and include the goals and service targets of the pharmacy practice model; the nature, type, and acuity of patients served; the scope of pharmacy services offered; the physical layout of the hospital facility(ies) and pharmacy locations; the order management methods (CPOE vs. pharmacist order entry); the level and type of automation (central or unit-based); the nature and scope of clinical information system integration and use by the pharmacy; regulatory requirements for pharmacist activities and supervision of technical staff; and local human resource policies. Collectively, these items and other factors create a unique environment and support the need for a thoughtful, institution-specific plan.

Although the development of a best practice-based model for staffing suggests that a uniform method for developing a staffing plan is achievable, the mix of services, layout, and unique application of systems and processes in each hospital leads to the need to develop a local plan. The plan should use benchmarks, best practices, and other targets to focus continued process review and system development to work toward specific goals set jointly by pharmacy and hospital leadership. Management metrics describing cost, efficiency, and effectiveness, including metrics that describe and measure quality, should be reviewed regularly to focus efforts in improving services.

The starting point for a staffing plan is the development, understanding, and validation of a practice model. Glazier[2] outlines eight key elements of a staffing plan statement. They clearly describe the unique local nature of the considerations that underpin a comprehensive staffing plan.

- What primary issues face the institution and the pharmacy department?
- What objectives or results are to be achieved?
- What are the benefits that underlie the objectives?
- What metrics and goal-realization thresholds will describe success?
- What methodologies should be used to collect, analyze, report, and act upon the data?

- What are the mechanisms (i.e., processes, programs, and services) by which the objectives will be fulfilled?
- What are the requirements for the management model, staffing, skill mix, scheduling, and training?
- How will pharmacy interact with the medical staff and other disciplines?

A pharmacy staffing plan can be built from the ground up through the use of an activity matrix, using commonly recognized work activities, such as the review of a medication order, preparation and dispensing of a dose, completion of a clinical intervention, or other activities. This method has the advantage of addressing staffing as a fully variable cost and allowing costs and productivity to be completely addressed. In practice, there are significant limitations to this method, including minimum staffing required to cover off shifts, satellite locations, and times where work does not present at a rate that fully uses staff resources (e.g., lower workloads on a weekend evening shift or in a small retail pharmacy). In addition, time and work values for some activities are not well documented—not all activities are easily identified and counted. This is particularly true for clinical services in which definitions vary widely. The greatest barrier to this method is the significant technical and time requirements for developing the model and plan in this fashion, combined with the continuing need to measure and monitor all of the inputs necessary to assess the plan's status. A staffing plan is often derived from more global statistics, including worked and paid hours per adjusted patient day and key performance metrics, such as doses charged and orders processed. These are reasonable starting points but should not be the sole basis for developing a complete working plan. Overall metrics should be applied to workload at a detailed level, including staffing needed to meet basic professional service; management and leadership activities; non-patient care time including education, business services, required regulatory activities such as controlled substances management activities, education, and training; and other activities. The goal of a staffing plan is to provide a map for the assignment of staff and to allocate the available resources in the most effective fashion. When the staffing plan is reduced to a master schedule or is used in budget development, the details of shift differentials, holiday pay, and the ratio of paid to worked time should be considered carefully and in detail. A well designed staffing plan also identifies the need for competencies in specific practice areas (e.g., specialty areas such as a clinical service or an ICU or operating room satellite pharmacy) and core resources to support the pharmacy's services, such as information technology and automation support, and core business services, such as maintaining pharmaceutical inventory. A staffing plan can serve as the basis for a master schedule, including skill mix, work shifts, holiday and off hours coverage, and other documents that support work assignments and flexibility as patient volumes and activity change over time.

Measuring or benchmarking the pharmacy's staffing plan and resources is an important component of understanding the performance of a pharmacy department. In addition to the statistical and mathematical models of staffing discussed in chapter 12, the scope, nature, quality, and details of a specific service or department can be benchmarked. Although there are a variety of proprietary datasets and standards available, published references and professional society practice standards remain among the most effective measures in this arena.[4–9]

Recruitment and Retention

Pharmacists and pharmacy technicians have been among the more difficult professionals to recruit and retain in the past several years. Growth in employment opportunities for pharmacists in retail pharmacy, the pharmaceutical industry, education, and other areas are significant competition for a hospital pharmacy department. Pharmacist compensation in the hospital sector is typically lower than other employment opportunities, making recruitment and retention a significant activity for pharmacy leaders. Estimates of the cost of recruitment vary widely but are generally agreed to be substantial.

A structured plan for recruitment, combined with a varied strategy for retention, is the most effective way to mitigate the costs associated with turnover and vacancies.[3] Costs for separating an employee either voluntarily or for cause include the costs incurred for exit interviews, the cost of administrative functions related to termination, separation and severance pay, and potential unemployment compensation. The costs of the resulting vacancy include the net cost (or potential savings) incurred due to increased overtime or temporary employees needed to complete the work of the vacant position. Replacement costs include the cost of identifying and attracting applicants, conducting screening interviews, testing or other assessment of competency, preemployment administrative expenses, travel and moving expenses, and perhaps recruitment or other incentive payments. Finally, the new employee may not become a fully functional contributor to the work of the pharmacy for a significant period, as formal and informal orientation and training will consume a significant percentage of their time for periods up to a full year.

In some organizations the budgeting process includes an adjustment factor for anticipated vacancies during the year. A thoughtful approach to this issue by a pharmacy manager will review the turnover for a given job category and address the need for temporary staffing or overtime to meet patient care needs. A simple application of the vacancy rate from the prior year without attention to interim coverage will generally prove inadequate to meet patient care and operational requirements for the coming fiscal year.

Although recruitment and retention costs are significant, they are generally not budgeted separately for a pharmacy department except in times of large-scale recruitment during expansion or when large scale and prolonged vacancies make recruitment and retention a significant issue. Quantifying the costs associated with the recruitment and training of new staff can provide a significant basis for understanding the value and compensation needs for current staff.

Compensation

A full-scale discussion of compensation methodology is beyond the scope of this chapter. Hospitals and health systems generally adopt a comprehensive compensation philosophy across their workforce, including the full range of positions. Compensation for key professional positions, such as nurses, pharmacists, radiology technicians, physical therapists, and others may be viewed separately based on their crucial place in providing the core services of the hospital, the extended and costly recruitment and training period for new staff, and the competitive marketplace.

The purpose of a compensation philosophy is to attract, retain, and motivate employees while allocating the available funds in the most effective manner. To accomplish this, a hospital uses a mixture of base pay, incentive pay and benefits, and other nonfinancial rewards. A pay philosophy is a blend of all three components and reflects the hospital's values and the resources available. Compensation for positions may be based on a systematic review of each position and job description or structured job analysis. In this system, jobs requiring greater autonomy, specific skills, or knowledge and entailing greater responsibility are graded higher, resulting in higher compensation. This structured method ensures internal equity, that is, the relationship between compensation for a variety of jobs within the hospital. However, this method is generally supplemented with market surveys, internal assessments, and other methods to derive the most appropriate compensation for each job. Internal equity within a compensation system may also include the status of pharmacists as salaried or hourly workers, the size and scope of shift differentials and other premium pay, the role of longevity and performance in determining annual increases, and the differential between levels of supervision (e.g., how much greater is a manager's pay than those he supervises). Compensation is also constrained by the organization's financial resources, and the finite funds for paying staff may be allocated unequally across the hospital's workforce to meet greater challenges in other areas in a given fiscal year. The organization's compensation philosophy may also address the role of performance, longevity, and other factors across the workforce. A full understanding of the organization's approach can inform an effective compensation plan for the pharmacy.

When compensation changes at the open or close of a budget cycle or during the year, adjustments should be made both to the operating expense and to the budget. Significant changes in compensation may lead to variance over the year simply based on the magnitude of the change.

The role of the pharmacy leader is to understand and identify the factors leading to turnover and to focus attention on appropriate compensation based on the hospital's compensation philosophy and methods. Most often, the proof of the adequacy of compensation is turnover, loss of offered applicants to employers offering better compensation, and in some cases comments and other feedback from employee surveys. Regular attention to compensation is important, and thoughtful advocacy on behalf of the department can maintain an effective and current compensation program in the pharmacy. The pharmacy director should develop a compensation plan and philosophy. A detailed conversation with the hospital's human resources department and compensation specialist is a necessary start to understand the overall framework and develop a compensation plan for the pharmacy department.

Legal and Regulatory Considerations

Salaries, premium pay, overtime, and work practices are governed by a variety of federal, state, and local rules and regulations. Where labor unions are a part of the equation, the details of the contract and specific work rules may direct the course taken by a manager in using staff to the greatest advantage. In addition to compensation, the focus on work performance and on errors and lapses in care delivery has also focused attention on work schedules, time off, and shift duration. In some cases, specific rules apply to these situations. Again, this text is not designed to address these considerations in detail. The manager's best guide to this complex area is a good working relationship with the human resources department.

Routine Financial Management of the Human Resource Budget

The regular review of financial management of human resources is based on the staffing plan, the budgeted time available, workload, and activity. Routine biweekly or monthly review of time and activity reports with a focus on the continuing match of work, work performance, and changes in hospital activity is a key role for managers and leaders. Active forward planning for scheduled work time, including management of time off, will ensure that resources are used effectively.

The use of overtime and other premium paid time should be regularly reviewed and the department's performance managed to meet goals and standards set by leadership. The fine balance between professionalism and meeting budget targets is often met when professional staff must choose between meeting productivity and time guidelines and addressing a pressing patient care or clinical issue. A continued dialogue will ensure that thoughtful, defensible choices that meet the organization's leadership and patient care philosophy are made at all levels. Monthly review of the responsibility summary must include a review of hours, salaries and benefits, and vacancies and account for changes in workload and patient care activities.

Conclusion

A detailed and comprehensive pharmacy staffing plan is a key component in the effective and financially responsible use of human resources. A staffing plan should address the local considerations of pharmacy service scope, professional practice standards and regulatory requirements, the skills and competencies of the pharmacy staff, the capabilities of automation and technology, and the support needs at practice interfaces in the medication use process. Regular monitoring and review to meet plan goals and objectives and the measurement against benchmarks and professional standards supports, and the inclusion of recruitment, retention, and compensation plans will provide a sound basis for effective financial management of the pharmacy's human resources.

References

1. Breland BD. Believing what we know: Pharmacy provides value. *Am J Health-Syst Pharm.* 2007; 64: 1284–91.
2. Glazier HS, Malen J. Pharmacy staffing and productivity. *Am J Health-Syst Pharm.* 2007; 64: 2320–23.

3. ASHP Guidelines on the Recruitment, Selection, and Retention of Pharmacy Personnel. http://www.ashp.org/s_ashp/docs/files/BP07/HR_Gdl_Recruit.pdf.

4. Bond CA, Raehl CL. Changes in pharmacy, nursing, and total personnel staffing in U.S. hospitals, 1989–1998. *Am J Health-Syst Pharm.* 2000; 57: 970–74.

5. Gupta SR, Wojtynek JE, Walton SM et al. Monitoring of pharmacy staffing, workload, and productivity in community hospitals. *Am J Health-Syst Pharm.* 2006; 63: 1728–34.

6. Pedersen CA, Schneider PJ, Scheckelhoff DJ. ASHP national survey of pharmacy practice in hospital settings: dispensing and administration—2005. *Am J Health-Syst Pharm.* 2006; 63:327–45.

7. Pedersen CA, Schneider PJ, Scheckelhoff DJ. ASHP national survey of pharmacy practice in hospital settings: dispensing and administration—2007. *Am J Health-Syst Pharm.* 2008; 65: 827–43.

8. Vermeulen LC, Rough SS, Thielke TS et al. Strategic approach for improving the medication-use process in health systems: The high-performance pharmacy practice framework. *Am J Health-Syst Pharm.* 2007; 64: 1699–1710.

9. Schumock GT, Butler MG, Meek PD et al. Evidence of the economic benefit of clinical pharmacy services: 1996–2000. *Pharmacotherapy.* 2003; 23: 113–32.

Cost Management Basics

John A. Armitstead
Ann R. Hamlin
Teresa Centers

Introduction

Standard Cost Accounting Background

Effective costing by individual products in the pharmacy environment can be challenging for the pharmacy manager who has limited experience with accounting principles. But the time spent in understanding costing by product line can be beneficial to the pharmacy manager and to the institution in the current environment of growing drug costs and the complex financial world of health system management. There have not been many documents in the literature on pharmacy standard cost accounting, also known as product costing. Previous publications on managing costs and cost accounting described building intermediate products using systems of the ratio of costs-to-charges method, or averaging costs by therapeutic classes. Most of these publications were written before the expansion of computer hardware and software that is available today. Authors commented on the need to weigh the potential value of additional data against the time and effort needed to collect the data. Systems today make product line much more easy to attain, but diligence to the system detail is needed.

A well-designed product costing system can serve as a tool to explain the department's performance, case performance, and service line performance or physician practices. Product line costing is a tool to manage and evaluate costs and utilization of products (e.g., what goes in, comes out). What product line costing does not do is determine whether the cost expended was appropriate—best practice. For example, product line costing for a proposed service line increase will describe the drugs and associated costs required to deliver the service, but it will not reveal whether the use of those drugs is the best practice for the service line.

Product Line Costing Applications

Within the hospital system, pharmacy services expenses can easily account for 8–10 percent of the total hospital budget. Any department with that amount of impact on the financial status of the institution will be on the radar for financial review. If a product line costing system is effectively implemented and maintained, it can be used not only to measure the financial performance of the pharmacy department against the annual budget (static budget) but can be used to explain costs incurred after the budget was completed. Flexible budgeting is central to a meaningful review of pharmacy costs throughout the year. With flexible budgeting, the key is not how far off target the actual expenses are compared to the annual (static) budget. The key question with the use of a flexible budget is, "Are the actual expenses incurred reflected in the flexible budget?"

If there is a significant difference in expenses and the flexible budget, this is the opportunity to investigate and correct problems. It is better to try and fix a small leak then to wait until the whole dam collapses!

Basic Principles of Product Line Costing

Costing in the health-care industry has many challenges. In the pharmacy environment this can be seen thru the HCPCS (Healthcare Common Procedure Coding System) requirements for billing when compared to how the drugs are purchased or dispensed. This can cause additional challenges with the costing environment, which must adjust to accommodate the new billing requirements each year. Before those factors are discussed, a review of the basics of costing and building intermediate products is in order. In the case of pharmacy, an intermediate product (IP) should represent the standard costs associated with dispensing one unit of a drug. These costs should include all resources of the institution related directly and indirectly to this drug.

Classification of Costs

All costs are first classified into direct or indirect cost. Direct costs are the costs that can be identified specifically to the intermediate product. This includes the cost of the drug, the labor associated with the preparation and dispensing of the drug, and specific devices used in the dispensing. The indirect costs are those costs that cannot be traced directly to a specific intermediate product. These would include costs such as the cleaning cost for the space, administrative functions, or accounting functions. How these costs are allocated depends on how the costing system is configured.

After determining the cost relationship to an intermediate product, the cost is then classed into either fixed or variable category. Variable costs change in proportion to changes in the intermediate product, whereas fixed costs do not change despite changes in the intermediate product. For example, if the pharmacy department purchases the drug ampicillin sodium, it is a variable direct cost because the pharmacy manager can directly associate this cost with the dispensing of the drug. The cost of the equipment used to dispense the drug, such as an automated dispensing device (i.e., Pyxis MedStation) is fixed cost because it doesn't change in relationship to the volume or mix of drugs dispensed.

Exhibit 7.1 outlines cost assignments that are typically used in product line costing. For most of this discussion, direct variable costs and direct variable labor costs will be the focus.

Building Intermediate Products

The pharmacy manager may wonder about the benefit of these classifications. The ultimate goal for this type of financial management is give a department the ability to build a flexible budget and the ability to benchmark. A flexible budget makes variance management more accurate and responsive. All organizations go through the establishment of a static budget each year. The static budget is based on a specific amount of

Exhibit 7.1. Types of Cost Assignments

Initials	Term	Description
FDE	Fixed Direct Equipment	Distribution of cost of the depreciation and maintenance of the equipment involved in the intermediate product
FDF	Fixed Direct Facility	Distribution of cost of the depreciation and maintenance of the facility involved in the intermediate product
FDL	Fixed Direct Labor	Labor that does not change in proportion to the changes in intermediate product
FDO	Fixed Direct Other	Other costs that do not change in proportion to the changes in intermediate product (such as benefits)
VL	Variable Labor	Labor that changes in proportion to the changes in intermediate product
VO	Variable Other	Other costs that change in proportion to the changes in intermediate product (such as benefits)
VS	Variable Supplies	Cost of expendable supplies that change in proportion to the changes in the intermediate product

volume and case mix and is not adjusted after it is finalized. A flexible budget is the result of the static budget adjusted to the actual volume and mix experienced during the period.

There are many methods to accomplish a flexible budget in an organization working with standards by intermediate product. The decision support system capabilities will determine what choices a pharmacy manager has in this process. In the pharmacy environment managers have the ability to establish standard cost by each intermediate product. Exhibit 7.2 shows how direct and indirect costs are used to build the standard cost for each intermediate product. This is accomplished through establishing a relative value unit (RVU) for the cost type and category for each intermediate product that is used in calculating the standard cost. Exhibit 7.2 shows the RVU assignment and the budgeted and actual cost for the drug alteplase per 1 mg inj 100 mg, excluding the labor component. In this example, the RVU for VS drugs is $25.75, which is the expected cost per the dispensed drug based on purchasing contracts. The actual cost of $18.84 is the result of the actual general ledger cost in association with the volume produced, which can be affected by potential rebates, lost or wasted product, charge processing issues, or invoice processing. The $23.64 is the budgeted cost, which can be affected based on anticipated rebates for volume purchasing non-product specific or base line cost from historical actual costing.

An intermediate product standard should represent the best practice and therefore a target standard cost. This is the second advantage to the department. This gives the pharmacy the ability to benchmark performance in several different ways. The manager can

Exhibit 7.2. Alteplase per 1 MG inj 100 MG

Dept	IP	Cost Type	Cost Category	RVU	Volume	Act	Std
1058732410	72144	FDE	DEP/SC	1.00000000	600	0.03	0.02
1058732410	72144	FDE	OTHER	1.00000000	600	0.12	0.07
1058732410	72144	FDF	0	1.00000000	600	0.00	0.00
1058732410	72144	FDL	0	0.00000001	600	0.00	0.00
1058732410	72144	FDO	BEN	0.00000001	600	0.00	0.00
1058732410	72144	FDO	OCE	1.00000000	600	0.02	0.02
1058732410	72144	VL	OTHER	0.00000001	600	0.00	0.00
1058732410	72144	VL	RN	0.00000001	600	0.00	0.00
1058732410	72144	VL	TECH	0.00000001	600	0.00	0.00
1058732410	72144	VO	0	0.00000001	600	0.00	0.00
1058732410	72144	VS	DRUGS	25.75260000	600	18.84	23.64
1058732410	72144	VS	IMP	0.00000001	600	0.00	0.00
1058732410	72144	VS	SUPPLY	0.00000001	600	0.00	0.00
1058732410	72144	FI	0	23.7531	600	4.79	8.29
1058732410	72144	VI	0	23.7531	600	0.09	0.12

	Act	Std
Variable Direct Cost	18.84	23.64
Fixed Direct Cost	0.17	0.11
Total Direct Cost	19.01	23.75
Variable Indirect Cost	0.09	0.12
Fixed Indirect Cost	4.79	8.29
Total Indirect Cost	4.88	8.40
Total Cost	23.89	32.15

use the budgeted standards to compare to actual experience and to run actual trending analysis across budget years for all products. This helps assess labor efficiency or productivity, contract costing, and product waste management.

Application of Intermediate Products to Budget: Calculated, Forced, Actual

Some decision support systems are limited to maintaining only one RVU per product and do not have the capability of time-date stamp for RVU assignments. These two factors are constraints that a pharmacy manager may have to overcome in the costing environment, but there are processes that can be developed to limit the impact of these restrictions. In a single RVU assignment environment, the standard is a result of the RVU assignment for the product times the budgeted volume. In Exhibit 7.3, an RVU of $59.00 times the budgeted volume of 50 results in a budgeted weighted volume of 2,950. This result is the weighted volume for the intermediate product, which can be budgeted as described previously. The relationship of the individual intermediate product weighted volume for a particular cost type-category in ratio to the overall department's weighted

Exhibit 7.3. Department 1058999990

CDM	IP	Description	VS RVU	Bud Vol	Budgeted Weighted Volume	Alloc %	Allocation Cost	Forced Budget RVU
5100000	45000	Product A	59.00	50	2,950	1.03%	2,580.88	51.62
5200000	45001	Product B	1,250.00	125	156,250	54.68%	136,699.27	1,093.59
5300000	45002	Product C	62.00	649	40,238	14.08%	35,203.23	54.24
5400000	45003	Product D	71.00	1027	72,917	25.52%	63,793.28	62.12
5500000	45004	Product E	536.00	25	13,400	4.69%	11,723.33	468.93

Total Weighted Volume   285,755   100.00%   250,000

Requested budget $ 250,000

Weighted Volume Variance   114.30%

Exhibit 7.4. Department 1058999990

CDM	IP	Description	VS RVU	Act Vol	Actual Weighted Volume	Alloc%	Allocation Cost	Forced Actual RVU
5100000	45000	Product A	59.00	75	4,425	1.79%	4,932.95	65.77
5200000	45001	Product B	1,250.00	81	101,250	41.04%	112,872.59	1,393.49
5300000	45002	Product C	62.00	700	43,400	17.59%	48,381.93	69.12
5400000	45003	Product D	71.00	952	67,592	27.40%	75,350.96	79.15
5500000	45004	Product E	536.00	56	30,016	12.17%	33,461.57	597.53
				Total Weighted Volume	246,683	100.00%	275,000	
				Actual Spending	$ 275,000			
				Weighted Volume Variance	89.70%			

volume for that cost type-category is used to develop a forced/calculated budget RVU or cost, depending on the cost type. In Exhibit 7.3 that product is shown. Product A has an anticipated RVU for variable supply of $59.00; however, when the weighted volume allocation to the static budget for variable supplies is used, the forced or calculated cost becomes $51.62. In some cases these gaps can become significant and must be worked through to resolution accordingly.

This allocation is then used to generate a similar calculation for the actual volume and cost. In Exhibit 7.4, when the actual volume and cost is applied, it generates the calculated actual cost per intermediate product from the budgeted RVU assignment. The lesson to take from this is that one incorrect RVU can drastically affect the entire process. Exhibit 7.5 shows how one product can result in three different costs. The first being the anticipated cost or the RVU; the second being the budgeted cost; and then finally the calculated actual cost. This can make the review challenging; however it also helps to tighten the costing process, because it pushes all three steps to work with each other.

Maintaining Intermediate Products

It has been proposed that pharmacy managers should set the RVUs annually and then never look back until the next budget year. If the pharmacy department is to have the most accurate cost per unit information, then the pharmacy manager must actively adjust the relative value units (RVUs) assigned to the intermediate product to reflect current costs and dispensing practice. Monthly updates of product data are a reasonable goal. Steps include adding any new products, updating supply cost RVUs to the most recent average cost based on purchasing changes, tightening labor standards to gain efficiency, and evaluating the actual results as compared to the original budget. To go a step further, maintaining a separate data set outside of the decision support system—including the budgeted standard and RVU alongside the actual RVU and cost—provides the ability to review the purchasing contracts compared to the initial expectation. The pharmacy manager can also compare benchmark standards to other organizations' internal standards.

How does a pharmacy department accomplish all of this to result in a successful flexible budget? Standards must be developed for each intermediate product. To accomplish this each cost type and category for the intermediate products must have a relative value unit (RVU)

Exhibit 7.5. Department 1058999990

CDM	IP	Description	VS RVU	Forced Budget RVU	Forced Actual RVU
5100000	45000	Product A	59.00	51.62	65.77
5200000	45001	Product B	1,250.00	1,093.59	1,393.49
5300000	45002	Product C	62.00	54.24	69.12
5400000	45003	Product D	71.00	62.12	79.15
5500000	45004	Product E	536.00	468.93	597.53

assigned. Depending on the cost type, this RVU can either be the actual cost per unit, labor minutes per unit, or a weighting factor that helps distribute the cost accordingly.

In certain costing environments it is recommended that like products in cost are grouped together into a single intermediate product to reduce maintenance. This may actually cause more problems because most users are not focused on getting products moved to the correct grouped product as costs change. Then, when the product is changed to a different cost group, it makes problems for analysis. Each intermediate product should be maintained separately to accomplish the most accurate costing. The only environment in which grouping of products may work is with pharmacy labor standards, which are reviewed in detail later in this chapter.

Pharmacy Billing Interface to Patient Accounts

Before the pharmacy manager begins the process for costing within the pharmacy department, he or she must understand how the billing system is setup and the data that will be used for the costing process. In most environments, the billing quantity is pushed from the pharmacy clinical system to the patient bill. Because of this, converting the purchasing cost for each intermediate product to match the billing cost is required, even though the pharmacy may purchase or dispense in a different quantity.

Our hospital made a decision to bill both inpatients and outpatients based on HCPCS quantities. This required that all doses dispensed be converted to HCPCS billing units. Working with the pharmacy department, the authors created a crosswalk that reflects all the charge description master codes along with the CMS (Centers for Medicare and Medicaid Services) factors and purchasing units. This is maintained throughout the year so that it accurately reflects the RVUs (Exhibit 7.6).

For drugs that do not have HCPCS codes assigned, the pharmacy assigns charge description master (CDM) codes based on the single-unit package size (2 ml, 5 ml, etc.). The pharmacy order entry system defines a number for each drug's National Drug Code (NDC). Based on the drug form code and the total package size, the pharmacy calculates the cost per metric unit that is used as the basis to build the drug RVU.

Exhibit 7.6 identifies how the drug alteplase per 1 mg inj 100 mg has an HCFA quantity of 1 mg, but is dispensed as 100 mg, so the HCFA factor is 0.01. This step is necessary to convert the dispensing cost (RVU) to the billing cost (RVU). In this example the RVU weight is converted to reflect the cost of 1 billing unit at 1 mg.

With this crosswalk the appropriate RVU for the drug cost is show to be $25.75 for this example. This crosswalk allows accurate assignment of the variable drug cost in accordance with how the drug quantity is being passed to the costing system.

Once the method for extracting the final intermediate product volume and transferred to the costing system is understood, the RVU assignments can be addressed to begin the costing process. The best way to accomplish this is to develop an RVU worksheet to compile the information. For large areas such as pharmacy this can be accomplished within a worksheet (Exhibit 7.7).

Product Line Costing—Labor RVU

In the conversion process the variable drug cost RVU assignment is developed; however, the RVU assignment for the labor component remains to be addressed. The labor associated with a drug is not reflected in the billing quantity but is more accurately reflected in the dispensing volume.

Current systems do not always extract a separate dispensing quantity to the hospital billing system. Because it is critical to have the dispensing volume to accurately measure the labor, consider a separate extract to obtain the dispensing quantity associated with the billed units. Instead of maintaining each individual drug for labor, grouping all drugs into labor groups (Exhibit 7.8) as defined by the pharmacy department based on literature reviews and observations of workflow can be considered.

In the example of the drug alteplase "per 1 mg inj 100 mg," it is assigned to intermediate product 44342, which represents IV preparation, and it has a 3.6 minutes per dispensing volume RVU. Loading the dispensing quantity to the above groups calculates the anticipated labor requirements (Exhibit 7.9).

The labor RVU components are maintained in minutes, so one hour would be reflected as a 60 for the RVU. Maintaining this same RVU under the variable other, which in the authors' organization represents the variable benefits associated with the salary, keeps the ratio between the two consistent.

To assign staff, determine how each title within the department should be classified. If the department has a Pharmacy Technician 1, then what is the required minimum staffing to open the pharmacy service and then beyond that what portion of a position is fixed versus variable? Determine what portion of the position is intermediate product specific and what portion is general or fixed functions. This is important to maintain as functions change within a position to accurately cost labor. An example of one of the pharmacy services' labor distribution is shown in Exhibit 7.10.

Fixed Costs Assignments to Intermediate Products

Use the same concept for the fixed direct labor using minutes and the same RVU assignment for fixed direct other-benefits. If no RVU assignment is maintained on a cost type, then all the cost is equally spread across products. For fixed labor in which minimum staffing is required, this is an option.

For the fixed direct equipment the pharmacy manager can use a weighting system that looks at any equipment that may be involved in intermediate product. If equipment is used for a specific product preparation, then the pharmacy manager can assign a weight of 10, versus a product that doesn't use anything but minimal equipment, which can be assigned a 1. This distributes the cost of the depreciation and maintenance of the equipment accordingly (Exhibits 7.11 and 7.12). This is sometimes overlooked, but Exhibits 7.11 and 7.12 illustrate how this aspect of cost can drastically change the costing of an intermediate product.

Once the pharmacy department has completed the RVU assignments, the manager will have the data necessary to calculate both the budgeted and actual cost. Before moving forward, the pharmacy manager must review how the budgeted weighted volume compares to the budgeted cost. Exhibit 7.13 highlights how this is done with the variable supply in total. Review each category to verify whether the budget assignments appear reasonable. Typically, the upcoming budget year is based on the actual cost per unit for the current

Exhibit 7.6. Pharmacy CDM Review Products with HCFA Quantity Assigned

CDM	CDM DESCRIPTION	hcfa quantitiy	RVU Update	product_id
11041242	ALTEPLASE PER 1MG INJ 100MG	1	$25.75	5614
11041292	ALTEPLASE PER 1MG INJ 50MG	1	$25.75	5617
11345212	BASILIXIMAB 20MG, INJ	20	$1,442.45	2180
11431012	BEVACIZUMAB, PER 10MG	10	$53.32	5401
11453252	BIVALIRUDIN INJ PER 1MG	1	$1.70	5442
11617232	CASPOFUNGIN 5MG	5	$23.00	4843
11622562	CEFAZOLIN SODIUM, 500MG, INJ	0.5	$0.87	2316
11631252	CEFTAZIDIME INJ PER 500MG	0.5	$2.75	4714
11634262	CEFTRIAXONE SODIUM, PER 250MG	0.25	$0.94	2340
11642062	CETUXIMAB INJ PER 10MG	10	$47.01	5406
11766022	CLOFARABINE 1MG/ML	1	$110.17	5554
11938712	DACLIZUMAB, PARENTERAL, 25MG	25	$170.83	2509
11989003	DAPTOMYCIN INJ PER 1MG	1	$0.32	5391
12007316	DARBEPOETIN (NON-ESRD) 1MCG	1	$2.35	5729
12007319	DARBEPOETIN (NON-ESRD) 1MCG	1	$2.35	5730
12218562	DOBUTAMINE HCL, PER 250MG	250000	$3.25	2650
12228232	DOLASETRON MESYLATE 10MG INJ	10	$3.78	5301
12515212	FILGRASTIM (G-CSF) 300MCG INJ	300	$156.27	2808
12515222	FILGRASTIM (G-CSF) 480MCG INJ	480	$248.97	2809
12674722	GEMCITABINE HCL, 200MG	0.2	$117.25	2887
12732302	GRANISETRON HCL, 100MCG, INJ	0 .1	$9.28	5476
13016520	IMMUNE GLOBULIN PER 500MG (GAM)	0.5	$29.49	5686
13016500	IMMUNE GLOBULIN PER 500MG (GAM)	0.5	$29.49	5685
13016410	IMMUNE GLOBULIN PER 500MG (POLY)	0.5	$27.18	5637
13009212	INFLIXIMAB, 10MG, INJ	10	$54.21	3053
14106332	OCTREOTIDE ACETATE INJ PER 25MCG	25	$1.20	5561
14106312	OCTREOTIDE ACETATE INJ PER 25MCG	0.025	$0.34	5562
14288872	PEGFILGRASTIM INJ PER 6MG	6	$2,068.24	5347
14484232	PIPRCLLN/TAZBCTM PER 1.125GM	1.125	$4.49	4920
14484212	PIPRCLLN/TAZBCTM PER 1.125GM	1.125	$4.72	4974
15751232	ZIPRASIDONE MESYLATE INJ 10MG	10	$19.01	5350
15760722	ZOLEDRONIC ACID INJ 1MG	1	$197.68	5257

Calculating hcfa factor:

1. If drug_form_code = 2, and strength_vol_prim >0; then hf = hcfa quantitiy/(strength_num_prim/strength_vol_prim).

2. If drug_form_code = 2, and strength_vol_prim = 0 or blank; then hf = hcfa quantity.

3. If drug_form_code = 1, and du_to_pu_factor >0; then hf = hcfa quantity.

4. If drug_form_code = 1, and du_to_pu_factor is 0 or is null; then hf = hcfa quantity/strength_num_prim.

Exhibit 7.6. Pharmacy CDM Review Products with HCFA Quantity Assigned (Continued)

generic_name	drug_form_code	du_to_pu_factor	hcpc	hcfa_factor	strength_num_prim	strength_unit_prim	strength_vol_prim	recalc hcfa factor	variance from database
ALTEPLASE	1		J2997	0.01	100	MG	0	0.01	0
ALTEPLASE	1		J2997	0.02	50	MG	0	0.02	0
BASILIXIMAB	1	20	J0480	20	20	MG	5	20	0
BEVACIZUMAB	2		J9035	0.4	25	MG	1	0.4	0
BIVALIRUDIN	1		J0583	0	250	MG	0	0.004	0
CASPOFUNGIN ACETATE	1		J0637	0.07	70	MG	0	0.071429	0.0006
CEFAZOLIN ADD-VANTAGE	1		J0690	0.5	1	GM	0	0.5	0.0000
CEFTAZIDIME	1	6	J0713	0.5	6	GM	24	0.5	0.0000
CEFTRIAXONE SODIUM	1	1	J0696	0.25	1	GM	10	0.25	0.0000
CETUXIMAB	2		J9055	5	2	MG	1	5	0
CLOFARABINE	2		J9027	1	1	MG	1	1	0
DACLIZUMAB	2		J7513	5	5	MG	1	5	0
DAPTOMYCIN	1	500	J0878	1	500	MG	10	1	0
DARBEPOETIN ALFA IN POLYSO	2		J0881	0	200	MCG	0.4	0.002	0
DARBEPOETIN ALFA IN POLYSO	2		J0881	0	500	MCG	1	0.002	0
DOBUTamine 500MG/250ML PREM	2		J1250	125	2000	MCG	1	125	0.0000
DOLASETRON MESYLATE	2		J1260	0.5	20	MG	1	0.5	0
FILGRASTIM	2		J1440	1	300	MCG	1	1	0
FILGRASTIM	2		J1441	1.6	300	MCG	1	1.6	0
GEMCITABINE HCL	1	1	J9201	0.2	1	GM	26.32	0.2	0.0000
GRANISETRON HCL	2		J1626	1	0.1	MG	1	1	0.0000
IMMUNE GLOB,GAM CAPRYLATE	2		J1567	5	1	GM	10	5	0.0000
IMMUNE GLOB, GAM CAPRYLATE	2		J1567	5	1	GM	10	5	0.0000
IMMUNE GLOBULIN S/D	1		J1566	0.05	10	GM	0	0.05	0.0000
INFLIXIMAB	1	100	J1745	10	100	MG	10	10	0
OCTREOTIDE ACETATE	2		J2354	0.05	500	MCG	1	0.05	0
OCTREOTIDE ACETATE	2		J2354	0.5	0.05	MG	1	0.5	0.0000
PEGFILGRASTIM	2		J2505	0.6	6	MG	0.6	0.6	0.0000
PIPERACILLIN/ TAZABACTAM VIA	1		J2543	0.25	4.5	GM	0	0.25	0
PIPERACILLIN/ TAZOBACTAM	1		J2543	0.5	2.25	GM	0	0.5	0
ZIPRASIDONE MESYLATE	1		J3486	0.5	20	MG	0	0.5	0.0000
ZOLEDRONIC ACID	2		J3487	1.25	4	MG	5	1.25	0

Exhibit 7.7.

| | | | | Variable Labor (VL) | | |
CDM	Description	IP Number	GL Key	RN	Tech	Other
1058732410	INPATIENT PHARMACY					
10500512	STERILE WATER IRRIG 1000ML	33578	50	0.00	0.00	0.00
10501422	STERILE WATER 1000ML	33580	50	0.00	0.00	0.00
10502752	SODIUM BICARB 5% 500ML	43442	50	0.00	0.00	0.00
10503432	ALCOHL 5%/DXTRSE 5% 100ML	67089	50	0.00	0.00	0.00
10505412	DEXTROSE 5%-LR 1000ML	33603	50	0.00	0.00	0.00
10505522	TPN PEDIATRIC	33604	50	0.00	0.00	0.00
10505552	ELECTROLYTE-A SOLN 1000ML	33606	50	0.00	0.00	0.00
10506412	TPN ADULT	33607	50	0.00	0.00	0.00
10511412	DEXTROSE 10% WATER 1000ML	41741	50	0.00	0.00	0.00

fiscal year multiplied by the projected volume for the upcoming budget year. If the RVUs are updated during the budget process, make certain that the formula is still within the expectation of 95 to 105 percent of target. Exhibit 7.13 shows how this grouping is slightly outside of the range at 114.30 percent. This calculation is based on the actual or budgeted weighted volume divided by either the actual cost or budgeted cost. In Exhibit 7.13 this would be $285,755 divided by $250,000, resulting in the 114.30 percent.

If the verification percentage is greater than 100 percent, then this could be a result of various reasons some of which may include the following:

Exhibit 7.8. Labor Grouping to Product

Product Type	Minutes
UD/Bulk Dose	1.4
IV Dose/Premix/AddV	2.2
Controlled Substance	2.8
IV Preparation	3.6
Oral Special	4.8
Nonformulary/PCA	5.0
Dose Packs	6.0
Dialysis Solutions	8.3
Chemo/Cardioplegia	10.0
IVIG Preparation	17.8
Special Handling	20.0
Compounded Item	20.0
Pediatric TPN	21.8
Adult TPN	25.5

Exhibit 7.7. (Continued)

| | Variable Supply (VS) | | Variable Other (VO) | Fixed Direct Labor | Fixed Direct Facility | Fixed Direct Other (FDO) | | Fixed Direct Equipment (FDE) | |
Drugs	Implants	General Supplies	Variable Other (VO)	Fixed Direct Labor	Fixed Direct Facility	Benefits	OCE	Depreciation/ Service Contracts	Other
$0.70	$0.00	$0.01	0.00	0.00	0.00	0.00	0.00	0.00	0.00
$0.74	$0.00	$0.01	0.00	0.00	0.00	0.00	0.00	0.00	0.00
$2.43	$0.00	$0.01	0.00	0.00	0.00	0.00	0.00	0.00	0.00
$7.64	$0.00	$0.01	0.00	0.00	0.00	0.00	0.00	0.00	0.00
$0.79	$0.00	$0.01	0.00	0.00	0.00	0.00	0.00	0.00	0.00
$35.01	$0.00	$0.01	0.00	0.00	0.00	0.00	0.00	0.00	0.00
$1.29	$0.00	$0.01	0.00	0.00	0.00	0.00	0.00	0.00	0.00
$37.21	$0.00	$0.01	0.00	0.00	0.00	0.00	0.00	0.00	0.00
$0.65	$0.00	$0.01	0.00	0.00	0.00	0.00	0.00	0.00	0.00

- The RVUs are overstated.
- Extra charges were processed (either incorrectly or outside of accounting period).
- Supplies were used that were purchased by another area.
- Bulk supplies were carried forward from last year.
- Invoice processing is inconsistent.
- There is a combination of any of the above reasons.

Had the variance been less than 100 percent, then the reasons would have changed to possibly one of the following:

- The RVUs are understated.
- Charges were not processed (or a major prior year correction was included in the volume).

Exhibit 7.9.

DEPT	CDM	VL IP	CHGS	Billing Qty	RX VL QTY
41	10500512		73.11	12	6
41	10501422		1118	167	124
41	10505522		34586.4	255	255
41	10506412		44504.65	107	107
41	10511412		839.52	99	96
41	10511422		124.22	16	16
41	10511432		4457.86	22	22
41	10520412		1582.22	187	170

Exhibit 7.10. Pharmacy Labor Table (capped/% fixed/% variable) Capped Positions:

| | | | | Shifts Covered | | | | | | | |
| | Pharmacy | Job | | | | | | | | | Total |
Cost Ctr	Area	Code	Position	M	T	W	Th	F	S	S	FTE
1058732410	Central	P0046H4	Pharmacist	3	3	3	3	3	3	3	4.2
1058732410	Central	T0181H0	Technician	6	6	6	6	6	6	6	7.88
1058732480	Pediatrics	P0046H4	Pharmacist	2	2	2	2	2	1	1	2.4
1058732480	Pediatrics	T0181H0	Technician	2	2	2	2	2	1	1	2.25
1058732480	Markey IP	P0046H4	Pharmacist	2	2	2	2	2	1	1	2.4
1058732480	Markey IP	T0181H0	Technician	2	2	2	2	2	1	1	2.25
1058732490	Markey OP	P0046H4	Pharmacist	1	1	1	1	1	1	1	1.4
1058732490	Markey OP	T0181H0	Technician	1	1	1	1	1	1	1	1.31
1058732900	KCP	P0046H4	Pharmacist	1	1	1	1	1	1		1.2
1058732900	KCP	T0181H0	Technician	2	2	2	2	2	2		2.25
Pharmacy Total		P0046H4	Pharmacist								11.6
Pharmacy Total		T0181H0	Technician								15.94

Job Code Assignments—Percent Variable Labor

Area	Job_Cd	Job Code Description	% Variable Labor	BUD FTE	V/L FTE
Central	N4059H0	PHARMACY TECH SR/ON-CALL/HOSPITAL	100%	0.90	0.90
	N4060H0	PHARMACY TECH/ON-CALL/HOSPITAL	100%	3.60	3.60
	N4064H0	PHARMACIST STAFF/ON-CALL/HOSPITAL	100%	4.80	4.80
	P0046H4	PHARMACIST CLIN STAFF/HOSP	50%	33.00	16.50
	P0052H4	PHARM CLIN STAFF/SJFT-BSD	100%	3.00	3.00
	P0184H4	PHARMACIST/HOSP	50%	0.30	0.15
	T0084H0	PHARMACY TECH LEAD/HOSP	100%	3.72	3.72
	T0181H0	PHARMACY TECH SR/HOSP	100%	22.32	22.32
	T0265H0	PHARMACY TECH/HOSP	100%	17.19	17.19
	X999999	BUDGET ADJUSTMENT – FPA	(blank)	–2.61	
Central Total				86.22	72.18
Markey IP	P0046H4	PHARMACIST CLIN STAFF/HOSP	50%	2.50	1.25
			100%	0.00	0.00
	T0181H0	PHARMACY TECH SR/HOSP	100%	1.86	1.86
	T0265H0	PHARMACY TECH/HOSP	100%	0.93	0.93
Markey IP Total				5.29	4.04
Markey OP	P0046H4	PHARMACIST CLIN STAFF/HOSP	75%	3.40	2.55
	T0265H0	PHARMACY TECH/HOSP	100%	2.73	2.73
Markey OP Total				6.13	5.28
Grand Total				97.64	81.50

Exhibit 7.11.

Equipment	Annual Dep/SC Cost	Procedure	Equip Used	Equip Cost	Equip Allocation	Weight
Equipment A	$2,000	Procedure A	C,E	$4,060	22.83%	2.28
Equipment B	$1,300	Procedure B	A,C,D	$5,064	28.48%	2.85
Equipment C	$2,060	Procedure C	B,E	$3,300	18.56%	1.86
Equipment D	$1,004	Procedure D	B,C,E	$5,360	30.14%	3.01
Equipment E	$2,000	Procedure E	None	$0	0.00%	0.00
	$8,364			$17,784	100.00%	10.00

Exhibit 7.12.

Procedure	Weight	Actual Cost	Even
Procedure A	2.28	$2,282.95	$2,000.00
Procedure B	2.85	$2,847.50	$2,000.00
Procedure C	1.86	$1,855.60	$2,000.00
Procedure D	3.01	$3,013.95	$2,000.00
Procedure E	0.00	$0.00	$2,000.00
	10.00	$10,000.00	$10,000.00

Exhibit 7.13.

Dept	CDM	Desc.	Budget Volume	VS RVU	Weighted Volume
9999	51000000	Product A	50.00	$59.00	$2,950.00
9999	52000000	Product B	125.00	$1,250.00	$156,250.00
9999	53000000	Product C	649.00	$62.00	$40,238.00
9999	54000000	Product D	1,027.00	$71.00	$72,917.00
9999	55000000	Product E	25.00	$536.00	$13,400.00

Tot Weighted Volume: $285,755.00
Tot VS Budget: $250,000.00
Weighted Vol. Variance: 114.30%

Exhibit 7.14. FY2007 Monthly Standard Review— Variable Supply Variances—November

CDM #	Description	IP Number	YTD Bud Volume	YTD Act Volume	Budget RVU	VS Drugs RVU
11111152	MISC MED OR	33731	2,842.30	1,562.00	$22.67	$3.21
11111132	NON-CHARGE	43486	10,637.03	12,043.00	$5.75	$5.75
11111112	MISC MED IN	33729	1,643.78	12,012.00	$9.11	$464.39
			3,541,167	4,434,891		

The flex budget is calculated from the relationship of the budgeted weighted volume to the budgeted cost.

$$\text{Flex Bud} = \frac{\text{Budget Wt. Vol.}}{\text{Budget VS}} \times \text{Act. Wt. Vol.}$$

- A bulk purchase occurred.
- Invoice processing is inconsistent.
- Another area used the supplies that the pharmacy department purchased.
- There is a combination of any of the above reasons.

One of the items that the pharmacy manager must look for when reviewing the resulted cost is the gap between it and the RVU. When working through this step, the pharmacy manager must evaluate to see whether issues are with invoice processing, billing, or truly with RVU assignment. If one product is incorrect, then all products will attempt to adjust to account for the incorrect RVU. To ensure that the pharmacy department is maintaining accurate costing, the pharmacy manager must work with the RVUs each month, adjusting when appropriate.

Exhibit 7.14. FY2007 Monthly Standard Review— Variable Supply Variances—November *(Continued)*

YTD Bud Drugs WV	YTD Bud Weighted Volume	YTD Act Drugs WV	YTD Act Imp WV	YTD Act Supply WV	YTD Act Weighted Volume
$64,427.27	$64,427.27	$5,014.02	$0.00	$0.00	$5,014.02
$61,176.75	$61,176.75	$69,247.25	$0.00	$0.00	$69,247.25
$14,971.55	$14,971.55	$5,578,252.68	$0.00	$0.00	$5,578,252.68
$5,750,959	$5,750,959	$12,218,024	$0	$4,256	$12,222,280

	VS Drugs	VS Imp	VS Supply	VS Total
Total YTD Actual Weighted Volume:	$12,218,024	$0	$4,256	$12,222,280
YTD Actual Variable Supplies:	$6,212,307	$0	#####	$6,375,457
YTD Actual Variance:	196.67%	0.00%	2.61%	191.71%
Total YTD Budget Weighted Volume:	$5,750,959	$0	$0	$5,750,959
YTD Budget Variable Supplies:	$5,848,911	$0	#####	$6,117,122
YTD Budget Variance:	98.33%	0.00%	0.00%	94.01%
Flex Budget:				$13,000,470
YTD Flex Variance:				$6,625,013

Pharmacy could have spent $6.6 million more???

Once all product RVUs and their relationship with the budgeted cost has been determined, the pharmacy manager can then monitor the relationship between the actual mix and volume levels. Sometimes what appears to work in the budget environment can encounter problems when working with the actual data. Much analysis should be conducted outside of the decision support system because of its limitations. Exhibit 7.14 is an analysis report reflecting the performance of a pharmacy areas and how the overall performance reflects both for budget and actual costing. The actual percent variance is 191.71 percent, but the budget percent variance is 98.33 percent. Why the gap?

This analysis resulted in a miscalculation in November of average costs for miscellaneous products, causing the standard to be overstated. It was the flexible budget analysis that recognized and resolved the problem. After the RVUs were corrected, the actual percent

Exhibit 7.15. FY2007 Monthly Standard Review—Variable Supply Variances—November

CDM #	Description	IP Number	YTD Bud Volume	YTD Act Volume	Budget RVU	VS Drugs RVU
11111152	MISC MED OR	33731	2,842.30	1,562.00	$22.67	$5.36
11111132	NON-CHARGE	43486	10,637.03	12,043.00	$5.75	$0.16
11111112	MISC MED IN	33729	1,643.78	12,012.00	$9.11	$3.79
			3,541,167	4,434,891		

variance as calculated to be 103.92 percent, which brought the variance within accepted limits of 95–105 percent (Exhibit 7.15).

Another example of flexible budget analysis is a situation in which the billing mapping was not updated when the hospital expanded services to the cancer center. The billing mapping is based on the area in which the patient is located when a dose is dispensed. When the cancer center was opened and a new nursing unit was added, the new nursing unit's billing defaulted to the central pharmacy account. This became apparent during a review of the flexible budget variance. The YTD flexible variance was calculated to be $965,402. This would imply that the cost center should have spent more money to provide the YTD

Exhibit 7.15. FY2007 Monthly Standard Review—Variable Supply Variances—November (Continued)

YTD Bud Drugs WV	YTD Bud Weighted Volume	YTD Act Drugs WV	YTD Act Imp WV	YTD Act Supply WV	YTD Act Weighted Volume
$64,427.27	$64,427.27	$8,372.32	$0.00	$0.00	$8,372.32
$61,176.75	$61,176.75	$1,926.88	$0.00	$0.00	$1,926.88
$14,971.55	$14,971.55	$45,525.48	$0.00	$0.00	$45,525.48
5,750,959	5,750,959	6,621,335	0	4,256	6,625,591

	VS Drugs	VS Imp	VS Supply	VS Total
Total YTD Actual Weighted Volume:	$6,621,335	$0	$4,256	$6,625,591
YTD Actual Variable Supplies:	$6,212,307	$0	$163,150	$6,375,457
YTD Actual Variance:	106.58%	0.00%	2.61%	103.92%
Total YTD Budget Weighted Volume:	$5,750,959	$0	$0	$5,750,959
YTD Budget Variable Supplies:	$5,848,911	$0	$268,211	$6,117,122
YTD Budget Variance:	98.33%	0.00%	0.00%	94.01%
Flex Budget:				$7,047,441
YTD Flex Variance:				$671,984

Discovered that invoices:
1) Billed by wholesaler to wrong account.
2) Invoices received by month-end were not accrued.

actual weighted volume (Exhibit 7.16). During the analysis of the product lines, it was discovered that many of the drugs were not usually dispensed from this cost center. On further investigation, it was discovered that these reported costs were from the new cancer center nursing unit that had not been set up to map to the cancer center pharmacy.

As part of the costing process, the pharmacy manager must recognize that to gain the most benefit he or she must analyze the results. This is where the results from maintenance will be achieved. Over the years, analysis may identify billing errors, outstanding invoices, incorrect RVU allocations, payroll issues, and purchasing contract issues. This demonstrates the power of using the standards on a regular basis as part of the analysis,

Exhibit 7.16. FY2007 Monthly Standard Review—
Variable Supply Variances—December

	Description	IP Number	Total Current RVU	YTD Bud Drugs WV
13009212	INFLIXIMAB, 10MG, INJ	34723	$54.21	$43,607.95
11924212	CYTOMEGALOVIRU IMM GLOB PER VI	34184	$828.50	$100,579.90
11065262	INFUSION, ALBUMIN 25% 50ML	52362	$24.60	$82,272.72
14816100	AHF, REC (RECOMBINATE) PER UNI	69691	$0.93	$63,457.54
12674722	GEMCITABINE HCL, 200MG	34561	$117.25	−$1,036.93
14828212	FLUOCINOLONE ACET 0.59MG (RETI	72583	$18,250.00	$19,162.50
12223712	DOCETAXEL, 20MG	34340	$310.10	$3,423.50
11111112	MISC MED INJ/CHEMO/CONTROL SUB	33729	$5.36	$18,286.95
12477100	FACTOR VIIA RECOMB. PER 1MCG	73114	$0.92	$0.00
14484670	PIPERACIL NA/TAZOBACT 1.125G	68241	$5.36	$8,988.05
11431012	BEVACIZUMAB PER 10MG	62862	$53.32	$11,049.79
12228212	DOLASETRON MESYLATE 10MG INJ	34342	$7.14	$204,294.76
13016410	IMMUNE GLOBULIN PER 500MG (PO	73117	$27.18	$0.00
12386212	ENOXAPARIN SODIUM, 10MG, INJ	34378	$4.56	$140,648.40
11249012	ARGATROBAN INJ PER 5MG	51930	$17.50	$68,058.10
14861712	RITUXIMAB 100MG INJ	35572	$460.56	$4,173.28
12777200	FACTOR VIIA RECOMB. PER 1MCG	73116	$0.92	$0.00
15343712	TRASTUZUMAB, 10MG	35815	$53.71	$3,441.60
14288872	PEGFILGRASTIM INJ PER 6MG	60692	$2,068.24	$8,920.63
				$6,919,893.02

Highlighted high volume drugs
not dispensed by this account.

Exhibit 7.16. FY2007 Monthly Standard Review— Variable Supply Variances—December (Continued)

YTD Bud Imp WV	YTD Bud Supply WV	YTD Bud Weighted Volume	YTD Act Drugs WV	YTD Act Imp WV	YTD Act Supply WV	YTD Act Weighted Volume
$0.00	$0.00	$43,607.95	$86,193.90	$0.00	$0.00	$86,193.90
$0.00	$0.00	$100,579.90	$91,963.50	$0.00	$0.00	$91,963.50
$0.00	$0.00	$82,272.72	$100,540.20	$0.00	$0.00	$100,540.20
$0.00	$0.00	$63,457.54	$102,936.12	$0.00	$0.00	$102,936.12
$0.00	$0.00	−$1,036.93	$109,042.50	$0.00	$0.00	$109,042.50
$0.00	$0.00	$19,162.50	$109,500.00	$0.00	$0.00	$109,500.00
$0.00	$0.00	$3,423.50	$112,256.20	$0.00	$0.00	$112,256.20
$0.00	$0.00	$18,286.95	$112,999.52	$0.00	$0.00	$112,999.52
$0.00	$0.00	$0.00	$123,648.00	$0.00	$0.00	$123,648.00
$0.00	$0.00	$8,988.05	$127,305.36	$0.00	$0.00	$127,305.36
$0.00	$0.00	$11,049.79	$133,300.00	$0.00	$0.00	$133,300.00
$0.00	$0.00	$204,294.76	$149,354.52	$0.00	$0.00	$149,354.52
$0.00	$0.00	$0.00	$150,033.60	$0.00	$0.00	$150,033.60
$0.00	$0.00	$140,648.40	$187,716.96	$0.00	$0.00	$187,716.96
$0.00	$0.00	$68,058.10	$204,750.00	$0.00	$0.00	$204,750.00
$0.00	$0.00	$4,173.28	$206,330.88	$0.00	$0.00	$206,330.88
$0.00	$0.00	$0.00	$216,377.56	$0.00	$0.00	$216,377.56
$0.00	$0.00	$3,441.60	$219,029.38	$0.00	$0.00	$219,029.38
$0.00	$0.00	$8,920.63	$270,939.44	$0.00	$0.00	$270,939.44
$0.04	$0.04	$6,919,893.10	$8,413,637.12	$0.05	$5,173.28	$8,418,810.45

	VS Drugs	VS Imp	VS Supply	VS Total
Total YTD Actual Weighted Volume:	$8,413,637	$0	$5,173	$8,418,810
YTD Actual Variable Supplies:	$7,799,336	$0	$186,390	$7,985,726
YTD Actual Variance:	107.88%	0.00%	2.78%	105.42%
Total YTD Budget Weighted Volume:	$6,919,893	$0	$0	$6,919,893
YTD Budget Variable Supplies:	$7,034,841	$0	$322,594	$7,357,435
YTD Budget Variance:	98.37%	0.00%	0.00%	94.05%
Flex Budget:				$8,951,128
YTD Flex Variance:				$965,402

Pharmacy account could have spent $1 million more?

Exhibit 7.17. Department 1058999990

CDM	IP	Description	VS RVU	Bud Vol	Budgeted Weighted Volume	Forced Budget RVU	Actual Volume	Flex Budget
5100000	45000	Product A	52.00	50	2,600	30.98	50	1,548.85
5200000	45001	Product B	1,080.00	125	135,000	643.37	125	80,420.97
5300000	45002	Product C	55.00	649	35,695	32.76	649	21,263.90
5400000	45003	Product D	65.00	1027	66,755	38.72	1027	39,766.68
5500000	45004	Product E	470.00	25	11,750	279.98	25	6,999.60

Total Weighted Volume	251,800	
Original Budget	$250,000	
Savings Expectation	$(100,000)	
Revised Budget	$150,000	

Total Flex Budget	150,000.00
Actual Spending	251,800.00
Flex Variance	(101,800.00)

Original Weighted Volume Variance	100.72%
Revised Weighted Volume Variance	167.87%

whether examining a department's performance, case performance, service line performance, or physician practices. The boundaries are unlimited if effort is invested in creating and maintaining accurate standards.

The flexible budget is calculated from the relationship of the budgeted weighted volume to the budgeted cost. This percentage is then applied to the actual weighted volume, as Exhibit 7.17 illustrates. This exhibit also shows how savings identified during the budget process that are not captured within the RVUs can drastically affect the flexible calculation. If savings are anticipated within the annual budget process, then planning on how to achieve the savings has to be captured within the RVU process.

Although the process of developing product line costing and flexible budgeting may appear overwhelming, it is straightforward as long as sufficient resources are allocated to the process. A budget is not something that can be partially done and accomplish satisfactory results. Developing a strong relationship between the finance and pharmacy divisions with dedicated staff working toward a common goal is critical to success. When the various reports are distributed, the business office in the pharmacy department must be responsive to analyzing the results and working to correct any identified issues. This chapter represents an abbreviated look at how product costing can be achieved within a pharmacy environment, and, although it can be time-consuming, the overall outcome is a significant advance to providing the financial information and efficiency management tools expected in a successful pharmacy department.

Glossary of Product Line Costing Terms

Term	Definition
Crosswalk	Table that contains values that allow two tables to be related for data analysis.
Direct costs	Costs that can be identified specifically to the product.
Fixed costs	Costs that do not change despite changes in the intermediate product.
Flex budget	Interactive budget that adjusts the static budget based on the actual volume and mix for a period of time.
Forced budget	The relationship of the individual intermediate product weighted volume for a particular cost type-category in ratio to the overall department's weighted volume for that cost type-category is used to develop a calculated (forced) budget RVU or cost. The forced RVU multiplied by projected volume provides the forced budget.
HCPCS	Healthcare Common Procedure Coding System.
Indirect costs	Costs that cannot be traced directly to a specific item.
Intermediate product (IP)	An intermediate product (IP) represents the standard costs associated with dispensing one unit of a drug. These costs include all resources of the institution related directly and indirectly to this drug.
Labor cap	Required minimum staffing to operate.
Relative value unit (RVU)	Depending on the cost type, this RVU can either be the actual cost per unit, labor minutes per unit, or a weighting factor that helps distribute the cost accordingly.
Static budget	Snapshot of expected costs; is not adjusted or altered after it is submitted.
Variable costs	Costs that change in proportion to the changes in intermediate product.

Budget Variance Analysis and Controlling Operating Results

James G. Stevenson
Alice Schuman

Why are drug supply costs going up? And what can the pharmacy department do about it? Pharmacy managers can use data from their monthly financial reports and their pharmacy dispensing system to develop answers to these questions. Monthly financial statements often compare the budget and actual values for the month and year-to-date. The differences between the budget and actual expense are referred to as variances and are shown as absolute dollars and percent differences (Table 8.1).

The information will be most useful if it is first organized by categories that match operational responsibility. For example, if there are two assistant directors and five managers reporting to them, the high-level report for the pharmacy department should be divided first into the two areas managed by each assistant director and then sub-divided by each manager's area of responsibility.

It is useful to present the information in layers: one page that summarizes the department as a whole, followed by supporting pages, one for each manager, in more detail. The ability to understand the drivers of expense are critical to managing budget variances (Table 8.2).

These reports need to be timely so that management staff can plan necessary changes and monitor the effect of changes already implemented. A common target is to have monthly financial reports available by the 10th of the following month.

The monthly financial statements should be reviewed by each manager to identify areas of concern that will need further analysis. Each institution will have its own level of tolerance for variance. Managers will often be expected to have tighter variances (0–1 percent) in areas over which they are perceived as having more control, such as staff expense. More tolerance may be given for higher variance in costs that are driven by factors partially outside the manager's control, such as blood factor costs. Variance tolerance may also be defined in absolute dollars. A $500,000 drug supply expense variance may be less than 1 percent of the pharmacy department budget, but still a concern to the hospital CEO.

Margin is revenue less expense. It is typically shown as a percent of revenue. It is often the first analytic tool used for financial data. Margin percent indicates the proportion of revenue that is left after expenses have been covered. Each department must contribute its share of margin to cover the hospital's overhead expenses and capital investment needs.

Table 8.1. Pharmacy Services—Budget vs. Actual

| | Inpatient Areas | | | |
	Admin	Investigational	Inpatient	Blood Factor
YEAR-TO\-DATE BUDGET				
Revenue	—	—	68,947,587	2,529,516
Salary	675,288	163,235	3,978,451	—
Supplies	30,520	23,412	15,249,656	1,302,389
Other	28,493	(187,321)	88,545	—
Benefits/Depr	221,055	51,302	1,369,093	—
Total exp	955,355	50,627	20,685,744	1,302,389
Gross margin %			*70%*	*49%*
YEAR-TO-DATE ACTUAL				
Revenue	—	—	67,832,801	2,219,122
Salary	642,758	168,762	3,958,036	—
Supplies	42,771	110,821	14,092,204	1,044,239
Other	26,846	(179,258)	243,096	—
Benefits/Depr	191,904	50,544	1,242,745	—
Total exp	904,278	150,869	19,536,081	1,044,239
Gross margin %			*71%*	*53%*
DOLLAR VARIANCE				
Revenue	—	—	(1,114,787)	(310,394)
Salary	32,530	(5,527)	20,415	—
Supplies	(12,251)	(87,410)	1,157,452	258,150
Other	1,648	(8,063)	(154,551)	—
Benefits/Depr	29,150	758	126,347	—
Total exp	51,077	(100,242)	1,149,663	258,150
PERCENT VARIANCE				
Revenue				−12%
Salary	5%	−3%	1%	0%
Supplies	−40%	−373%	8%	20%
Other	6%		−175%	0%
Benefits/Depr	13%	1%	9%	0%
Total exp	5%	−198%	6%	20%

Table 8.1. Pharmacy Services—Budget vs. Actual *(Continued)*

Outpatient Areas		Pharmacy Total	Area Summaries	
Retail	Infusion		Inpatient	Outpatient
9,214,082	44,987,344	125,678,529	71,477,104	54,201,425
583,391	671,715	6,072,079	4,816,974	1,255,105
5,843,708	13,767,152	36,216,836	16,605,976	19,610,860
30,187	899	(39,198)	(70,284)	31,086
203,108	213,669	2,058,226	1,641,449	416,778
6,660,394	14,653,435	44,307,944	22,994,115	21,313,829
28%	67%	65%	68%	61%
9,502,406	41,066,849	120,621,178	70,051,923	50,569,255
589,624	613,179	5,972,358	4,769,556	1,202,803
6,504,945	12,269,803	34,064,782	15,290,034	18,774,748
28,518	2,115	121,317	90,684	30,633
209,364	165,325	1,859,883	1,485,193	374,690
7,332,451	13,050,422	42,018,340	21,635,466	20,382,873
23%	68%	65%	69%	60%
288,324	(3,920,495)	(5,057,351)	(1,425,181)	(3,632,170)
(6,233)	58,536	99,720	47,418	52,302
(661,236)	1,497,349	2,152,055	1,315,942	836,113
1,669	(1,216)	(160,514)	(160,967)	453
(6,256)	48,344	198,343	156,256	42,088
(672,057)	1,603,013	2,289,604	1,358,648	930,956
3%	−9%	−4%	−2%	−7%
−1%	9%	2%	1%	4%
−11%	11%	6%	8%	4%
6%	−135%			1%
−3%	23%	10%	10%	10%
−10%	11%	5%	6%	4%

Table 8.2. Pharmacy Services, Inpatient Area—Budget vs. Actual

	Month			
	Budget	**Actual**	**Variance**	**Var %**
Inpatient Revenue	13,064,240	12,435,878	(628,363)	−5%
Outpatient Revenue	721,967	768,764	46,796	6%
Total Operating Revenue	13,786,207	13,204,641	(581,566)	−4%
Management Staff	8,916	18,140	(9,224)	−103%
Clinical Pharmacist	101,472	94,570	6,901	7%
Pharmacists Regular	476,251	447,253	28,998	6%
Pharmacists OT	3,862	7,026	(3,164)	−82%
Pharmacists Temp	4,391	4,781	(390)	−9%
Residents	2,917	3,582	(666)	−23%
Tech Regular	204,750	203,276	1,474	1%
Tech OT	1,966	15,090	(13,123)	−667%
Tech Temp	2,635	4,130	(1,496)	−57%
Total Salary	798,244	779,709	18,535	2%
Office and Misc Supplies	14,714	12,115	2,599	18%
Med Surg Supplies	111,882	157,012	(45,130)	−40%
Pharmacy Supplies	4,131,727	3,511,501	620,226	15%
Pharmacy Supplies Recharged	(1,199,520)	(1,980,093)	780,573	
Total Supplies	3,058,803	1,700,534	1,358,268	44%
Other Expense	6,458	8,104	(1,646)	−25%
Telephone	1,370	1,500	(130)	−9%
Equipment Expense	9,381	7,636	1,744	19%
Travel Expense	500	69	431	86%
Total Other Expenses	17,709	17,309	400	2%
Total Benefits	274,424	254,298	20,127	7%
Total Operating Expense	4,149,180	2,751,851	1,397,329	34%
	Budg Hrs	**Act Hrs**	**Hrs Var**	**Var %**
Management Staff	173	359	(185)	−107%
Clinical Pharmacist	2,082	1,945	137	7%
Pharmacists Regular	10,400	10,030	370	4%
Pharmacists OT	78	157	(80)	−102%
Pharmacists Temp	85	105	(20)	−23%
Tech Regular	14,196	13,665	531	4%
Tech OT	93	694	(601)	−644%
Tech Temp	128	310	(183)	−143%
Total	27,062	26,907	155	1%

Table 8.2. Pharmacy Services, Inpatient Area—Budget vs. Actual *(Continued)*

Year-to-date

Budget	Actual	Variance	Var %
65,336,884	63,975,326	(1,361,559)	−2%
3,610,703	3,857,475	246,772	7%
68,947,587	67,832,801	(1,114,787)	−2%
44,062	86,792	(42,729)	−97%
501,448	457,070	44,378	9%
2,342,207	2,145,447	196,761	8%
20,210	48,953	(28,743)	−142%
20,914	25,626	(4,711)	−23%
14,583	19,213	(4,630)	−32%
1,012,187	1,006,137	6,051	1%
10,290	136,134	(125,844)	−1223%
12,549	32,665	(20,117)	−160%
3,934,388	3,871,244	63,144	2%
68,033	60,853	7,180	11%
517,067	798,011	(280,944)	−54%
20,663,595	21,050,449	(386,854)	−2%
(5,999,040)	(7,817,109)	1,818,069	
15,249,656	14,092,204	1,157,452	8%
32,292	187,869	(155,577)	−482%
6,850	5,786	1,064	16%
46,903	49,156	(2,253)	−5%
2,500	285	2,215	89%
88,545	243,096	(154,551)	−175%
1,369,093	1,242,745	126,347	9%
20,641,681	19,449,289	1,192,392	6%

Budg Hrs	Act Hrs	Hrs Var	Var %
867	1,673	(806)	−93%
10,409	9,444	965	9%
52,000	47,787	4,213	8%
413	1,115	(702)	−170%
410	498	(88)	−21%
70,980	68,695	2,285	3%
495	6,658	(6,162)	−1245%
615	2,611	(1,996)	−324%
135,322	136,806	(1,485)	−1%

A margin percent that is at expected levels also indicates that billing is being done correctly. If margin percent variances are noted, the manager must investigate to determine the cause. It may indicate problems with waste, loss or diversion, or unusual inventory changes.

Budget Variance Analysis Techniques

The first layer of budget variance reporting shows the difference between budget and actual by location (by area, type of expense, etc). It takes further analysis to discern what caused the difference. All financial variance, for both revenue and expense, is driven by some combination of changes in price per unit, overall patient volume, and/or the mix of items purchased/dispensed.

This section will describe three detailed methods for doing variance analysis. The first two methods, box analysis and stepwise, are shown to demonstrate the underlying process and problems associated with variance analysis. The third method, formulas built into a spreadsheet, will be the method most often used in practice. In the simplest possible variance analysis, one product has one change, in price:

Budget Drug A 40 vials $\times$ $15/vial = $600
Actual Drug A 40 vials $\times$ $20/vial = $800
                Total Variance ($200)

The price variance of $5 additional cost per vial ($20/vial less $15/vial) multiplied by the 40 vials used is the cause of the $200 expense variance.

In the next level of complexity, one product has two changes, in price and volume.

Budget Drug A 40 vials $\times$ $15/vial = $600
Actual Drug A 50 vials $\times$ $20/vial = $1,000
                Total Variance ($400)

We can use the box method to calculate and display the variances (Table 8.3).

Table 8.3. Box Method Variance Analysis, One Drug with Volume and Price Change

	$15 Budget Price	$5 Extra Price
40 Budgeted Vials	$15 $\times$ 40 = $600, Original expected cost	$5 $\times$ 40 = $200, Price variance on budgeted quantity
10 Extra Vials	$15 $\times$ 10 = $150, Volume variance at budgeted price	$5 $\times$ 10 = $50, Variance from the combination of extra price & extra quantity

Table 8.4. Stepwise Method Variance Analysis, One Drug with Volume and Price Change

Budget Volume × Budget price	Actual volume × Budget Price	Actual Volume × Actual Price
40	50	50
×	×	×
$15	$15	$20
$600	$750	$1,000
	$150 Volume Change Variance	$250 Price Change Variance

In this example, $200 of the variance is being caused by a price increase, $150 of the variance is being caused by a volume increase, and $50 of the variance is being caused by a combination of both factors. This last item, a combination of both factors being analyzed, is referred to as the corner.

An alternate method is to use a stepwise analysis. This method lines up all the factors being analyzed, starting with all factors at their budgeted level. Then, at each step in the analysis, one of the factors is shown at its actual level rather than budgeted level. In this case, we will calculate volume variance first, and then price variance as shown (Table 8.4).

In this analysis, we still describe $150 of the variance as being caused by a volume increase, but this analysis method says that the variance from price changes is $250. In effect, the corner has been absorbed into the price variance. In the stepwise method, the corner will get absorbed into whichever step we choose to make the last step.

The final (and most common) level of complexity is to analyze changes in the expense of a group of drugs. In addition to price and volume, we need to consider the impact of changes in the mix of drugs used. The volume changes in each drug are caused by a combination of overall volume changes (more patient days or discharges), changes in the mix of patients (types of illnesses), and changing practice patterns (using more of one drug and less of another to treat the same type of patient). Each new variable is another step in the stepwise analysis method.

There must be common unit of measure for quantity to do mix analysis. For example, orthopedic patients typically incur lower medication expense than cardiac patients do. Even if drug prices and the hospital's total number of patients remain the same, if the percent of cardiac patients increases and the percent of orthopedic patients decreases, overall drug costs will rise. A mix analysis that observes changes in patient mix will use discharges or days as the common unit of measure across the medical services. On the

Table 8.5. Sample Data for Analysis with Volume, Mix, and Price Changes

Budgeted Amounts

	Volume Doses	Mix Percent	Price Cost/Dose	Total Cost
Drug A	60	60%	15	900
Drug B	40	40%	35	1,400
Total	100			2,300

Actual Amounts

	Volume Doses	Mix Percent	Price Cost/Dose	Total Cost
Drug A	105	70%	20	2,100
Drug B	45	30%	32	1,440
Total	150			3,540
Drug A Change				1,200
Drug B Change				40
Total Cost Change				1,240

other hand, if a change in antiemetics is being evaluated, a common dose equivalent must be decided upon for analytic purposes. For example, 16 mg of ondansetron, 100 mg of dolasetron, and 1 mg of granisetron could each be considered one dose in a mix analysis. Simplification of actual clinical practice is necessary to keep the analyses from being too complex. These equivalents can be useful, even if they do not match clinical practice exactly.

To illustrate, one data set (Table 8.5) can be analyzed using the box method (Table 8.6), the stepwise method (Table 8.7), or with spreadsheet formulas (Table 8.8). The sample data show the budget and actual values for two drugs that have changes in price, overall volume, and mix.

Adding a third factor or mix changes the box method from a four-box analysis (Table 8.3) to an eight-box analysis (Table 8.6). The total volume for each drug is now made up of four parts:

- The original budget
- The increase in that drug resulting from the overall hospital volume increase
- The increase of the original volume from mix changes
- The increased volume because of a combination of the overall volume and mix changes

The price increase (or decrease) is then applied to each of these sections of the volume change. This is clearly too unwieldy for practical use.

Table 8.6. Box Method Variance Analysis
Two Drugs with Volume, Price, and Mix Changes

Drug A

	$15 Budgeted price	$5 Extra price
60 doses, budgeted quantity	$15 × 60 = **$900**	$5 × 60 = $300
30 doses, quantity increase due to overall volume increase (50%)	$15 × 30 = $450	$5 × 30 = $450
10 doses, quantity increase due to mix change on original volume (10% of 100)	$15 × 10 = $150	$5 × 10 = $50
5 doses, remaining quantity increase due to mix change on increased volume (10% of 50)	$15 × 5 = $75	$5 × 5 = $25

Drug B

	$35 Budgeted price	($3) Decreased price
40 doses, budgeted quantity	$35 × 40 = **1,400**	−$3 × 40 = −$120
20 doses, quantity increase due to overall volume increase (50%)	$35 × 20 = 700	−$3 × 20 = −$60
Minus 10 doses, quantity decrease due to mix change on original volume (10% less of 100)	$35 × −10 = −350	−$3 × −10 = $30
Minus 5 doses, remaining quantity decrease due to mix change on increased volume (10% less of 50)	$35 × −5 = −175	−$3 × −5 = $15

	Drug A	Drug B
Bold Type—Budgeted Cost	**900**	**1,400**
Blue Shading—Volume Variance	450	700
Yellow Shading—Mix Variance	225	(525)
Green Shading—Price Variance	525	(135)
Total Actual Cost	2,100	1,440

The stepwise method folds these corners into the three main factors: volume, mix, and price. Each step considers the effect of that factor on the remaining amount of the variance. If only volume had changed, the variance would be $450. After that is taken into account, if only mix had changed there would be an additional $225 variance. Price is the only remaining factor, so all of the remaining variance, $525, must be from price changes (Table 8.7).

Even though the corners are neatly tucked away in a stepwise analysis, the pharmacy manager must remember that they are there and that because of them the order of the stepwise analysis matters. If we changed the order of the stepwise analysis and analyzed price, then volume, then mix, the variance for Drug A would be price $300, volume $900, and

Table 8.7. Drug A: Detailed Analysis Using Stepwise Method with Volume, Mix, and Price Levels

Budget total volume × Budget % for this drug × Budget price	Actual total volume × Budget % for this drug × Budget price	Actual total volume × Actual % for this drug × Budget price	Actual total volume × Actual % for this drug × Actual price
100 doses	150 doses	150 doses	150 doses
60%	60%	70%	70%
$15	$15	$15	$20
$900	$1,350	$1,575	$2,100
$450 Volume change variance	**$225** Mix change variance	**$525** Price change variance	**$1,200** Drug A total change

mix $300. The recommended order of analysis is to place the least controllable factor first. In the hospital setting, overall volume is not in the pharmacy department's control. The mix of patients is not under pharmacy control, but the mix of medications can be influenced by pharmacy, because drug price negotiations and drug usage patterns are generally considered the responsibility of the pharmacy department.

The stepwise analysis formulas can be built into a spreadsheet (Table 8.8). This makes it easier to analyze a long list of drug categories, medical services, and so forth. It also provides a more compact format to display the results of the analysis.

Budget Variance Analysis Process

It is not always necessary to do a full, detailed, variance analysis to understand the expense or revenue picture for pharmacy services. The first step after reviewing financial statements is to conduct high-level adjustments and then do volume/mix/price analysis if needed on specific drugs or drug categories that seem problematic (typically high-cost or high-volume drug categories).

The high-level adjustments for medication expense and/or revenue can include the following:

1. Adjust total spend for high-level volume change (patient days or discharges) in excess of budgeted increases.

2. Adjust for overall estimated price increases (inflation level) in excess of budgeted increases.

3. Adjust for one-time occurrences (drug loss from power outages/floods, drug shortage forcing higher-cost substitution).

4. Confirm that the variance is real: check for inventory fluctuations, or wholesaler getting behind on drop ship charges.

5. Separate the highly variable expensive medications, such as blood factor, from all other medications.

If there is still a significant unexplained variance, do budget versus actual comparison (or a year-over-year comparison) by drug category, or for the top 20–50 drugs. Select the drugs and/or categories that are driving the variance. Drill down into them with a full volume/mix/price analysis.

Table 8.8. Stepwise Variance Analysis in Spreadsheet Format with Formulas

	A	B	C	D	E	F	G	H	I	J	K
1		Budgeted Doses	Budg $/dose	Total Budg $	Actual Doses	Actual $/dose	Total Actual $	Volume Variance	Mix variance	Price Variance	Total Variance
2	Drug A	60	$15	$900	105	$20	$2,100	$450	$225	$525	$1,200
3	Drug B	40	$35	$1,400	45	$32	$1,440	$700	-$525	-$135	$40
4		100		$2,300	150		$3,540	$1,150	-$300	$390	$1,240
5											
6											

Volume Variance Formulas
Actual volume × Budgeted mix × Budgeted price less
Budgeted volume × Budgeted mix × Budgeted price

Cell H2 = (E$4*(B2/B$4)*C2)−(B$4*(B2/B$4)*C2)
Cell H3 = (E$4*(B3/B$4)*C3)−(B$4*(B3/B$4)*C3)

Mix Variance Formulas
Actual volume × Actual mix × Budgeted price less
Actual volume × Budgeted mix × Budgeted price

Cell I2 = (E$4*(E2/E$4)*C2)−(E$4*(B2/B$4*C2))
Cell I3 = (E$4*(E3/E$4)*C3)−(E$4*(B3/B$4*C3))

Price Variance Formulas
Actual volume × Actual mix × Actual price less
Actual volume × Actual mix × Budgeted price

Cell J2 = (E$4*(E2/E$4)*F2)−(E$4*(E2/E$4)*C2)
Cell J3 = (E$4*(E3/E$4)*F3)−(E$4*(E3/E$4)*C3)

Staffing expense variance is also driven by volume (change in total number of staff or staff hours), mix (between staff pharmacists, clinical pharmacists, technicians, and administrative staff) and price (salary or wages for each category, overtime usage). It can be useful to calculate the staff expense related to non-productive time (training, paid time off, medical leave, etc.), especially if the non-productive percent of salary expense has changed from historic or budgeted levels.

Special Variance Analysis Topics

Variance analysis can be done based on actual vs. budget or as "this year actual" vs. "last year actual." "Actual vs. budget" may be the specific question the pharmacy manager has to answer for upper management, but in most cases budgets will not have been done at the individual drug level, so there will be more detail available when comparing "this year vs. last year." Clinicians will often respond better to analyses that tie to their actual behavior changes or to actual changes in patient mix, rather than to hypothetical budget targets.

Flexible budgeting is used at some hospitals. It adjusts all budgets by some common factor, usually volume. For example if discharges are up 4 percent over budgeted levels for the first half of a fiscal year, the budget for the first half of the year for expenses that vary by patient volume will be increased by 4 percent. In effect, the volume variance is controlled for before the monthly financial statements are issued. Pharmacy managers will still need to do further analysis to explain the impact of mix or price changes.

Budget variance data come from financial data sources, but detailed information about cause often comes from clinical data sources. For example, dispensing system data will be needed to identify which medical services are prescribing specific medications. These two data sources do not always show the same picture. Financial data may show the expense for stockpiles of drugs that have been purchased in anticipation of specific shortages or for waste because of expired medications. Details drawn from dispensing system data will have more creditability if a reconciliation is done to show what is driving the differences between usage data and the overall financial data.

Communication of Financial Results and Budget Variance Analysis

The pharmacy manager will need to communicate financial results and budget variance analyses to two very different audiences. Upper management wants to know whether the variance is expected to continue and what the pharmacy manager is planning to do to help control it. Internal managers want to know how they can help control the budget variance. Upper management may ask for reports when they perceive a problem with current financial reports. Reports are often requested when variances exceed some institutionally established threshold, incorporating a dollar value, a percentage, or both. Internal managers should receive reports monthly so that they can continuously plan for and manage process improvements.

Key indicators are an effective way to monitor changes in financial operations over time. The pharmacy manager should be clear about the intent of each measure selected. They can be used to identify areas of concern, to clarify the source of cost, or to measure success of management initiatives. There are a variety of ratios that can be used (Table 8.9). The manager should choose ones that are most meaningful for measuring and monitoring current issues. The key indicators should be reviewed at least annually to be sure that the reports and ratios focus on the current main issues.

Choose measures carefully to drive efforts in the correct direction. For example, additional medication costs in an outpatient retail pharmacy should generate additional revenue and improve the hospital's bottom line. The key measure for a retail pharmacy would be a margin percentage that meets or exceeds the goal. On the other hand, in the inpatient setting, additional medication costs do not usually result in additional revenue. The key measure in the inpatient setting is one that monitors drug or overall pharmacy cost.

Data can be shared either in graphs or in data tables. For most audiences, a combination of the two will be the most effective form of communication. See Table 8.10 for a sample monthly dashboard that could be used by internal pharmacy managers.

Managing Variances

Once a manager has recognized and understood the causes for variances, the expectation is that they will either take actions to correct those factors that are under their control or identify other actions that will produce operating results as close to the projected budget as possible.

Personnel Expense Variances

Often personnel expense variances are considered more within the control of the pharmacy manager than supply expenses. Pharmacy managers are normally expected to manage within budgeted personnel dollars. If expenses are greater than budgeted, this is often a result of factors such as poor management of overtime, inadequate recruitment and retention strategies, or lack of oversight of scheduling patterns. After identifying the specific reasons for the personnel budget variance, the pharmacy manager should develop a plan to bring personnel expenses back in line with budget targets. Strategies to do this include improving recruitment and retention of existing personnel (thus reducing the need for overtime to cover vacancies), streamlining and consolidating processes to reduce needed manpower to accomplish department objectives, and carefully reviewing all department processes to determine those that may be cut or reduced without significantly impacting the primary goals and mission of the department or compromising patient care or safety. As new processes are introduced, managers may neglect to identify those activities that are now obsolete and can be modified or reduced.

On the other hand, if budget variances are a result of factors such as patient care volumes that are greater than anticipated or changes in service demands, the manager should be prepared to explain why the budget variance is justified and must continue. In either case, the pharmacy manager is expected to take a responsible position to either adjust or defend the use of personnel resources.

Table 8.9. Sample Financial Ratios and Measures

Category Ratio	Description	Purpose
Variance Measurement		
Budget vs. Actual	Can do for both revenue and expense, at high level or by line item.	Identify significant differences between amounts planned and amounts actually incurred.
Last Year vs. This Year	Can do for both revenue and expense, at high level or by line item.	Identify significant year over year changes. Especially useful if budget was not done at required level of detail (medical service or specific drug).
Medication Supply Cost Analysis		
Drug expense per discharge or Drug expense per day	Overall or by clinical service category. Can be done by discharge or by patient day.	Controls for volume changes, can be used to track the effect of mix and price changes over time.
Drug expense per dispensing system vs. Financial report drug expense	Compares medication expense from two different sources: financial reports and pharmacy department dispensing system.	Identifies the cost of medications purchased but not yet dispensed, either because of inventory value changes or because of waste and/or diversion.
Inventory Efficiency Analysis		
Inventory Turn Rate	Total medication expense for selected time period/Inventory value at one point in time during that time period.	Higher turn rate values indicate that medication supplies are being purchased as needed rather than having excess supplies on the shelf.
Inventory Stock-Out Rate	Unfilled pick requests for selected time period/ total pick requests for same time period.	Low stock out rates indicate adequate medication supply one hand.

Note: These two measures are at opposite ends of a spectrum. Improving turn rates too much can lead to unacceptable stock out rates and vice versa.

Staffing Expense Analysis		
Staff Turnover—Annual	Number staff leaving department in last year/ Total budgeted positions (overall or by type of staff–technician, staff pharmacist, etc.).	One measure of staff satisfaction, either with scope of work or working conditions.

Staff Vacancy Rate	Number open positions/Total budgeted positions (overall or by type of staff).	Measures recruiting effectiveness; may indicate salary levels that are not market competitive.
Staff Percent On-line	Hours worked/total hours paid.	Highlights percent of salary payments for non-productive time, such as training, vacation, sick time, etc.
Staff Expense (or hours) by Category	By staff pharmacists, clinical pharmacist, technician, administrative, etc.	Clarifies staffing mix for one time period or changes over time.
Staff Expense (or hours) per Patient Day	Overall or by staff category.	Controls for volume changes can be used to track changes in staffing mix and price over time.

Table 8.10. Inpatient Pharmacy Services Dashboard

Current Year Budget vs Actual:

	Budget	Actual	% Diff
Revenue	71,477,104	70,051,923	−2%
Salary	4,816,974	4,769,556	−1%
Supplies	16,535,152	15,380,718	−7%
Benefits & Other	1,641,449	1,485,193	−10%
Total exp	22,994,115	21,635,466	−6%
Gross margin %	*68%*	*69%*	

Comparison to Prior Year Performance:

	Last Year	This Year	% Diff
Revenue	68,961,434	70,051,923	2%
Salary	4,411,156	4,769,556	8%
Supplies	15,469,527	15,380,718	−1%
Benefits & Other	1,304,086	1,485,193	14%
Total exp	21,184,768	21,635,466	2%
Gross margin %	*69%*	*69%*	

Hospital Patient Volume Indicators:

	Last Year	This year	% Diff
Discharges	18,229	18,168	0%
Patient Days	105,676	107,123	1%
LOS	5.8	5.9	2%
Percent Occupancy	82%	84%	

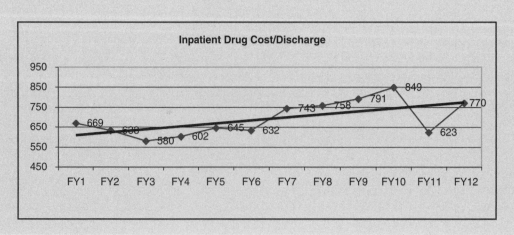

Inpatient Drug Cost/Discharge

Table 8.10. Inpatient Pharmacy Services *(Continued)*

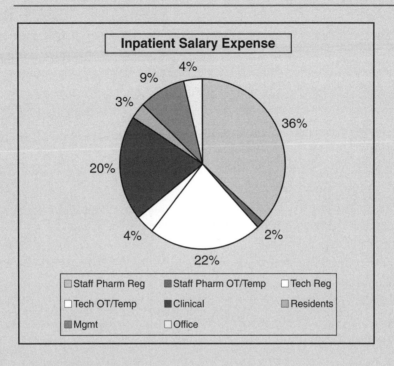

Staffing Indicators:

Total percent above (below) budget	−1%
Total percent above (below) prior year	8%
Technician turnover rate, last 12 months	14%
Pharmacist turnover rate, last 12 months	6%
Current vacancy rate	8%

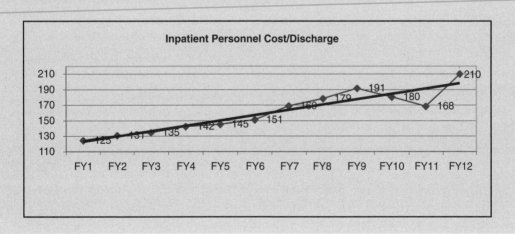

Drug Expense Variances

As mentioned previously, drug expense variances may be better tolerated than personnel cost variances because drug expenses may be considered less within the direct control of the pharmacy manager. However, an effective pharmacy manager will have a strong command of the reasons contributing to supply expense variances and will develop clear plans to influence this variance to the degree possible. Because drug expenses are typically 75 to 80 percent of the operational expense of a hospital pharmacy, this area should receive significant attention.

There are major challenges in developing a pharmacy supply budget because of the many uncertainties that must be integrated into the annual drug budget. These include lack of certainty around factors such as (1) which new drugs will be approved, (2) when they will be approved, (3) how much they will cost, and (4) what will be their usage. Similarly, there is nearly as much uncertainty about drugs that will be losing patent exclusivity because it is difficult to predict where the future price point will stabilize when these products become available generically and to anticipate the impact of patent-extension strategies by manufacturers. Changes in drug use are also sometimes difficult to predict. Newly published data on existing drugs may have a significant impact on their usage—either to significantly increase or decrease their use.

The role of the pharmacy manager is to assure that drugs are used in the safest, most appropriate, and cost-effective manner. Therefore, when a negative variance in drug expenses is identified, several considerations must be made.

First, the manager must determine which drugs are contributing to the budget variance and must examine those factors causing the variance. Is the variance a result of an unanticipated change in pricing or of increased use? If it is use, can the increased use of the drug be justified on clinical grounds? Perhaps new information has been published that demonstrates that a particularly expensive drug produces superior outcomes to a less expensive alternative that was previously the standard of practice. In these cases, the positive outcomes preclude any efforts to change usage. In these instances the manager is left with considering contracting strategies to attempt to reduce the unit cost of the medication or simply accepting the increase and explaining why it is justified. However, if the situation indicates that other alternatives that may be equally or more cost-effective exist, then the responsible manager works on contracting to achieve the best unit cost and on influencing usage. This may be achieved by a variety of means, including educational initiatives targeted at key physicians, drug use evaluations, or pursuing guidelines or restrictions on use through the pharmacy and therapeutics committee.

Another factor that may contribute to drug expense variance is lax inventory management. Failure to follow sound inventory management principles can result in thousands of dollars in increased expenses that are not commensurate with changes in actual use. Managers should ensure that there are adequate inventory processes in place to prevent this from happening or to recognize when inventory control may need to be reestablished. Although conducting full counts of physical inventories is one method of determining the cost of inventory, it may be more feasible to do a limited physical inventory of top dollar products on a more frequent basis. Automated inventory and dispensing systems may also allow an estimate of inventory levels on a regular basis. When a budget variance is a result of an inventory management problem, appropriate attention to re-establishing inventory management principles will normally produce a one-time savings that should assist in reducing the budget variance.

If factors beyond the control of the pharmacy manager contributed to the negative supply variance, it may be impossible to mitigate the impact of the specific drug. However, a fiscally responsible pharmacy manager will look for other opportunities to control drug expenses. These include examining opportunities to use strategies such as moving market share within a therapeutic category to achieve favorable contract pricing (because pricing is often predicated on market share), identifying therapeutic equivalence scenarios as a means of exerting leverage in contracting, and pursuing other opportunities to use clinical pharmacists to influence the appropriate and cost-effective use of medications.

One tool is the use of therapeutic interchange to modify the market share of drugs in a specific therapeutic class rapidly. By moving market share toward one product, manufacturers will often provide preferential pricing. This is an important strategy in identifying cost-containment opportunities in hospitals. Examples of therapeutic categories in which interchange programs may be considered include antiemetics, antimicrobials, and erythropoietic growth factors.

Therefore, even if the primary driver of a negative drug expense variance must be accepted because the use of the drug is clinically appropriate based on current evidence, there may be opportunities to use clinical pharmacists, pharmacy and therapeutics committee actions, or contracting strategies to influence the use and costs of other agents. These actions may assist in controlling the overall drug expense variance even though these drugs were not directly contributing to the variance.

In summary, managing budget variances starts with having systems in place to measure and recognize trends in both personnel and supply costs. When variances do occur, the manager must have the ability to diagnose the situation by using data on costs and activity volumes. Inventory levels must also be considered if there are negative supply cost variances. After gaining a thorough understanding of the drivers of a budget variance, the pharmacy manager must develop a plan to explain why the variance is appropriate or inappropriate and to outline what measures will be taken to help mitigate the impact of the variance throughout the budget year. Strategies can normally be considered in the areas of contracting; inventory management; drug use policies; or restrictions targeted at utilization, education by clinical pharmacists regarding appropriate use, or therapeutic interchange programs to move market share of specific agents rapidly and effectively.

Financial Aspects of Pharmaceutical Contracts and Supply Chain Management

Wayne Russell
Fred J. Pane

Group purchasing organizations (GPOs) are organizations whose primary service is the development of purchasing contracts for product and nonlabor service agreements that their membership can access.[1] By pooling, or aggregating the purchases of their member hospitals, GPOs can negotiate lower prices from suppliers and manufacturers.

According to the Health Industry Group Purchasing Association (HIGPA), hundreds of hospital GPOs exist, but only about 30 GPOs negotiate sizable contracts. These large GPOs are the result of mergers in the mid-1990s. Premier, Inc., for example, was the result of a merger between SunHealth Alliance, American Healthcare Systems, and Premier Health Alliance. Novation, LLC, was the result of University Hospital Consortium (UHC) and Voluntary Hospitals of America (VHA) combining their supply chain operations into one GPO. Premier and Novation are currently the largest GPOs, based on purchasing volume in dollars. Other GPOs include Consorta, MedAssets, Health Services Corporation of America, Amerinet, Broadlane, and many others.[2]

GPO Services

GPOs typically offer contracts for most products used in a hospital or physician's office, including pharmaceuticals, medical and surgical supplies, laboratory supplies and equipment, food, and capital equipment. Services contracted outside of product contracts include consultative services, risk insurance, educational services, technology and safety programs, and comparative data to assist organizations in benchmarking and cost-reduction strategies. Some GPOs also offer private label programs, whereby they contract with a manufacturer to provide products that have the GPO's private label on them. NovaPlus, one of the largest private label programs, is offered by Novation and provides hundreds of products, ranging from pharmaceuticals to medical supplies.

GPOs are typically funded by one of two mechanisms. Either the membership pays a fee to belong to the GPO and to access the contracts the GPO offers, or the manufacturer or supplier of the product pays administrative fees. Administrative fees typically range from 1–3 percent of the purchase price of the product. The Social Security Act, amended in 1986, allows GPOs to collect administrative fees from those suppliers with which the GPO has developed a contractual relationship, and are not considered "kickbacks." In order to not be considered a kickback, administrative fees must be disclosed in an agreement between the GPO and each participating member. The agreement must state that the fees are 3 percent or less of the purchase price of the product.[3] If the fees are higher, the amount each vendor will pay must be disclosed in writing at least annually, along with the amount received by each vendor from purchases made by the member. Most GPOs keep their administrative fees at 3 percent or less; however, several GPOs collect fees above this amount and must disclose the additional fees. Most GPOs subtract operating expenses from the administrative fees and return the remainder of the fees to their membership each year. The percentage returned to the member hospitals varies among GPOs. These monies are called patronage fees.

GPO membership varies depending on the type of GPO (nonprofit or for-profit). Many nonprofit GPOs have owner hospitals that own stock in the GPO. They can also have regional group affiliate members, which are smaller regional GPOs that can access the larger GPOs contracts, and affiliate hospital members that are sponsored by owners or regional groups. Group purchasing organizations sometimes offer contracts to providers outside of acute care hospitals, which might include physician offices, retail pharmacies, clinics, and other nonacute care sites, long-term care facilities, home care agencies, and other alternate sites of care.

GPO Contracting

Several studies have been conducted in the past few years that examine the benefits of GPOs on product costs. Most of these studies have shown that GPOs typically decrease hospital supply costs by 10 percent, and that the absence of GPOs would lead to higher prices of 10–35 percent.[4] Thus, GPOs provide a competitive advantage and benefit to hospitals by reducing costs by allowing suppliers to bid for higher volume sales in return for price reductions.

A typical GPO pharmaceutical portfolio contains 10,000–12,000 individual items and represents contracts with 150–200 suppliers. The contracts represent products and prices used in the acute care class of trade (hospital inpatients and outpatients) as well as other classes of trade (typically nonacute nonretail, long-term care, managed care, home care, physician office, and retail pharmacy). With the Medicare Modernization Act of 2003, GPOs also contract for disproportionate share hospitals on inpatient-priced products. These hospitals use 340(b) pricing for their outpatient purchases.[5] The inpatient portfolio is called "Disproportionate Share Hospital (DSH) inpatient" to differentiate from the acute care pricing or 340(b) outpatient pricing.

GPOs typically conduct a bid every three years (some do this every two years, others have contracts that last up to five years) on their portfolio of pharmaceuticals. The GPO bid process is very labor intensive because products and pricing must be compared to current products on contract in generic drug categories. Nonfinancial attributes are considered in the bid process, such as barcodes, unit dose, latex-free packaging, alcohol-free solutions, and so forth. Most GPOs conduct the bid via a Web-based tool. The contract terms and conditions must be renegotiated in the bid process, and this function usually takes more time and effort than the analysis of products and pricing. Sole-source manufacturers typically submit a price, but, because their product does not have generic competition, there is less ability to negotiate the price when compared to generic products.

However, sole-source contracts may contain other features, such as firm pricing for a specified period, caps on price increases, market share considerations for performance-based programs, and other benefits that lead to negotiation during the bid process. In the generic market, intense competition and product pricing occurs, and product attributes are extremely important.

GPOs must also consider whether a manufacturer is able to supply the market, especially in the generic marketplace, because products are launched by manufacturers who cannot supply enough product for the entire market. This situation leads to a separate strategy regarding whether to award a manufacturer the contract solely or to award the contract to multiple suppliers who have access to the GPO membership. A "market competitive" clause often exists in generic contracts that allows for price reductions if competitors within the generic class offer a lower price to GPO members. A GPO must have a mechanism for monitoring pricing in the marketplace, which is often done by analysis of pharmacy wholesaler data representing the GPO members' purchases through contract, noncontract, and off-contract. Noncontract purchases occur when neither the GPO nor the member has a contract. Off-contract purchases occur when the member does not purchase through the GPO agreement but through an individual contract with the supplier or another GPO or distributor agreement with the supplier.

Various contracting strategies exist as part of the bid process. A GPO typically seeks to have sole-source products on contract because they may not have competition (e.g., oncology drugs) or they may have competition within a therapeutic class. Selecting one product within a therapeutic class to have on contract at the exclusion of all other products within the same therapeutic class is very difficult, especially for large GPOs that represent a large number of hospitals, each with their own pharmacy and therapeutics committees and clinicians with a wide spectrum of opinions. Thus, a GPO will typically contract for all sole-source products within a therapeutic class, like quinolone antibodies, to allow their members to choose which products represent the clinical needs of that particular organization and its patient population. This strategy does not hold true for generic products. Some GPOs limit the number of generic products within a category to increase the market share and contract compliance of the supplier product on contract at the exclusion of other generic suppliers with the same product. Other GPOs tend to contract for multiple generic products with the same chemical entity to give their members the widest selection possible, in the hope that it will drive contract compliance.

Contract compliance and volume are critical factors to a generic supplier. Better pricing can be achieved if the GPO limits the number of suppliers on contract with the same product so that they can implement measures to enhance volume, market share, and contract compliance with the supplier(s) on contract. Two GPOs (Novation and Amerinet) have private label programs with suppliers that aim to drive contract compliance toward the contracted product. Additional fees and rebates are provided to members who purchase the private label product. Premier has developed an autosubstitution program that allows the contracted product to be ordered at the wholesale level, even if another similar generic product was ordered. The contracted product is "automatically substituted" for any noncontracted generic. The hospital member must agree to participate in this program by signing a letter of commitment, and the member can select a percentage of products in the autosubstitution portfolio that they do not want substituted for clinical or safety reasons.

The Bid Process

The bid process that occurs approximately every three years usually encompasses the majority of the pharmaceutical portfolio. However, during the course of the year, "minibids" for specific items are conducted if the awarded supplier decides they cannot continue to be price competitive on a specific generic drug or contract. The GPO will conduct a minibid for the generic product and guide suppliers of that product through a process that takes on average one month to determine a new contract awardee that is market competitive. This process can also occur if the contract awardee cannot supply product to the GPO membership and the membership must obtain a competitor product off-contract. The GPO will conduct a minibid if continued or prolonged product supply or quality issues cannot be resolved in a timely manner (usually stipulated in the terms and conditions of the contract). Other contract strategies include negotiations (no bid), which frequently occur with proprietary sole-source products that do not have a competitor in the marketplace.

Another contract strategy is a reverse auction. This process has been employed in other industries (automotive, chemical, lumber) in which multiple suppliers bid for a contract through an electronic auction process. Three or more suppliers must participate so that, although the suppliers can see the prices submitted by their competitors, they cannot determine which competitor represents any given price. The price is driven down through the auction process (hence the term *reverse auction*) rather than driven up. Auction rules include the stipulation that the competitors must be able to supply the marketplace a given length of time so that competitors do not drive down the price without the intention to continue to stay in the market at the auction price. Suppliers participating in a reverse auction must agree to the GPO contract terms and conditions prior to the auction, so once a contract award is made there is no further negotiation of contract terms and conditions. This allows the product to be launched on contract in the market very quickly.

Many pharmaceutical suppliers do not want to participate in a reverse auction because they believe the market competitiveness of the generic marketplace will determine the ultimate price. Many suppliers also believe this process does not promote a sustainable relationship with the GPO or members. A hypothetical advantage of a reverse auction is that it allows prices to decrease more rapidly than they would under normal market conditions. This may also be viewed as a disadvantage because the rapid decrease might drive some suppliers out of the market entirely and thus create product supply issues. If a single generic supplier remains in the market, the price may escalate because of a lack of a competitive threat. Therefore GPOs must monitor the generic market closely and ensure that competition continues to exist, so generic products with multiple suppliers do not become sole-source generic drugs; acting like proprietary drugs (sole-source, brand name drugs), leading to price escalation. There are multiple examples of this occurring, and in each case the price of the generic increased dramatically.

No standard electronic bid tool is used across the GPO industry for conducting bids. Each GPO has developed its own homegrown system. The major challenge in conducting a bid is negotiating contract terms and conditions and ensuring that the product and price data submitted by the manufacturer is accurate so that, when the contracts are awarded, the process of notifying the pharmacy wholesalers and members can be accomplished in a timely manner. Wholesalers typically need 30–45 days to accurately load a new pharmacy portfolio and to change existing pharmaceutical stock in their distribution centers to accommodate the GPO membership. Usage data and communication with pharmacy distributors and suppliers on the GPO contracts is essential to a smooth transition from the exiting portfolio to the new portfolio. If the portfolio transition process is not managed well, the installation of the new contract portfolio contract will be prolonged and membership will be dissatisfied because of the charge-backs and rebills associated with incorrect products and pricing.

Contract Types

GPOs encounter a variety of contract types with the pharmaceutical industry. Listed below are the various types and features of each:

- Base contract
- Base contract with rebate
- Bundled contract
- Performance contract based on market share, total units purchased, or total dollars purchased with or without a rebate

Contracts used to be simple base contract pricing, whereby the products and prices were listed for each class of trade. The price might vary based on the class of trade; however, with generic drugs the pricing is usually the same across all classes of trade. The net price paid by the provider was the contract price plus or minus the wholesaler markup or markdown. In today's environment, most hospitals receive a markdown from the wholesaler for GPO-contracted products, so the next price, for example, might be contract price minus 2 percent. The pharmacy distributor markup or markdown is often based on the amount of purchases per month in total dollars, the payment terms, and the number of deliveries per day or per week to the facility. The more purchases per month, the less deliveries per week, and the more timely the payment terms results in a better cost of goods through the pharmacy distributor.

Many generic suppliers now offer a base price contract with an additional rebate that is paid either quarterly, semiannually, or annually. The rebate is a percentage of the total purchase cost of the product. Rebates are meant as an incentive to purchase more product. Rebates are also used to "hide" the actual price of the product from either the pharmacy distributor or other competitors. Pharmacy distributors also have their own generic product line (especially in the retail market, but now also in the hospital market), and generic manufacturers will use a rebate in the GPO contract so that the true price of the product in not known except to the GPO and the GPO's membership.

Bundled contracts are contracts for multiple products produced by a single manufacturer. If a pharmaceutical manufacturer wants to encourage contracts for multiple products with the GPO to maximize their production runs and to minimize manufacturing costs, they will offer lower pricing for one or more products if the GPO contracts for all the products included in the bundle. This type of contract is usually anchored by a key product in a competitive market, along with several other products for which the manufacturer has competition from other suppliers. A good example is propofol, which is currently manufactured by four pharmaceutical companies. These suppliers have many other product lines, and, to entice the GPO to put their propofol on contract, they bundle it with several other products that may or may not have competitors.

Performance agreements are typically used by proprietary manufacturers for sole-source products in defined therapeutic categories. Good examples of drugs with performance contracts include erythropoietin, proton pump inhibitors, and glycoprotein IIb/IIIa inhibitors. These contracts are meant to reward providers for increased use of a specific product within a therapeutic class. Performance agreements typically have multiple tiers, each of which is associated with a product price. Tiers are differentiated based on a market share percentage scale, total number of units purchased, total dollars spent, or a combination of these attributes. The price a member pays for a contracted product decreases as the market share percentage for the product increases, the total units purchased increases, or the total dollars spent increases. Another variable used in some performance agreements (typically antibiotics) is days of therapy. Performance agreement calculation of market share is usually based on a market basket of competitive products, whereby the contracted product usage is divided by overall usage of all other products in the market basket. This calculation can be complex when products are not dosed or provided in the same strength, thus leading to conversions necessary to compare actual amounts of product used.

Sometimes the comparison is based on dollars purchased, and, to equilibrate the calculation, the actual cost of goods is not used. Instead, wholesale acquisition cost (WAC) is compared among products within a given therapeutic class. Many performance-based contracts are created to penalize the provider if the manufacturer's product is not used the majority of the time (i.e., high market share percentage). If a member falls below a certain market share percentage by using multiple products within the defined therapeutic class or market basket, the WAC discount will be a very small percentage. These programs by definition are designed to reward contract compliance and performance.

Many performance programs have letters of commitment (LOCs) that the pharmaceutical supplier requires the provider to sign in order to access the program. These LOCs may be managed by the GPO, to track membership enrollment in the program, or by the pharmaceutical supplier, in which case the GPO may not be able to reliably track which members have enrolled in the program. This latter situation leads to members not receiving the pricing agreed to by the program because of a communication breakdown between the manufacturer and the pharmacy distributor regarding the assignment of the tier (pricing) to the hospital member. Many GPO agreements require that the GPO manage any performance-based agreement in which a LOC is required so that the GPO can assist the members in determining if they are receiving the correct pricing based on the tier assignment and also in notifying the member when they are close to achieving the next tier (better pricing). Some GPOs have developed sophisticated calculation tools to allow members to determine how they are performing in these contracts so appropriate decisions can be made regarding procurement, formulary status, and clinical utilization of specific products.

Other Contracts

GPOs contract for other types of products and services used in hospital pharmacy departments. Examples of these contracts are service agreements with pharmaceutical distributors; reverse distribution agreements; auditing services; specialty distributor agreements; agreements for pharmacy technology and equipment such as IV hoods, medication administration cabinets, robotics, and carousels; as well as contracts for consulting services that usually do not focus on labor reduction but on operational design and improved medication usage and standardization. Sometimes the consulting services are agreed to "at risk," or "success-based," meaning that an agreed-upon savings target is built into the contract. If the consultant's assistance does not result in the hospital achieving the agreed-upon savings, then the GPO will reimburse the facility the difference between the actual amount saved and the target amount in the contract.

Most GPOs have advisory committees comprised of GPO membership that assist the GPO-contracting staff in product and supplier selection and in other strategic initiatives and goal setting. In the pharmacy area, a national pharmacy committee usually implements a strategy and sets goals. Other advisory committees might include a contracting committee to assist with the bid process and individual contract and product decisions; a clinical committee to assist in setting practice guidelines and sharing best practices among members; a safety committee to monitor adverse events and share knowledge related to safe medication practices; and an advocacy committee to work on issues related to pharmaceutical pricing, reimbursement, revenue cycle management, and other issues that could affect overall product pricing, availability, and usage in various practice settings. Multidisciplinary committees assist in contract negotiations for products used throughout the health-care system such as IV fluids, IV pumps and sets, medication administration cabinets, bedside barcode technology, and so forth.

Providers expect much more today from their GPOs than in the past, when GPOs primarily provided contracts for goods and services. Although contracting is still the primary role of GPOs, many now provide additional services to their members to differentiate themselves to suppliers in the marketplace and also to provide the additional value their membership expects. Hospitals expect the following from GPOs:

- Price-competitive goods and services
- Price protection on contracts for specified lengths of time, especially in commodity markets
- Ability to assist members in driving costs out of their systems through improved contracting and improved resource usage
- Provision of decision-support tools and reports that assist the organization in more appropriate use of resources as well as up-to-date information on best practices
- Information that allows the members to benchmark themselves against other organizations of similar characteristics
- Consulting services (whether fee-based or in-kind) to assist in contract pull-through as well as standardization and best practice initiatives
- Contracts that cover the breadth of products and services a hospital would need and contracts that are competitive and representative of different facets of the membership

• Ability to support the members in innovative contracting exercises, such as regional aggregation to obtain better pricing than the standard agreement

Suppliers expect GPOs to assist them with contract uptake after a product(s) is added to the contract. They also ask GPOs to assist in member education on clinical issues related to their products. Suppliers want access to GPO leadership. They view GPOs as an avenue to certain markets and, in the case of generic products, a necessity to survive in a very competitive landscape. Some suppliers expect the GPO to assist them in enrolling members into their performance programs and have structured administrative fees on a sliding scale to encourage GPO support. This activity can create ethical issues for the GPO if a competitor's products are also on contract. Purchase data is also important to suppliers in very competitive markets, and GPOs are often asked to provide purchase data at the aggregate level, to calculate market share for performance agreements, and to provide this data to the manufacturer.

Getting the Most from a GPO

Pharmacy distributors work closely with GPOs to provide purchase data and to stock appropriate quantities of products under GPO contracts. Group purchasing organizations also contract separately with pharmacy distributors to offer price matrices that allow members competitive pricing on contract and noncontracted purchases. Pharmacy distributors expect the GPO to assist them in inventory management at the distribution center level by assisting with member communications regarding estimated supply and demand reports. Pharmacy distributors also work with GPOs to provide repackaged products, in which the manufacturer only supplies the product in bulk quantities. Hospitals need unit dose and barcoded products, and GPOs contract with subsidiaries of the pharmacy distributors to provide these products. Group purchasing organizations also contract with pharmacy distributors to provide technology such as robotics, medication administration cabinets, and so forth, so the relationship between the GPO and pharmacy distributors crosses many product lines and services.

Pharmacy directors and managers must maximize the value of their GPO relationship, and pharmacy management should consider the following areas of focus regarding contract pricing:

• Develop communications with the pharmacy staff at GPO corporate offices. A pharmacy manager can do this by meeting with GPO pharmacy staff at national meetings or by participating on pharmacy advisory committees. Consider scheduling time to visit the corporate or regional office.

• Volunteer to serve on pharmacy advisory committees. Committees devoted to pharmaceutical contracting, pharmacy distributor relationships, or overall GPO/hospital strategy are the most appropriate committees on which directors of pharmacy and management should serve so that they understand the contracts and meet the contract staff at the GPO office.

• Volunteer to be involved in the committee that oversees the portfolio bid process and is involved in product selection. This allows the member to have input into the product criteria (both financial and nonfinancial) as well as input into final product selection.

- Designate an individual in the organization to be responsible for GPO contracts, pharmacy procurement, and supply chain operations. Many large health systems have developed a corporate pharmacy director position to oversee supply chain responsibilities for the entire system and to work with each local pharmacy director to develop supply chain efficiencies and standardization. This individual should also be involved as a member of a GPO committee focused on contracting and should have an excellent understanding of the GPO contracts, both pharmaceutical and pharmacy distributor agreements. The individual should also be proficient in running a variety of reports that depict departmental or health system pharmaceutical spend by therapeutic and generic class and by on and off-contract purchases and in comparing GPO to pharmacy distributor pricing to ensure the correct price is paid across the organization. If the organization is a disproportionate share hospital, this individual should also understand the regulations affecting 340(b) pricing and product procurement and inventory control.

- Many manufacturers require GPO declaration forms to be signed before they recognize an organization has joined a specific GPO and allow that organization access to the contract price. Ask the GPO if they have posted the GPO declaration forms that the manufacturers require on a Web site and if they assist the member in signing these forms. This requirement would also hold true for the letters of commitment that some manufacturers require to participate in specific performance-based contracts. Sign these documents and send copies to both the manufacturer and the GPO, but also keep a copy. If the pricing is incorrect, this copy will serve as documentation to ask for credit/rebills from the pharmacy distributor and the affected manufacturer.

- Understand all the performance contracts available through the GPO. If rebate agreements are included, some GPOs can have 70 or more performance-based agreements. Analyze each one within specific therapeutic classes to determine which contract offers the best pricing based on usage of competing products within that therapeutic class. Many organizations do not monitor which tier they qualify for within a specific performance agreement or how close they are to the next tier, which offers better pricing. Understanding the LOC and how the performance agreement tiers are measured will allow the pharmacy director to engage their physicians and clinical staff in discussions regarding appropriate usage, which affects the overall cost.

- Monitor pricing through the pharmacy distributor to ensure that the GPO-contracted products are not being substituted but also that the correct price is being invoiced. If a GPO-contracted item cannot be obtained through the distributor, contact the GPO to allow the GPO staff to determine why the product is not available and to seek a remedy.

- Communicate with the GPO if a supplier offers a price below the GPO-contracted price. Suppliers who are not awarded the GPO contract may try to work around the contract award by offering selected hospitals a lower price for a generic or branded product. Most generic contracts awarded by GPOs have a market competitive clause, so, if the GPO is aware of this activity in the marketplace, the GPO can get the contracted supplier to lower their price to become competitive. It is in the best interests of the hospital member to remain contract compliant if possible to demonstrate to the awarded suppliers that the GPO contracts are influencing market share and offering value to the membership.

- Recognize specialty programs or services the GPO offers and assess their applicability to their respective health system. For example, private label programs or autosubstitution programs offer additional savings beyond the contracted acute care price. Electronic tools provided by the GPO assist in product selection, product standardization, and education and are valuable to pharmacy staff in controlling overall costs through appropriate usage. Consulting services may be offered to GPO members on a limited basis in-kind versus fee-for-service, and the hospital pharmacy director should consider when to take advantage of the expertise the GPO can offer. Benchmarking tools are also a valuable product many GPOs offer to understand where opportunities to improve may exist.

- Take advantage of educational programs many GPOs offer to assist members in keeping up-to-date on regulatory and other issues affecting pharmacy practice. Some may be local, Web-based, or held in conjunction with national meetings.

- Be aware of communication tools the GPO offers to provide timely information. Assign staff in the department the responsibility of monitoring the information disseminated by the GPO, which includes communications on contract updates via e-mail newsletters, clinical abstracts and reviews, patent expiration information, Joint Commission information, product safety information, reimbursement and revenue cycle management information, GPO declaration forms and LOCs, performance-agreement contract abstracts, and electronic toolkits that assist in determining the best product for a specific facility within a therapeutic class. All are examples of information provided by GPOs.

When organizations are considering changing from one GPO to another, questions frequently arise in the discussion and analysis. Listed below are examples of questions to consider if this situation occurs:

- Will the GPO assist the organization in portfolio conversion if changing GPOs?
- Does the GPO offer Web-based diagnostic tools for the organization to employ in identification of cost strategies?
- Does the GPO have field-based staff to assist the organization in contract usage and optimization opportunities and are these staff pharmacists?
- Does the GPO offer consultative services?
- Does the GPO offer local and national networking opportunities?
- How does the GPO manage contracted product pricing, and how is this information communicated to the membership?
- Does the GPO offer budget forecast analyses to assist with pharmaceutical cost projections that affect the hospital pharmacy budget?
- What programs are in place to assist the member with procurement of products in short supply?

Issues GPOs face today are multifaceted. They must deal with government scrutiny of the safe harbor anti-kickback statues, membership commitment to contracts, development of large integrated delivery networks (IDNs), or large heath systems, that want to contract selected products for themselves; reporting capabilities; governmental setting of pricing formulas that affect competitive pricing; market competitiveness; and erosion of GPO contracts by either pharmacy distributors or nonawarded manufacturers or both. It is not within the scope of this chapter to go into detail on all of the above issues; however, several should be discussed.

Many hospitals have integrated into large IDNs, usually anchored by one or two large hospitals (many times a teaching hospital) and several smaller community or rural hospitals, clinics, and other alternate sites of care. Some of these organizations have created positions such as a corporate director of pharmacy or a supply chain executive, whose focus is to drive costs out of the system. One of the methods employed to do so is to develop individual contracts specific only to that organization. This activity does not benefit the entire GPO membership unless the pricing terms offered to the IDN are offered to others within the GPO who meet the same qualifications. Some GPOs now assist their large IDNs in developing contracts that allow other GPO members to qualify if contract criteria (market share requirements, purchase volume requirements, etc) can be met. In other words, a new pricing tier is created for these large organizations. This activity also benefits the manufacturer by demonstrating contract compliance and enhanced volume to them in return for a contractual relationship with the GPO. Manufacturers typically do not want hundreds of individual contracts with separate organizations; in fact, many manufacturers have very small contracts departments because, through GPOs, a single contract can be in effect for hundreds of hospitals. The contracting functionality of the GPO has brought efficiency to the supply chain by reducing the administrative burden on the manufacturer and the individual hospital.

As a result of the Medicare Modernization Act of 2003, hospitals, physician office practices/clinics, have been affected by the enactment from Centers for Medicare and Medicaid (CMS), through the implementation of the Average Sales Price (ASP) reimbursement formula for Medicare Part B drugs, since 2005 in the Physician setting and 2006 in the Hospital Outpatient setting. The movement away from a percentage of AWP (Average Wholesale Price) model to the ASP + % model, has decreased Medicare payments for drugs, but placed an increasing financial strain on health-care organizations. In some cases, the reimbursement for selected drugs may be less than the acquisition cost of the drug and when the manufacturers submit quarterly ASP's to CMS, it takes 6 months (two quarters) for the ASP to be adjusted. In 2008, drugs are $60 receive a package payment and won't be reimbursed individually, unless they are part of a Special Package Rule (e.g. anti-emetics). One outcome of the ASP formula is that it discourages proprietary manufacturers from negotiating competitive pricing with a GPO, because, if they lower the price for one organization, they have to raise the price to another to keep the average the same. Some product prices have also increased to allow the ASP to increase and thus increase the reimbursement to physicians who administer selected products in their office setting. Hospitals have put pressure on their GPOs to obtain competitive pricing for oncology products and immune globulins in particular, which are affected by ASP reimbursement, yet manufacturers of these products have been reluctant to reduce the acquisition cost of the product, knowing that it will adversely affect the reimbursement rate. Group purchasing organizations need to continue to work with CMS, private payers, and other organizations, to understand the impact of governmental pricing and reimbursement for drugs, develop new innovative ways to contract for these drugs, and to assist their membership with reimbursement and revenue cycle management.

Pharmacy distributors have their own generic products under contract that in the past have been sold primarily in the retail markets. Recently pharmacy distributors have attempted to expand their generic presence into the hospital markets, where GPO contracts have traditionally provided this support. This competitive friction in the generic marketplace has created an awareness of the various options hospital members have for contracting certain segments of their pharmaceutical portfolio. However, hospital pharmacy directors should ensure that they thoroughly understand the costs associated with this activity and should analyze the financial impact to their budget, including loss of patronage fees if they use non-GPO contracts. Monitoring product pricing over time is strongly encouraged because in the generic marketplace the pricing of products and selection of products on-contract can be volatile.

Conclusion

In conclusion, GPOs have been in existence for many years. Publications on GPOs first appeared in the mid-1970s in the *American Journal of Health-System Pharmacy*. The concept of aggregation of purchasing volume to obtain lower pricing has existed in many manufacturing markets outside of pharmaceuticals. Yet pharmaceuticals are somewhat unique in that they are affected by sole-source manufacturers who may not have competition in the marketplace within a therapeutic class, generic manufacturers who exist in a highly competitive market, and the impact of governmental pricing on overall manufacturer pricing and contracting strategies. Group purchasing organizations are being asked to provide many more services outside of contracting in today's health-care environment. Consulting, reporting, advocacy, and educational activities are just a few services GPOs are expected to provide to their membership today as demands on health systems and hospitals continue to increase.

References

1. Hovenkamp H. Competitive Effects Of Group Purchasing Organizations' (GPO) Purchasing and Product Selection Practices in The Health Care Industry. http://www.higpa.org/pressroom/hovenkamp.pdf, April 2002, pp 4 (accessed 5 June 2008).
2. Hovenkamp H. Competitive Effects Of Group Purchasing Organizations' (GPO) Purchasing and Product Selection Practices in The Health Care Industry. http://www.higpa.org/pressroom/hovenkamp.pdf, April 2002 pp 4 (accessed 5 June 5 2008).
3. 42 CFR Section 952.1001(j).
4. Hovenkamp H. Competitive Effects Of Group Purchasing Organizations' (GPO) Purchasing and Product Selection Practices in The Health Care Industry, http://www.higpa.org/pressroom/hovenkamp.pdf, April 2002 (accessed June 5, 2008).
5. Medicare Prescription Drug, Improvement, and Modernization Act of 2003, Public Law 108–173, Section 1002. http://www.cms.hhs.gov/MMAUpdate/downloads/PL108–173summary.pdf (accessed June 5, 2008).

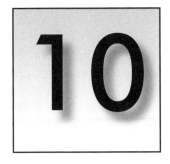

Budgeting Revenue

James A. Jorgenson
Kristin Fox-Smith
Paul J. Conlon

Introduction

Health care in the United States today is big business. In 2004, total national health expenditures increased 7.9 percent, which was over three times the rate of inflation. Total spending was $1.9 trillion and represented 16 percent of the gross domestic product.[1] Hospitals, as part of this equation, operate in many ways akin to normal business. A typical 500-bed hospital might represent $500 million dollars annually in gross revenue. However, revenue management in the hospital setting is markedly different from a normal business. Most commercial business operations offer products or sell services at a competitive price intended to generate an acceptable return on investment or profit. A typical business today might expect a 10–20 percent annual operating margin (net revenue minus expenses). The majority of hospitals operate as not-for-profit entities under section 501(c)(3) of the Internal Revenue Code and qualify for tax-exempt status.[2] This means that they try to produce a positive annual operating margin, but, unlike normal business enterprises, this profit is not dispersed to owners or shareholders. Instead, operating profit is reinvested in the hospital to purchase capital equipment and to fund building initiatives. The operating margin for most hospitals is also considerably smaller than a normal business, with the majority of hospitals working in the 0–6 percent range. Approximately 26 percent of hospitals actually post a negative operating margin.[3]

Because of the nature of health-care provision and payment, pharmacy is an essential component of an effective revenue management strategy. Although most hospital departments focus on expense management, the pharmacy must effectively manage both expense and revenue to support the financial operation of the hospital. Most services, such as nursing, housekeeping, facilities, and accounting, do not directly generate revenue and represent expense only. It falls to pharmacy, radiology, the operating room, and laboratory to generate the majority of the operating revenue for the facility. As reimbursement patterns for hospitals have changed, senior leadership has stressed expense management, because every dollar saved on the expense line produces an equal gain in operating margin. Revenue management is often seen as a less effective tool for margin improvement because contractual allowances and discounts present in reimbursement formulas dictate that the amount charged will not be the amount collected and thus the incremental gain in margin will be less than "dollar for dollar," as in the case of expense reduction. Yet it remains imperative that the pharmacy have a solid plan for revenue management, because overall dollars will still be significant. It is also important to note that reimbursement differs by service and payment location (e.g. inpatient versus outpatient).

An effective revenue budget strategy should not be a mad scramble once a year during budget season. Rather, planning for pharmacy revenue should be a continuous process that occurs throughout the fiscal year. It should consist of regular financial reviews with established benchmarks and financial indicators, as well as regular reviews of contracts, payers, patient mix, coding/reimbursement changes, and collection rates. This process should be coordinated with the organization's budget office so that, when it is time to prepare revenue projections for the coming budget cycle, a clear and consistent path is already established.

Planning for Revenue

To initiate planning for pharmacy revenue, a workload unit measure must be established. On the inpatient side, patient days, numbers of admissions, and discharges are common measures. On the outpatient side, patient visits, such as emergency room or clinic visits, are common indicators. For those organizations that provide traditional retail prescription services, prescription volume would be a common measure. Because payment will differ between patient types, this information must be further analyzed to determine the actual composition of patients. For example, a medical oncology patient will generate more pharmacy revenue than a surgical oncology patient, and an infusion clinic visit will generate more pharmacy revenue than a pediatrics clinic visit. Historically, most organizations use a revenue/patient day, revenue/clinic visit, or revenue/prescription figure as a key financial indicator. This will be a valid tool for budget projection and financial analysis only if the patient mix remains stable. If anticipated changes to the composition of the patient population are expected, this must be factored into the revenue equation. Once a solid foundation has been established for expected revenue per workload unit, it is possible to build on this for the next budget cycle. Changes in workload units will move the revenue projections up or down, assuming all other factors remain constant.

Pricing strategies can then be applied to meet organizational revenue requirements. Most pharmacy pricing structures traditionally involve a cost base with an applied markup. The average wholesale price (AWP) is often used as the cost base. This number is readily available and has been a recognized number by most payers. However, recent changes in government reimbursement have moved away from using AWP as a cost base for reimbursement, with the acknowledgment that AWP has no direct relationship to the actual cost of manufacturing a drug or the actual sale price of that product in the market. Commercial entities have also started to move away from AWP to other drug cost benchmarks. Regardless of the cost basis and pricing structure chosen by the pharmacy, a consistent and defensible pricing strategy is needed that can be readily explained to payers. A formula based on actual acquisition cost plus markup may be more defensible as the basis for a pharmacy pricing formula and would be an alternative to traditional AWP-based strategies. The markups applied to the cost base may also be variable and reflect the amount of effort that is required to prepare the dosage form for administration to a patient. Different categories of fee structures, such as unit dose, large volume parenteral, total parenteral nutrition, and chemotherapy, may be established. Total revenue generated from these categories can be monitored and adjusted by looking at volume, changes to base costs, and the final markup applied.

The pharmacy leader must understand how final patient charges will appear in the market place. The final pricing strategy selected should be competitive with the local/regional market and must be accepted by the primary payment sources. For traditional retail Rx business, this process is generally much easier, because virtually all business outside of cash transactions are at an established payment rate and structure. Each payer will negotiate a payment contract that generally follows the formula AWP − % Discount + Fee. Pharmacies have the opportunity to negotiate the discount rate and the fee to establish the overall reimbursement with that payer. Depending on the number of payers in the area, an average pharmacy may have over 100 different payer contracts loaded into their retail computer system. Budgeting for retail pharmacy revenue is a matter of tallying Rx volume by contract and average reimbursement per Rx within each contract; adjusting for any change in volume, Rx mix, or contract parameters; and projecting the final revenue totals. The contract volume forecast and the complexities of mix and contract parameters illustrate the importance of coordinating with the organization's contracting personnel. The pharmacy department should carefully analyze any contract that involves pharmaceuticals for its overall impact on pharmacy revenue.

When planning for pharmacy revenue, the pharmacy leader must distinguish between gross revenue and net revenue. Gross revenue is the total amount of revenue billed based on the established charging structure. Net revenue is the actual amount of revenue collected less contractual adjustments, discounts, and bad debt. For inpatients, the pharmacy will typically not know how much is actually collected on each line item for pharmaceuticals that are billed. The hospital's accounting department will send out the bills, work the collections, and then perform a reconciliation to understand what was billed and what was paid. The difference between gross and net revenue will then be written off by the organization and will form the basis for the organization's overall contractual and discount rate. This is the number that is generally provided to the pharmacy for budgeting purposes and that appears on the monthly operating statement. This number represents the total amount written off on all charges, not just pharmacy charges, and, when applied to pharmacy revenue, provides a reasonable estimate of net revenue.

A variety of payment sources contribute to the overall contractuals and discount rate. Government programs, such as the prospective payment system, use established payment rates per diagnosis-related group. Many private payers have also followed suit with capitated payment plans. The majority of remaining payers use some type of discounted fee for service contracts in which a negotiated discount from the normally charged rates will be established. The remaining patients will be self-pay, with a percentage of those being indigent, meaning there will be no (or limited) cash collections. It is important to work with the finance department to understand the organization's payer mix because this forms the basis for the contractual and discount rate that will be used to estimate pharmacy net revenue from gross revenue.

When budgeting revenue the organization will generally set a target for pharmacy net revenue contribution required to produce the organizational bottom line, or operating margin. The pharmacy must understand what changes need to occur in gross revenue to produce the required changes in net revenue. Outpatient pharmacy revenue or traditional retail Rx business is generally easier to plan for because this will not require planning for contractuals and discounts in the same fashion as inpatient revenue. All of this business is either cash or an established payment rate with a third party. These net numbers can be directly projected, and the only variable is a specific line item for bad debt (this generally includes uncollected co-pays and problem payments from insurers).

For projections to be meaningful, the pharmacy leader must understand how the organization actually records or "books" this revenue. This can happen either on a cash basis or an accrual basis. In the cash model, although Rx's are dispensed, the revenue does not appear on the pharmacy operating statement until it is actually collected and deposited. In an accrual system, the full value of the Rx will be booked at the time that the claim is adjudicated. The accrual system will produce a more stable revenue pattern for budgeting purposes because it is based on Rx's dispensed rather than when the actual payment arrives. With either system, a solid reconciliation process must be established to ensure that payment actually matches Rx's dispensed and contracted rates. This will be discussed in more detail later in this chapter.

Monitoring Financial Performance

Building the budget should be a continuous process of analyzing and updating existing financial information. A key component of this analysis is the monthly pharmacy operating statement. This document is prepared by the finance department and details the pharmacy's performance against revenue, expense, workload, and additional selected indicators.

Pharmacy services use several indicators to monitor financial performance. Each indicator is important, but, when used in combination, a clear picture of financial strengths and weaknesses is formed. For example, if the number of prescriptions filled are increasing while revenue and drug expenses are decreasing, one might reasonably conclude that a higher volume of lower price/cost drugs are dispensed now than in the past. This assumption may be correct. However, scrutiny might reveal that the drug costs loaded in the billing system are outdated, causing an unintentional discount to sales and a reduction in revenue. Closely monitoring financial indicators can identify potential problems and help to provide timely resolutions.

One of the most important indicators is workload units (WLUs). Identifying what the WLU should be varies by organization and even by the type of pharmacy within a system. An outpatient pharmacy may use the number of prescriptions filled (regardless of the number of doses dispensed), whereas an inpatient pharmacy may use adjusted patient days. The WLUs allow the manager to break the business down to the lowest common denominator. In fact, when building the budget for a new fiscal year, the first item commonly identified is the number of WLUs, or volume. One glance at total WLUs from a year-over-year perspective can foretell what the new fiscal year will bring and can be used to compare similar pharmacies. For example, if the WLU trend is flat or only modestly decreased/increased, then the new fiscal year will likely be similar to the last. A significant increase might be explained by the completion of a planned expansion, such as a newly remodeled hospital outpatient pharmacy that can handle a larger volume than in prior years. Conversely, a pharmacy with decreasing WLU volume may decide to discontinue an unprofitable service line, such as a remote telepharmacy service that provides a high volume of commonly prescribed medicines with low profit margins. Workload unit indicators allow managers to compare similar pharmacies of varying size on a level playing ground. Two different-sized retail pharmacies with similar patient and location demographics will have similar financial indictors per WLU, even though one store may have double the volume and revenue. An astute manager will use WLUs to benchmark pharmacies within the system to determine best practices.

Workload unit-based indicators used by pharmacies include the following: revenue, salaries and benefits, and drugs and medicines. Workload unit-based indicators may vary widely between pharmacies depending on the medical specialty practiced at the location. The infusion pharmacy at a cancer hospital may have revenue per WLU of approximately $450, whereas the retail pharmacy, located in the same building, averages $115 per WLU. An inpatient pharmacy, which uses adjusted patient days for WLUs, may average approximately $420 per WLU. By recognizing the unique characteristics of each pharmacy and maintaining a working knowledge of the revenue per WLU of each, a manager will be able to identify potential problems quickly.

Here is an example. At the beginning of a new fiscal year, a pharmacy's actual revenue did not increase as budgeted but remained unchanged. The pharmacy manager assessed WLUs for volume changes. More patients were being treated, and the number of drugs dispensed had increased. The pharmacy manager then calculated the pharmacy's revenue per WLU, which had remained unchanged from the prior year. When the budget was built for this pharmacy, an increase in the cost of drugs had been factored into the revenue calculation. However, the cost of the drugs used to calculate revenue had not been updated, and several drugs had gone generic, causing overall revenue to remain unchanged, although WLU volumes increased. By comparing year-over-year revenue per WLU, the pharmacy manager identified and corrected the revenue shortfall.

In any given year, the cost of drugs purchased by a hospital pharmacy service accounts for approximately 75–85 percent of its operating expenses and is the primary revenue driver. If a an error or incorrect estimate is made projecting drug expenses, the entire expense/revenue budget will be off for the year. Drugs are difficult to budget because of the dynamics of the market. Every year new drugs, and often more expensive drugs, are introduced to the market. New drugs sometimes replace older drugs, and patents expire, allowing some drugs to be sold in cheaper generic versions. The total cost of drugs purchased in a system can increase by up to 15 percent or more annually, and there may be large variances based on business type. General hospital pharmacy expenses may increase 8–9 percent annually, retail pharmacy may have only a minor year-over-year increase of 3–4 percent, and a cancer specialty hospital pharmacy may easily experience regular double-digit increases. The financial statement will only show the total dollar cost of drugs increasing significantly every year. However, calculating drug costs at the WLU level allows for scrutiny of the actual inflationary increase.

Building revenue budgets can be an overwhelming experience, with moving financial targets, new or expanded lines of service, and drug formularies that are in a constant state of flux. A consistent game plan for the budget process is essential. Each pharmacy in an organization should be planned separately. A good starting point is to break each line item on the financial statement down to the revenue and expense per WLU level. For comparative purposes, use different time frames to calculate the WLU base. Systems often use a rolling thirteen-month average, or the total financial results for the last thirteen months. It is also possible to use year-to-date actual numbers, depending on how much time has progressed in the current year when beginning the budget. If the system allows, compare the projected budget to the last two full years. Breaking down revenue and expenses to the lowest common denominator provides a base upon which to build the budget with current year assumptions. In budgeting terminology, the "rate" for doing business for each line on the financials has just been calculated.

Revenue and drug expenses use the base WLU amount (rates), multiplied by the projected number of WLUs (volume), to give projected base numbers. If nothing else changed, these numbers would be the budget for revenue and drug expense for the next fiscal year. However, because change is a constant element of doing business, each pharmacy must be reviewed to determine and to quantify any changes to business for the new fiscal year. Changes can include new lines of services, such as an anticoagulation business, or an increase in the number of infusion stations, or moving the pharmacy from the back of a clinic to the front for better exposure. Once quantified and annualized, the business change numbers are then added to the earlier projected base numbers.

Perhaps the most important piece in the budget process is identifying the inflationary increase in the cost of drugs. Understanding the discount rate on billed charges is important to accurately project contribution margin. With a 50 percent discount rate, when the cost of a drug is increased by $1, revenue must be increased by $2 to maintain the same contribution margin. Retail pharmacies are usually easier to predict because of the relatively static mix of drugs sold. In this setting, a 2 percent increase in the cost of drugs with a 4 percent increase in revenue to maintain the contribution margin is a good rule of thumb. Inpatient and cancer pharmacies are somewhat different because of several factors: the higher cost mix of drugs, the high potential for cost fluctuation, the algorithm used to calculate patient prices, and the contractual adjustment. Given these additional factors related to pricing inpatient drugs, for every 1 percent increase in cost, it may require a budgeted 1.2 percent increase in gross revenue. If we project an 8 percent cost increase, then we could expect approximately a 9.5 percent increase in revenue to maintain the same contribution margin.

The final step in the budget process spreads the totals for each line by month for the new year. Several methods can be used to determine how to spread the budget, including seasonal trends, open business days, number of days in the month, and historical trends. Selecting the appropriate method depends largely on the type of service the pharmacy provides. Retail pharmacies may use the number of open business days. Inpatient pharmacies may use seasonal or historic trends if certain months have proven to be more or less busy than other months. The number of days in the month is the most commonly used method for spreading budgets.

Reimbursement Sources

Government[4-7]

The pharmacy leader must identify patient population and mix by payer type to establish estimated revenue and payment cycle dates. Having an accurate estimate of the number of Medicare, Medicaid, and commercial-covered lives within the institution annually will allow accurate forecasting of revenue that should be received. Medicare Parts A and B, which provide hospital and outpatient reimbursement for Medicare-covered enrollees, reimburses a fixed percentage rate based on the type of service identified within the billing. Medicaid also has fixed reimbursement rates based on the designation of service. Know what these reimbursements are and update them annually. Creating a billing and reimbursement system that estimates revenue based *only* on the insurance allowable will produce limited contractual adjustments and more accurate reporting of expected revenue.

With the implementation of electronic billing, Medicare Parts A and B should be billed weekly, bimonthly, or monthly (at a minimum), and payment can be expected within 14 days of receipt of a clean claim. It is important to designate a patient's Medicare status prior to rendering service, because this will determine the level of documentation needed when providing service in order to secure payment. When a patient receives Medicare Part B-covered service, such as diabetic supplies, immunosuppressive medications, nebulizer solutions, and anti-cancer medications, proper documentation is essential to receiving accurate reimbursement. It is often necessary to determine if Medicare is primary or secondary to a commercial carrier or Medicaid, because many patients have dual coverage. Billing requirements vary, and the documentation necessary when Medicare is primary is not always the same as when Medicare pays as a secondary for an identical service. Information not typically gathered in an outpatient pharmacy setting, such as diagnosis, patient's length of time on a specific drug or using a specific product, patient's employment status, height of the patient, and weight of the patient, is often necessary for accurate Medicare billing. Although electronic billing is possible for Medicare Part B-covered services, there is no point-of-sale system for Medicare Part B reimbursement. This requires all billing to occur *after* the time of dispensing, which is a potential liability. Gather as much information as possible up front, and verify Medicare eligibility before allowing a patient or medication to leave the pharmacy.

Medicare Part D allows for online adjudication of outpatient pharmacy charges or take-home medications, and payments are received on a 30-, 45-, or 60-day cycle. Verify whether Medicare Part D is primary or secondary to another carrier, because billing windows for Medicare Part D are small, typically no more than 90 days, and it is difficult to correct online adjudication of claims *after* a service has been rendered. To complicate matters, patients are not always clear about their coverage order. It is also important to know if an individual is retired or actively working if over the age of 62. For a dual-eligible individual covered by Medicare Part D and Medicaid, Medicaid is *always* the payer of last resort. However, if a patient receives a medication not covered by Medicare Part D, Medicaid can be billed directly. Many items covered by Medicare Part B are also covered by Medicare Part D, based on individual patient circumstances. If patients are receiving anti-cancer medications, anti-emetics, nebulizer solutions, or immunosuppressive agents, Medicare Part B coverage is likely available and should be billed before trying to access coverage from Medicare Part D.

Unfortunately, many pharmacies that accept Medicare Part D patients are *not* Medicare suppliers and may need to refer patients to pharmacies that can accurately access a patient's Medicare Part B benefit. If a Medicare Part B-covered item is billed to Medicare Part D and is adjudicated online, documentation must be kept on file indicating *why* Medicare Part D was billed. These are frequent targets for audits, because Medicare Part D plans are often billed for expensive, high-dollar items that should be accessed through a patient's Medicare Part B benefit.

Medicare enrollees with limited resources are often eligible for additional federal assistance through Medicare's Limited Income Subsidy (LIS) benefit. This additional help can increase patient's cost savings by paying part of their monthly premium, annual deductibles, and monthly prescription co-payments under the Medicare Part D program. This extra assistance can be worth as much as $3700 annually per patient.

Medicaid also allows for online adjudication of all outpatient pharmacy services, and payments are turned around weekly. Identify dual-eligible patients at the time of service if secondary billing to Medicaid is necessary. Most state Medicaid plans allow online adjudication and receipt of claims as a secondary payer, and no paper or manual billing is necessary. If a pharmacy does not have the ability to process multiple payers electronically, gather a copy of the patient's primary insurance card and any other documentation necessary for a clean secondary billing to Medicaid by HCFA 1500 or UB-04. A more extensive reimbursement tracking system is needed for these claims, because payment should not be applied until the Medicaid remittance advice is received for verification of accurate coinsurance and co-payment reimbursement. Medicaid reimbursement is typically processed and issued weekly, which allows for timely correction of unpaid claims if necessary.

Commercial Sources

Commercial insurance plans provide pharmacy cards that allow for convenient, online adjudication of outpatient pharmacy services. Verify if a patient has any other coverage *before* processing an electronic claim, because billing requirements vary if a commercial carrier is the primary or secondary insurer. If an individual has access to Medicaid coverage in addition to commercial coverage, Medicaid would be secondary to the commercial plan.

Reimbursement Reconciliation

The importance of identifying patient mix is made clear when establishing reimbursement time frames and follow-up dates. All outpatient pharmacy services rendered to a patient with Medicare Part D, Medicaid, or commercial insurance plans should always be paid no later than 60 days from the date of service for a clean claim. Consistent reimbursement follow-up and research of unpaid claims allows for timely resolution and payment on denied claims and underpaid claims, which are common when working with Medicare, Medicaid, and many commercial programs.

Reimbursement mechanisms vary from an inpatient setting to an outpatient setting. Many inpatient systems are linked to hospital and medical billing and may not allow for line item reconciliation. A stand-alone pharmacy billing department is beneficial, because this allows for a more accurate statement of cost of goods, billed charges, anticipated reimbursement, and actual revenue. Inpatient pharmacy billing should also be isolated from outpatient pharmacy billing if possible, because contracts, reimbursement rates, billing systems, and types of expertise vary between inpatient and outpatient models.

Outpatient pharmacy settings processing high-dollar/high-volume receivables should consider a relationship with an information management vendor, who can provide accurate financial and information management. Vendors currently processing pharmaceutical claims and data are able to effectively provide line item reimbursement and claim detail for single pharmacies or large pharmacy chains. This link to finance allows for forecasting of reimbursement based on patient population, payer mix, prescription volume, and contract rates.

In addition to an inpatient and outpatient reimbursement process, Medicare Part B volume must be separated, which requires more involved documentation, reimbursement tracking, and patient follow-up. Because Medicare Part B claims cannot be adjudicated or reconciled at point of sale, this line of business must be kept separate from any information management process, because the dollars can only be recorded on the back end.

Uncompensated Care

Budget and Oversight

Uncompensated care is an unavoidable cost of doing business in the health-care sector. Many medical and catastrophic plans have high out-of-pocket maximums or low pharmacy benefit maximums that further restrict patient access to necessary pharmaceuticals. With the emergence of Medicare Part D in 2006, which allows pharmacy coverage for more than 43 million individuals, medication affordability became a reality for a large percentage of the disabled and senior patient population. Although large deductible amounts, co-payments, and out-of-pocket costs still exist for many patients, the number of federal programs and prescription manufacturers offering various levels of subsidies and assistance are increasing. Underinsured patients are becoming as common as uninsured patients, and it may be difficult to differentiate between the two in an outpatient pharmacy setting in which no coverage is available. Inpatient pharmacy benefits and maximums often mimic medical coverage, which allows for a broader range of coverage availability than many outpatient pharmacy benefits. The pharmacy leader should identify an institution's total percentage of unfunded and underfunded patients to establish a realistic budget and reimbursement goal for pharmacy services.

Medications/Indigent Care Programs

Manufacturer-sponsored patient assistance programs provide millions of dollars of inpatient and outpatient prescription drugs annually. More than 200 manufacturers provide some level of patient assistance, and all programs result in some level of patient savings. Requirements vary by manufacturer (must be a U.S. resident, can have no insurance coverage for outpatient pharmacy services, income level must be below state/federal poverty guidelines, etc.), as do levels of medication assistance. A well-trained pharmacy staff can navigate the hurdles of manufacturer and financial requirements to assist your institution's underfunded and unfunded patient population. This vulnerable population often has no access to computer equipment, software, or technology that allows them to connect with these drug manufacturers, and an intermediary familiar with patient assistance requirements can often eliminate the confusion and hassle.

Medicare Part D not only dramatically changed the landscape of patient assistance availability through drug manufacturers, it also opened more windows. Patients without access to medication coverage before Medicare Part D who are still unable to afford their Medicare Part D deductibles, co-payments, and coinsurance often qualify for special assistance programs that offer drug coverage during these times of hardship. This is another opportunity to screen patients for Limited Income Subsidy, available through Social Security. If a patient's annual income is below $14,700 for an individual and $19,800 for a married couple, he/she may be eligible for free or reduced Medicare Part D premiums, deductibles, and co-payments. A successful patient assistance team should use state and federal poverty guidelines, along with a minimum level of documentation necessary across all patient assistance providers (tax returns, Social Security earnings statements, paycheck stubs), to generate a standardized form for individuals interested in patient assistance. This often alleviates frustration for patients. All necessary information can be gathered once, but multiple vendors and patient assistance opportunities can be explored based on a patient's individual needs.

Pharmacist Services

The Medicare Prescription Drug, Improvement, and Modernization Act of 2003 (MMA), includes a section on medication therapy management services (MTMS). Although not limited to pharmacists, the description of MTMS states that "drug therapy management may be furnished by a pharmacist."[8] No other professional is mentioned as a provider of MTMS. The MMA provides MTMS to Part D-eligible individuals who (1) have multiple chronic diseases, (2) are taking multiple drugs, and (3) are likely to incur expenses that exceed a level specified by the secretary of the Department of Health and Human Services.

Medication therapy monitoring programs could include managing and monitoring drug therapy in patients receiving treatment for cancer or chronic conditions, such as asthma and diabetes; consulting with patients and their families on the proper use of medication; conducting wellness and disease prevention programs to improve public health; and overseeing medication use in a variety of settings, such as home care settings, hospitals, ambulatory care settings, long-term care facilities, clinics, and intensive care units. Pharmacists currently have three nationally recognized codes to bill third-party payers for medication therapy management services. Current Procedural Terminology (CPT) codes 0115T, 0116T, and 0117T describe pharmacist-provided MTMS and recognize the initial face-to-face encounter, subsequent visits, and any appointment lasting beyond 15 minutes.

Strategies to Offset Uncompensated Care

It is important to offset or reduce uncompensated pharmacy services when it is possible to do so. Many state Medicaid programs have spenddown provisions, which allow for individuals who are not fully Medicaid eligible because their income or resources are above the state poverty thresholds to reduce their income or resource liabilities by applying past and current medical and pharmacy bills to offset their income. Although many patients have medical bills that allow them to surpass this poverty guideline, others may be on the threshold or within $0–$250. In many instances, it is financially worthwhile for an institution to cover an individual's spenddown amount instead of allowing the patient to be completely unfunded because of resources and income over the Medicaid limit. Clear guidelines must be established, but it may be feasible to offer Medicaid spenddown payment assistance for individuals within a specific dollar amount of qualifying for full Medicaid coverage. The pharmacy leader should identify the institution's access to medical and pharmacy reimbursement for the given individual and whether ongoing medical and pharmacy care will be needed for the patient in question. Medicaid is often willing to allow for retroactive Medicaid coverage in catastrophic illness or injury situations for patients who were unfunded at the time of admission to an institution, once medical bills total a specified dollar amount.

Individuals receiving medical and pharmacy coverage through COBRA plans often run into financial difficulties while trying to maintain the high cost of COBRA premiums, in addition to large deductibles, co-payments, and out-of-pocket costs. Individuals who have the opportunity to receive COBRA benefits but are unable to afford premiums to qualify for this coverage may seek charity care or assistance from the institution. In many instances, it is more cost effective for an institution to gain access to a patient's medical and pharmacy benefit by paying the COBRA premium than it would be to provide charity or uncompensated care.

Conclusion

Regular monitoring of financial performance will give a pharmacy manager an early opportunity to identify and correct potential problems within the pharmacy system. A review of indicators such as WLUs, revenue per WLU, and expense per WLU on a monthly basis, with benchmark comparison against prior months and similar pharmacies will quickly bring attention to areas of concern. A comprehensive reconciliation program to evaluate billed charges and rates versus actual amounts paid and a regular review of this process will ensure that all available revenue is maximized. A regular review of government and commercial regulations regarding payment will support a comprehensive budget and revenue management plan. Tracking financial indicators will be beneficial to managers at budget time, helping them to develop a realistic and workable revenue budget that supports organizational goals and objectives.

References

1. Smith C, Cowan C, Sensing A et al. National Health Spending in 2004. *Health Affairs*. 2006; 25(1): 186–196.
2. The Levin Group. Analysis of American Hospital Association Annual Survey Data. www.aha.org/aha/trendwatch/2006/cb2006chapter4.ppt (accessed 2007 February).
3. Tracy K. Know the effects of not-for-profit conversions—includes related information on Section 501c3. March 1991. *Healthcare Financial Management*.
4. United States Department of Health and Human Services. Centers for Medicare and Medicaid Services. www.cms.hhs.gov (accessed 2007 February 18).

5. Levinson DR. Identifying Beneficiaries Eligible for the Medicare Part D Low-Income Subsidy, OEI-03-06-00120. http://oig.hhs.gov/oei/reports/oei-03-06-00120.pdf (accessed 2007 February 18).

6. United States Social Security Agency. Help with Medicare Prescription Drug Costs—Information for Organizations. http://www.ssa.gov/medicareoutreach2/index.htm (accessed 2007 February 18).

7. Goldfarb D. Medicare and Medigap Insurance Policies: Maximizing the Benefits. http://www.seniorlaw.com/medicare.htm (accessed 2007 February 17).

8. Cost and Utilization Management; Quality Assurance; Medication Therapy Management Program. SEC. 1860D–4.(c) (2) (A) (i) The Medicare Prescription Drug, Improvement, and Modernization Act of 2003, P.L. 108–173. Enacted 2003 December 8.

Pharmaceutical Reimbursement

Philip E. Johnson

Overview of the Medicare Program

The Medicare program's authority and requirements are established by the U.S. Congress through legislation (e.g., the Medicare Prescription Drug Improvement and Modernization Act, Balanced Budget Act, Title XVII of the Social Security Act). The Centers for Medicare and Medicaid Services (CMS) establishes program policies in accordance with congressional mandates through regulations, transmittals, and directives to regional and state Medicare contractors that are referred to as fiscal intermediaries (FI). These contractors establish local policies in accordance with CMS directives and provide clarification about coverage and billing issues as needed; this clarification reflects medically accepted local practices.

The Medicare program has three parts (A, B, and D) that pertain to pharmaceutical reimbursement (Figure 11.1). Part A covers hospital inpatient and outpatient services, nursing home care, home health care, and hospice care. Part B covers physician services, medical supplies such as durable medical equipment, some oral cancer chemotherapies, and end-stage renal disease services. Hospital outpatient services are administered through Part A Outpatient Prospective Payment System (OPPS), but Part B rules are followed. Efforts are under way to merge Parts A and B. Currently, Part A coverage is automatic, but Part B coverage is optional and requires payment of monthly premiums. Part D covers outpatient prescription drugs. Minimal benefits are guaranteed through Part D.

A durable medical equipment regional carrier (DMERC) license is required for outpatient prescription pharmacies that dispense oral chemotherapy and other oral drugs covered under the DMERC provisions of Part B. In the near future, the oral drugs that are currently covered under Part B DMERC provisions will be covered under Part D.

In the past, reimbursement policies at the state level were referred to as *local medical review policies*. The current term is *local coverage determinations* (LCDs); however, the two terms often are used interchangeably.

In the future, 15 regional Medicare Administrative Contractors (MACs) will replace the 50 state Carrier Advisory Committees (CACs). The first regional MAC began in 2007 as the Rocky Mountain region.

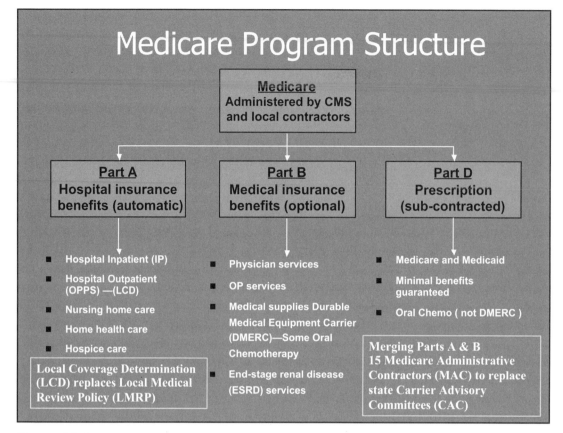

Figure 11.1.

Overview of Process for Changes in CMS Rules

CMS is a dynamic organization that is constantly changing; therefore it is important to keep three things in mind when evaluating Medicare or other CMS rules. First, CMS follows requirements established by Congress, after which local or regional Fiscal Intermediaries develop rules that may vary. Second, CMS must adhere to a budget that is approved by the U.S. Congress; therefore all internal changes must be budget neutral, meaning if they pay more for Part A drug benefits, they have to pay less for something else. Finally, CMS has a systematic plan to make regular changes to achieve long-term goals. They follow a process of issuing proposed rule changes (typically in July), followed by a period of open response, followed by advice from their advisory committee's Ambulatory Payment Classification Group (APC) and Medicare Coverage Advisory Committee (MCAC), followed by another open response period, followed by an announcement of the final rules (usually in October) to be implemented in the first part of January. When evaluating rules and assigning codes, be sure that you are following the most current rules. The examples that follow are for a specific year, and will undoubtedly have changed by the time you read this chapter. Please refer to the CMS Web site, ASHP Reimbursement Resource Center Web sites, and other more current references for advice before undertaking a project focusing on reimbursement.

Pharmaceutical reimbursement rates have consistently declined over the past several years for Part A hospital OPPS (outpatient) providers (Table 11.1). Drugs with "pass through"

Table 11.1. Changes in the Basis for Pharmaceutical Reimbursement Rates by Medicare, 2003–2008[a]

	2005	2006	2007	2008
OPPS Part A UB04/CMS 1450	83% AWP 68% AWP 46% AWP	1.06 ASP—or – 95% AWP until HCPCS-Code	1.06 ASP - Package <$55	1.05 ASP - Package <$60 - No pay for 21 NQF Never Events
IP PPS	DRG	DRG 10 Quality Indicators	CS-DRG (Severity Adjusted) Optional 21 Quality Indicators (3.4%)	CS-DRG (Severity Adjusted) Required 21 Quality Indicators (3.4%) P4P
Part B CMS 1500	1.06 ASP	1.06 ASP – or – CAP	1.06 ASP – AMP if < ASP - CAP option - No Package - 5–6 Quality Indicators (1.5%, start 7/1)	1.06 ASP – AMP if < ASP - CAP option - No Package - 5–6 Quality Indicators (1.5%)
Part D Outpatient Rx Benefit	Discount cards	Schedule – or – Contract	- Tiers changed - Gap increased	- Tiers changed - Gap increased

[a]AMP = average manufacturer price; ASP = average sales price; AWP = average wholesale price; CAP = competitive acquisition program; CS-DRG = consolidated severity-adjusted diagnosis related group; DRG = diagnosis related group; GAO = Government Accountability Office; OIG = Office of Inspector General.

status, meaning they have an assigned HCPCS code, went from being reimbursed at 95 percent of Average Wholesale Price (AWP) in 2005, to Average Sales Price (ASP) plus 6 percent in 2006, to ASP plus 5 percent in 2008. When daily drug costs (based on ASP) in this setting fell below the threshold of $60 (in 2008), their costs were packaged (i.e., bundled) into the reimbursement for an associated drug that was covered by Ambulatory Payment Classification (APC), a diagnostic classification analogous to an outpatient diagnosis related group. Those drug costs were not reimbursed separately, with 5-HT$_3$-receptor antagonists being an exception. Reimbursement rates differed for the physician office setting under Part B (in 2008), with reimbursement set at ASP plus 6 percent, and packaging of daily drug costs not required. For example, diphenhydramine is bundled under Part A coverage with no reimbursement, while it was reimbursed under Part B coverage. Proposals for 2009 will attempt to equalize both Part A and Part B drug reimbursement at ASP plus 4 percent, and standardize reimbursement for drug administration. It is unclear what is proposed for the discrepancy related to bundled drugs.

In 2007, reimbursement based on the consolidated severity-adjusted diagnosis related group (CS-DRG) was introduced for the hospital inpatient setting. As a pay-for-performance (P4P) initiative to compensate high-quality care, a 3.4 percent premium is paid if 21 quality indicators are reported. A provider has the option to collect and report the indicators;

however, failure to report them results, effectively, in a 3.4 percent penalty. CMS will evaluate the impact on both outcomes and cost over a 3 year span to determine the impact of this program and whether it should be expanded, modified, or eliminated.

Several proposed changes in CMS rules and rates are expected from 2009–2010 that are likely to affect pharmaceutical reimbursement. For the hospital inpatient prospective payment system, an increase in the number of CS-DRGs from 526 to 861 has been proposed to address total costs associated with differences in severity for some CS-DRGs (e.g., low, moderate, and high severity).[1] For the hospital outpatient perspective payment system (OPPS), reporting of 25 quality indicators to avoid loss of a 3.4 percent premium had been proposed, analogous to the 2007 change for the hospital inpatient setting, and unique indicators for specialty practices are being considered.

Decreased payment for cases involving medical errors was proposed during a May 2006 Senate hearing as a form of pay for performance.[2] No payment will be made for additional care that is required as the result of one or more of 27 "never events" identified by the National Quality Forum (NQF) in 2007. Two of these 27 events are pharmacy related: severe injury or death due to contaminated medication or medication error.

Other changes being considered for the future include modifications in drug administration codes and rates to provide more detailed and accurate reporting. CMS has attempted to address inequity associated with the way drug handling costs are reimbursed considering ASP plus X percent is insufficient in most providers' opinion. CMS is considering developing handling tiers that will sort drugs into several categories based on complexity resulting from compounding or clinical management complexity. In 2007, seven categories were proposed, in 2008, three categories, and for 2009, two categories. It remains to be seen if this strategy will actually be implemented.[3]

In a July 9, 2007, memorandum CMS proposed Average Manufacturer Price (AMP) as an option to ASP in certain situations. Recently using Widely Available Market Price (WAMP) or creating an altogether new cost base have been discussed because, while more reliable than AWP, it is clear that ASP is inconsistent and still creates situations where providers lose money on some drug items. For example, ASP always lags real world prices by six months, and ASP does not include 340B or CAP prices. However, for 2008 CMS reimburses new drugs at ASP plus 6 percent regardless of setting or AMP if it is less than ASP for Part B providers. This special pricing will last for two years for each new drug, at which time pricing will revert to the current formula being used for established drugs. For perspective, in 2008 this affected only 13 new drugs.

CMS Accountability

The American Society of Health-System Pharmacists (ASHP) and other pharmacy associations and stakeholders frequently contact CMS with concerns about pharmaceutical reimbursement through established advisory committees. Although CMS is receptive to these concerns, the agency is accountable to Congress and seeks to maintain neutrality in the federal budget. Advisory committees provide CMS with input about policies; the two committees that play key roles in pharmaceutical reimbursement policymaking are the Ambulatory Payment Classification Groups (APC) Advisory Panel and the Medicare Coverage Advisory Committee (MCAC). The

MCAC is responsible for advising on the scope of medical coverage provided and the rationale for clinical decisions. As such they are responsible for recommending the compendia that is used to support medical decisions. The APC is responsible for advising the method and level of payment for services provided. Both are open to input from the pharmacy profession and typically include pharmacists as volunteer committee members.

In pay-for-performance initiatives, CMS is collaborating with various public and private organizations whose common goal is to improve quality and avoid unnecessary health-care costs.[4] These organizations include the National Quality Forum (NQF), the Joint Commission, National Committee for Quality Assurance, the Agency for Healthcare Research and Quality, and the American Medical Association (AMA). The collaborative relationship with CMS gives these organizations some influence with the agency.

Billing

New drugs are often approved by the FDA prior to CMS establishing a HCPCS code. Until a billing code is established there are three billing options. The original code J9999 will result in documenting the use of a drug and enable the provider to bill an administration code, but there will be no reimbursement for the drug. Later, billing code J3490 was established that reimbursed a fixed rate (in Florida it is $160 in 2008) that varies by state and year. Considering that many new biotech drugs are more costly, code C9399 was established that reimburses at wholesale acquisition cost (WAC) or ASP plus 6 percent, whichever is less. Once an HCPCS code is established the current billing rules apply. CMS has a strong financial incentive to promptly assign HCPCS codes once a drug receives FDA approval, because payments for drugs with these C, J, and Q codes are less than 106 percent of WAC or ASP. In the past, six to nine months often elapsed between FDA approval and assignment of HCPCS codes, but this time frame has shortened. Drugs without HCPCS codes must be billed manually, which adds to the processing cost for both the provider and CMS. The availability of HCPCS codes eliminates the need for manual billing for the drug, but this advantage comes at a cost of reduced revenue.

Preauthorization for drug therapy is not available from Medicare, but it is possible to ascertain whether Medicare covers the therapy for a patient's condition based on the International Classification of Diseases, Ninth Revision (ICD-9) code. This is done by using "scrubber" software that compares the patient claim with the indications approved by each Fiscal Intermediary. Each Fiscal Intermediary should be able to provide a list of software vendors they collaborate with, and some sell software themselves. Claim denials often can be anticipated (e.g., for an off-label use of a drug). If the therapy is not covered by Medicare for the patient's ICD-9 code, the patient must sign a CMS form called an Advance Beneficiary Notice (ABN) that explains alternative treatment options, quality-of-life issues, and the patient's obligation to pay for the therapy if the claim is not approved by CMS. The ABN may be completed by a physician's designee, but it must be signed by the physician providing services and the patient. The patient must disclose any coverage or financial assistance from secondary insurance providers, medication assistance programs, patient assistance programs, or charities. If the bill is denied, the health-care provider can appeal, but only if an ABN was signed by the patient.

Many institutions use case managers to facilitate the ABN process. They have also found that the ABN process has a favorable impact on physician financial accountability and physician-patient communication because physicians tend to be more aware of financial issues associated with care, and patients have opportunities to ask more questions of physicians about their therapy. Some commercial insurers have adopted the ABN process, utilize CMS forms, and follow the reimbursement policies established by CMS for accepted drug uses.

Pharmacists can play a role in the ABN process by screening drug orders for Medicare beneficiaries to ascertain whether the use is consistent with CMS-approved compendia. Another strategy is to include indications for use that are supported by CMS-approved compendia when preparing preprinted medication order forms. If the prescriber uses the drug outside of the listed indications, they will be required to document justification for use, and obtain an ABN.

Health-care providers may appeal a denied claim by providing clinical rationale for use and resubmitting the claim. The FI has 30 days to determine if the appeal is valid and 90 days from the time of the appeal to make a decision. The result may be a request for additional information, notification of denial, or notification of acceptance of the appeal and subsequent reimbursement. It is also possible to request a change in the Local Coverage Determination (LCD) for a specific drug, requesting approval for a previously unapproved indication. To do this an appeal is made directly to the FI, and in most cases they will require a real case with a patient who has signed an ABN. The FI will consider evidence, place their proposed decision in a public domain for 30–60 days for feedback, and then implement a final decision.

When the FI denies a claim, they are obligated to provide an Explanation of Benefits (EOB) that gives the specific reason for the denial. The provider should always ask for an EOB. If the problem is related to the way the claim was processed (wrong or missing codes are most common), the provider should correct their system. In other cases the provider should determine if they have valid support to reverse the denial based on evidence based clinical rationale that has been published or documented in phase 3 trials.

Expanding Compendia and Off-Label Uses

In 2008 the MCAC evaluated compendia that are used to make therapy decisions. They also openly solicited and received input that led to significant changes in compendia that is approved. Beginning in 2008, CMS will consider several new compendia to substantiate off-label drug use (uses not approved by FDA). The following were established in 2008: (1) Drug Dex by Thompson Micromedex, (2) Clinical Pharmacology by Elsevier Gold Standard, (3) AHFS-DI, (4) NCCN Drugs and Biologics Compendia, (5) published phase 3 clinical trials data, and an additional 21 specific peer-reviewed medical journals. The 21 accepted journals include, among others, *American Journal of Medicine, Annals of Internal Medicine, JAMA, Journal of Clinical Oncology, Blood, Drugs, New England Journal of Medicine*, and the *Lancet*. Compendia can also be added at the local level by petitioning a fiscal intermediary.

The use of genetic markers to provide targeted therapy in individual patients (personalized medicine) is a trend that CMS has started to consider. Eventually, the ability to individualize therapy on the basis of gene expression may make compendia-based reimbursement decisions that rely on population-based data obsolete. Genomic tests are not yet routinely covered by CMS; however, there are some instances where positive genome expression is required for use of specific drugs.

To optimize pharmaceutical reimbursement, pharmacists should stay abreast of changes in CMS rules. Information from recognized compendial sources should be incorporated into the drug-ordering process (e.g., on computer screens or in standardized drug order forms or clinical notes) to ensure that the justification for off-label use is documented, preferably in an automated manner, using computers to the extent possible. This documentation is particularly important when primary therapy has failed and alternative therapy that might be challenged by CMS has been used. Fiscal intermediaries should be contacted and educated about issues that affect patient care, leading to requests for expanded coverage through the approval of new LCDs.

Cost Base for Reimbursement

The use of ASP began in 2006 with ASP plus 6 percent (i.e., 106 percent of ASP) as the basis for pharmaceutical reimbursement that was intended to cover the acquisition cost of the drug plus the cost of handling the drug. Results of an analysis published in 2005 demonstrated that pharmacy handling and overhead costs are not insignificant, accounting for 26 to 28 percent of total direct drug expenses.[5] Challenging the validity of this finding, CMS insisted that 106 percent of ASP is more than adequate to cover handling costs, as Government Accountability Office data have suggested that 103 percent of ASP should suffice. Pharmacy groups rebuffed that argument, using survey data suggesting that reimbursement rates up to 50 percent higher than the drug acquisition cost are needed to cover handling and overhead costs, including clinical services.[5] In an attempt to negotiate reimbursement rates that more accurately reflect acquisition and handling costs, ACCC, ASHP, HOPA, and some group purchasing organizations presented survey data and proposed a rate based on ASP plus 14 percent as more reflective of actual costs. However, to maintain budget neutrality, the final rule for 2006 and 2007 allowed for only ASP plus 6 percent, and for 2008 only 5 percent for Part A and 6 percent for part B providers. The inequity between Part A and Part B has never been rationalized, and for 2009, CMS is proposing ASP plus 4 percent for both, except for new drugs with pass-through status that will continue to be reimbursed at ASP plus 6 percent.

CMS calculates ASP on the basis of manufacturer-reported sales data for hospitals, pharmacies, physician offices, wholesalers, and others.[6] ASP reflects manufacturer promotions, discounts, and rebates, but it does not reflect 340B pharmaceutical procurement program discounts or data from competitive acquisition program (CAP) providers (a program for CMS Part B providers). ASP is updated quarterly on the basis of data for the previous two quarters, and it may not accurately reflect current sales prices because of inflation and contract changes. For example if the inflation impact for two quarters is 2 percent, the reimbursement rate is in effect reduced to ASP plus 4 percent instead of ASP plus 6 percent.

Receiving reimbursement for handling costs is one of the biggest issues for pharmacists. CMS recognizes the need to collect data and provide fair reimbursement. Part A and Part B providers need to provide data on their direct and indirect costs. Direct costs include compounding labor, supplies, and direct costs associated with meeting mandatory USP chapter 797 requirements for sterile product compounding. Direct costs also include clinically related costs associated with patient monitoring and management. Indirect costs include institutional overhead that can be provided by a hospital's business office.

Differences in the amount of handling (both compounding and clinical) required for different drugs have been recognized by CMS. The agency has considered the use of specific C codes and a rating system for the amount of handling required for certain drugs to build a database of information that could be used to determine fair reimbursement rates for handling costs. In 2006 seven codes were proposed, and in 2007 three codes were proposed; however, none were implemented. Whether CMS can develop a method to differentiate the cost required for complex drugs versus simple drugs has not yet been determined.

Many pharmacies will need to change the cost base in their pricing formulas. Published information about the relationships between different cost bases is available from the Office of the Inspector General.[7] For example, a pharmacy with a pricing formula based on AWP can switch to WAC as the cost base, knowing that the WAC is 16 to 22 percent lower than the AWP (i.e., choosing 19 percent as the middle of the range, an AWP of $100 translates into a WAC of $81). Similarly, because ASP has been found to be 26 to 30 percent lower than AWP, a $100 AWP translates to an ASP of $72 if a reduction of 28 percent at the middle of the range is chosen.

Paying for Health Care

Understanding the health-care revenue stream can provide insight into the forces that cause change. At the beginning of this stream, employers purchase health-care benefits. Employer concerns include costs, lost workdays and productivity, and employee satisfaction. Chronic low back pain is the most common reason for lost workdays.[8]

Patients are responsible for copayments and deductibles. Additional costs are incurred by uninsured patients. All patients pay for health care indirectly through taxes. Patient concerns include cost, access to care, quality of care, and personal outcomes, including quality of life.

Payers (e.g., CMS, commercial insurers) act as agents for employers and patients by processing money and establishing the rules that determine what care is delivered by providers. Payer concerns include enrollee (i.e., patient) retention and their net margin.[9] High turnover rates among enrollees account in part for payer reluctance to cover preventive medicine, from which benefits may not be observed in the short-term.

Providers receive payments for services and are liable for substandard care and therapeutic failures. Provider concerns include patient outcomes, provider liability, and their net margin.

Distributors and group purchasing organizations receive a fee for their service. The net margin and providing support to providers are their main concerns.

Finally, health-care manufacturers earn profits for shareholders and reinvest some of those profits in research and development of new products. Manufacturers have been the target of criticism from FDA, payers, politicians, and the public in recent years. Manufacturers'

Table 11.2. Pharmaceutical Reimbursement Information Sources

ASHP Pharmaceutical Reimbursement Resource Center
- http://www.ashp.org/s_ashp/cat1c.asp?CID=490&DID=532
- Provides education and guidance for pharmacists responsible for pharmaceutical reimbursement in their institutions

Centers for Medicare and Medicaid Services Medicare modernization update
- http://www.cms.hhs.gov/MMAUpdate/
- Provides information about recent changes in the prescription drug provisions of the Medicare Prescription Drug Improvement and Modernization Act

Centers for Medicare and Medicaid Services Hospital Outpatient Prospective Payment System
- http://www.cms.hhs.gov/HospitalOutpatientPPS/
- Provides information about ambulatory payment classifications and other topics

Centers for Medicare and Medicaid Services Medicare Coverage Center
- http://www.cms.hhs.gov/center/coverage.asp
- Provides information for pharmacists and other providers about the Medicare coverage process

Centers for Medicare and Medicaid Services Medicare Learning Network
- http://www.cms.hhs.gov/MLNMattersArticles/
- Provides information for providers about new or changed Medicare policies

Centers for Medicare and Medicaid Services Medicare Prescription Drug Coverage
- http://www.medicare.gov/
- Provides information for patients about prescription drug plans, formularies, and other topics

concerns include their market image, satisfying the demands of owners and shareholders, their net margin, market competitiveness, and patient outcomes.

Collaboration among participants in the health-care revenue stream—purchasers, patients, payers, providers, and pharmaceutical manufacturers—is needed to improve the health-care delivery system. Stakeholders need to make their voices heard by CMS, and they need to deliver a consistent message that is logical and well supported by data. Collaborative summit meetings are needed to develop consensus rules for pharmaceutical reimbursement for consideration by CMS before the agency imposes rules that are untenable. The resources listed in Table 11.2 may be helpful in these efforts.

Research into clinical outcomes, quality of life, and the actual costs of care is needed. Patient productivity on the job and employee absenteeism, along with their economic impact also should be addressed, because the main portion of the revenue stream starts with employers purchasing health-care benefits. With this information, perhaps a more compelling argument can be provided to support the way drug use is approved and reimbursement justified.

Conclusion

An understanding of the complexities of Medicare pharmaceutical reimbursement can help pharmacists improve the financial viability of their institutions, and expand their scope of service to improve the health care provided to patients. The pharmacist has always been a patient advocate for safe and effective therapy, and that includes ensuring that financial issues do not serve as a barrier to adequate care.

Notes

1. Centers for Medicare and Medicaid Services. Medicare program; proposed changes to the hospital inpatient prospective payment systems and fiscal year 2007 rates; proposed rule. 42 CFR Parts 409, 410 et al. April 25, 2006. http://a257.g.akamaitech.net/7/257/2422/01jan20061800/edocket.access.gpo.gov/2006/pdf/06-3629.pdf (accessed 2007 Jul 10).

2. Centers for Medicare and Medicaid Services. Eliminating serious, preventable, and costly medical errors—never events. http://www.cms.hhs.gov/apps/media/press/release.asp?Counter_1863 (accessed 2007 Jul 9).

3. Proposed Rule: Medicare Hospital Outpatient Prospective Payment System for CY2009, *The Federal Register,* CMS-1404-P, July 18, 2008.

4. Centers for Medicare and Medicaid Services. Medicare pay for performance (P4P) initiatives. http://www.cms.hhs.gov/apps/media/press/release.asp?Counter_1343 (accessed 2007 Jul 10).

5. Medicare Payment Advisory Commission. Report to the Congress: issues in a modernized Medicare program. http://www.medpac.gov/documents/June05_Entire_report.pdf (accessed 2007 Jul 10).

6. Johnson PE. Changes in reimbursement rates and rules associated with the Medicare Prescription Drug Improvement and Modernization Act: introduction. *Am J Health-Syst Pharm.* 2006; 63(suppl 7): S2–6.

7. Department of Health and Human Services Office of Inspector General. Medicaid drug price comparison: average sales price to average wholesale price. http://oig.hhs.gov/oei/reports/oei-03-05-00200.pdf (accessed 2007 Jul 10).

8. Guo HR, Tanaka S, Halperin WE et al. Back pain prevalence in US industry and estimates of lost workdays. *Am J Public Health.* 1999; 89: 1029–35.

9. Wood SD. Strategies for improving health plan member retention—1999 HFM Resource Guide. *Healthc Financ Manage.* December 1998. http://findarticles.com/p/articles/mi_m3257/is_12_52/ai_53450277/pg_1 (accessed 2007 Jul 11).

This chapter is adapted from Johnson PE: Pharmaceutical reimbursement: An overview. *Am J Health-Syst Pharm.* 2008; 65 (suppl 1): S4–10. It is based on the proceedings of a symposium held June 23, 2007, during the ASHP 2007 Summer Meeting and Exhibition in San Francisco, CA, and supported by an educational donation from Amgen. It was updated in August 2008 to current CMS rules and proposals.

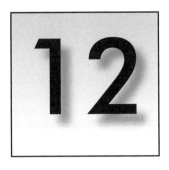

Benchmarking and Productivity Analysis

Steve Rough
Chad Stashek

Introduction/Definitions

The purpose of this chapter is to summarize the current state of pharmacy department productivity monitoring systems, limitations of these systems, and strategies to help overcome these limitations. This chapter will help the reader to understand internal and external benchmarking and practical approaches in monitoring pharmacy workload.

Benchmarking is the continuous process of measuring products, services, and practices against the company's toughest competitors, or those companies identified as industry leaders to find and implement best practice.[1,2] Similarly, *operational benchmarking* (also commonly referred to as external benchmarking and external productivity monitoring) is a system whereby hospitals submit department-level data (usually on a quarterly cycle) into a vendor-managed financial and operational comparative database to compare departmental, operational and financial performance to peer organizations. This comparison provides a process of measuring costs, services, and practices against the organization's peers or "best in class" organizations. In contrast, *internal benchmarking* (i.e., internal productivity monitoring) is a process of measuring one's self (i.e., department) against one's self over time, comparing current and future department performance against prior department performance.[3-5]

A *full-time equivalent (FTE)* is a full-time employee who works 2,080 hours per year. A *peer group* is a grouping of like hospitals or departments. A reported metric (e.g., volume statistic, expense, revenue, etc.) within a productivity monitoring system is often referred to as a *data element.* A *percentile* is a relative ranking of how one is performing versus a compare (peer) group. In operational benchmarking, percentiles range from 0 to 100 percent, and better performance is typically signified with a lower percentile ranking. For example, if a department ranked at the 25th percentile, that means that it is performing better than 75 percent of the compare group and worse than 25 percent in that category of performance. A ranking of 50th percentile indicates that the department is an average performer. A ranking of 75th percentile indicates that the department is better than 25 percent of its compare group.

Acuity is a measure of severity of illness. Productivity ratios or metrics are often reported with an "acuity adjustment" to modify the reported ratio for severity of illness. *Case mix index (CMI)* is the average diagnosis related group (DRG) weight for all of a hospital's Medicare volume.[6] It can be used to adjust the average cost per patient (or day) for a given department or hospital relative to the adjusted average cost for other hospitals by dividing the average cost per patient (or day) by the hospital's calculated CMI. The adjusted average cost per patient would reflect the charges reported for the types of cases treated in that year. CMI is an approximate measure of the relative costliness and expected total resource consumption of patients treated within a facility. This CMI weight reflects the average level of total resources consumed for an average Medicare patient in a DRG, relative to the average level of resources for all Medicare patients. The standardized charge for each DRG is calculated by summing the charges for all cases in the DRG and dividing that amount by the number of cases (discharges) classified in the DRG. Thus, statistical outliers are eliminated.

Weighting is a method used to recombine a department's varied work outputs equitably to produce a single figure that represents the department's entire output. Weighting can also be defined as a measure of time to perform one unit of each department output. Units of output can be classified in terms of a *workload unit (WLU)*, which is equivalent to one minute of time for an activity or the amount of labor resources measured in time increments. The difference between how a department is actually performing and targeted or budgeted performance is referred to as the *variance*, which is often used as a measure of department achievement and how well staff hours are being managed. A productivity ratio is a measure of productivity (output/input). Productivity ratios are often divided into *labor productivity ratios* (e.g., hours worked or paid per unit of output, hours worked per 100 orders processed, doses dispensed per hour worked) and *cost-based productivity ratios* (e.g., expense per unit of output, drug cost per 100 orders processed, total pharmacy cost per patient discharge).

A *characteristic* is a feature or aspect of service provided by a department that describes a distinguishable trait. More specifically, a *characteristic survey* is a profile of questions designed to identify characteristics of each participating department to assist departments in identifying a meaningful peer or compare group for benchmarking purposes. *Adjustment* in pharmacy, typically referred to as a *revenue adjustment*, is a modification to reported metrics for characteristics that can affect variance in measures. In pharmacy operational benchmarking, a revenue adjustment is most commonly used as a multiplier to adjust for pharmacy-specific outpatient activity to approximate true inpatient expense. Vendors use the revenue adjustment to report labor and cost ratios that are adjusted for pharmacy-specific outpatient activity based on reported gross and inpatient pharmacy charges. This ratio is necessary because most commercially available vendor software systems require that organizations report inpatient pharmacy expenses in the same benchmarking department as expenses that are incurred in ambulatory clinics, infusion centers, and procedure areas. The revenue adjustment is a ratio of pharmacy department gross (inpatient plus ambulatory) revenue/pharmacy department inpatient revenue. This adjustment helps to provide an approximation of actual inpatient pharmacy expense based on revenue adjustments, because the actual inpatient expense is not reported separately into the system. *Normalization* is a movement or transfer of reported costs, volumes, and hours from one department to another for the purposes of assuring that these statistics are reported and combined in the same way by each participating hospital. Normalizations are meant to allocate specific expenses into the most appropriate operational department across all organizations, thus they enable more pure "apples to apples" comparisons among dissimilar organizations. A *time standard* is the mean time required to perform a task, whereas a *volume indicator* is the frequency with which activities occur, often reported as a mean frequency when non-automated sources are used to provide the frequency.[4–6]

Background

Benchmarking has benefits, but it also has specific limitations. Benchmarking works well when the process being benchmarked is essentially the same across the multiple units participating in the exercise. It may be useful to compare the cost of producing the same drug dose, taking the same kind of customer order, or processing the same type of benefit claim across multiple companies. However benchmarking is not informative when it is used to compare fundamentally different processes or products. Differences in care delivery systems and automation produce variances that may limit the value of benchmarks where resources and processes differ significantly. Benchmarking of departments that do not offer similar services, levels of service, and quality to customers will result in an incomplete, incorrect or erroneous comparison.

Today's health-care executives must manage their operations more effectively than ever before, ensuring quality of care while keeping costs under control.[7] Mounting pressure for improved operational performance has prompted health system administrators to turn to benchmarking vendors and consultants for assistance in determining the appropriateness of allocated departmental staffing resources. Operational benchmarking provides health-care administrators with a tangible means of comparing financial and operational data at the departmental and organizational level to target areas for cost control, performance improvement, and ideally for improvements in efficiency. However, today's benchmarking systems provide little to no specific data on which efficient practices are in place at similar facilities to produce desired results. Although the key to effective health-care operational benchmarking is to draw comparisons across similar organizations and departments, this comparison is not always an easy task.

Little content in the literature describes the application of external benchmarking in health care. Although articles exist that assert that benchmarking in health care has resulted in breakthrough improvements, objective data is not reported in the literature to support these claims. The inability to measure workload and productivity effectively has been a longstanding problem for the hospital pharmacy. A gold standard in the literature does not exist to measure pharmacy productivity. Although many recommended pharmacy productivity workload ratios have been published, most are based on simple labor efficiency metrics that are tied to orders processed, doses billed, and FTEs per discharge.[8–13] Inclusion of clinical and other professional services provided is not included in most cases. Likewise, limited data exist to assist pharmacy directors in understanding the advantages and disadvantages of various hospital pharmacy workload and productivity monitoring metrics and systems.

In summary, the goal of benchmarking in pharmacy is to determine value and effectiveness of pharmacy services. This goal helps provide an effective management tool for quantifying how much time is spent on types of cognitive work, and to provide a comparison with similar institutions to identify problems and to establish appropriate, attainable goals. Benchmarking may assist with improving overall pharmacy department performance, but it is not currently maximized for this purpose, and there is very little pharmacy or health-care literature supporting its use for this purpose.

Commercially Available External Benchmarking and Productivity Monitoring Systems

The goal of external benchmarking in health care is to implement the best practices of peer organizations.[14–16] Although it is possible to identify variation in performance across a group of peers through external benchmarking and to identify targeted opportunities to improve efficiency and cost management, today's external benchmarking systems present significant challenges.[7] Commercial vendors and consultants who lack expertise in defining and measuring successful pharmacy practice may provide benchmarking metrics and packages that lack sufficient scope, depth, and understanding of pharmacy to adequately characterize the range of services and the quality of pharmacy services. Today's commercially available systems are typically rigid, not reflective of current pharmacy practice, and leave much to be desired. They usually focus on quantifying dispensed doses or orders, not quality. They produce productivity ratios that do not fully measure clinical workload or performance in patient care and service, and do not assess the overall impact of pharmacy services on patient outcomes and total cost of care.

Most firms specialize in operational benchmarking to assess pharmacy productivity and value compare staffing or workload ratios based solely on measures of product distribution. Rarely do they assess the extent to which evidence-based clinical pharmacy services are implemented nor the overall impact of pharmacist patient care services on patient outcomes and total cost. Both excessively rigid and overly casual use of cost and labor metrics create significant problems in assessing the value and utility of reported metrics. Too often, operational benchmarking results are used inappropriately in the budgeting process, and consulting vendors as well as hospital administrators often recommend (or mandate) reductions in pharmacy staffing to meet targeted labor productivity ratios, which, taken without context, do not provide a complete and thorough measure of overall pharmacy performance. Pharmacy is a unique hospital department. Often less than 20 percent of total department costs are for personnel, compared to greater than 60 percent for other hospital departments. Medications often account for more than 80 percent of total pharmacy department expense. A tradeoff can exist between lowering pharmacy labor costs and corresponding increases in drug expense. Pharmacy labor reductions may ultimately result in higher hospital drug expenditures, higher overall hospital costs, higher incidence of medication errors and preventable adverse drug events, and reduced quality of patient care. Pharmacy directors must understand that production-related productivity statistics do not correlate on a one-to-one basis with clinical activity needs, so pharmacy staffing ratios based on dose production trends will not address the need for effective clinical services.

External Benchmarking to Compare Operational Performance and Productivity

Data Elements

Data elements that are reported to external vendor productivity monitoring software systems provide the foundation for productivity reporting. Frequently reported elements are listed in Table 12.1. Data are generally reported from several areas of the organization, such as the general ledger (e.g., supply expenses), payroll system (e.g., paid hours, worked hours), chargemaster (e.g., procedure and other workload volumes), monthly financial reports (e.g., revenues), manual statistics supplied from departments (e.g., orders processed), and billing and coding data (e.g., revenues).

Table 12.1. Examples of Frequently Reported Pharmacy Data Elements

Staffing Configuration

- Paid FTEs
- Overtime hours
- Skill mix: % pharmacist
- Skill mix: % management
- Skill mix: % technicians
- Skill mix: % other

Facility Information

- Admissions
- Facility-wide drug expense
- Patient days
- Case mix index
- Pharmacy intensity score
- Discharges
- Clinic visits

Operating Statistics

- Gross drug charges
- Clinical service workload units
- Drug expense (can be broken down by drug classes and reported in aggregate)
- Paid hours
- Worked hours
- Orders processes
- Doses administered
- Labor expense
- Supply expense
- Inpatient gross drug charges
- Gross charges

Limitations of Commercial Vendor Productivity Monitoring Systems

Commercially available operational benchmarking systems used to monitor pharmacy labor efficiency and financial performance have significant pitfalls. Table 12.2 lists the most serious weaknesses inherent in many commercial vendor productivity monitoring systems. Benchmarking software and consulting vendors have an obligation to improve their systems to a level that does not identify high quality metrics performers as poor efficiency performers and vice versa. Understanding the limitations of current systems is necessary to explain potential causes leading to alleged poor performance. Examples of productivity measures commonly used by benchmarking vendors and consultants in evaluating pharmacy services are provided in Table 12.3.

Strategies for Deriving Value from an External Productivity Monitoring System

Strategies to assist pharmacy directors with effective implementation and use of an external operational benchmarking software system include understanding all functional elements of the system, such as required and optional data elements, characteristic questions, and normalizations. Spending time navigating the system and understanding data element reporting options will help determine how to build or modify a selected comparison peer group. Spend time with the hospital (fiscal) data coordinator to understand exactly where the department's reported data elements are derived. Work to find ways to automate the data submission as much as possible, and routinely follow reported data through the system to ensure accuracy, especially in reporting metric outputs. Such auditing work is a good task to delegate to a pharmacy budget manager. Review all available labor productivity and cost metrics (key indicators or ratios) within the system.

Take time to understand the definitions and mathematical formulas behind each productivity ratio. Understand which metrics represent the department favorably (and unfavorably), and understand the root causes behind these explanations. Develop systems to measure inpatient drug expense separately and accurately from other hospital drug expense. Work with the data coordinator to make sure this expense is reported per vendor reporting instructions. Developing a good relationship with the hospital's data coordinator is strongly suggested. Select a meaningful peer comparison group. If the hospital has already selected a peer group, start here, but spend time investigating whether this peer group is appropriate for the pharmacy department. The goal should be to limit the peer group to 15–20 organizations that are most like one's department. Evaluate available characteristic survey data from these peer organizations, and call the pharmacy director in each organization to determine whether their pharmacy services reflect the implementation of best practice for achieving quality and safety. If an organization is dramatically different in terms of type or quality of pharmacy service provided, eliminate that hospital from the peer group. The key is to learn everything possible about 15–20 hospitals that represent a peer group. Keeping this peer group small will make the job of understanding how each peer group department operates more manageable. Be sure to understand the clinical services they offer, their practice model, distribution services, hours of service, how they report their required data elements, and so on. Compare the services in terms of implementation of best practices. If the peer group has been preselected by hospital administration and some do not seem appropriate,

Table 12.2. Weaknesses of Commercial Vendor External Productivity Monitoring Systems

1. Drug expenses are not reported and broken down in meaningful groupings with clear definitions to incorporate areas of major drug expenses.
   a. This lack of clarity makes true peer group identification difficult.
2. The case mix index (CMI) is routinely used to approximate patient acuity. This is a flawed method for measuring pharmacy-specific patient acuity.
   a. Although CMI may be accurate from an overall perspective of hospital resource consumption in adjusting for patient acuity, it does not work well for pharmacy department comparisons. It assigns similar acuity ratings to patients who require vastly different levels of medication resources and pharmacist patient care services to achieve a positive outcome.
   b. Overall resource consumption does not usually match medication and pharmacy labor resource consumption.
3. Department definitions and breakouts do not allow for data to be submitted in a manner which allows for meaningful comparisons.
   a. Inpatient drug expense is reported in the same department as clinic, infusion center, retail pharmacy, emergency department, and sometimes retail pharmacy expense.
   b. Pharmacy departments with large infusion centers and high-cost procedure areas are negatively affected by having this drug expense lumped in with inpatient.
   c. Because inpatient drug expense is not reported "purely" in its own department, today's inpatient department ratios require the use of a flawed revenue adjustment to approximate inpatient costs. This creates inaccurate winners and losers.
   d. The above confusion results in inaccurate reporting by many customers and thus flawed productivity and cost reports.
4. Characteristic questions do not reflect current pharmacy best practices and do not assist customers with easily identifying meaningful peer groups.
   a. Questions are often yes/no questions without regard to the extent of best practice implementation.
   b. Questions are vague and misleading.
   c. Best practices for patient safety, quality outcomes, and drug cost reduction are not measured.
5. Clinical activity (workload performance) measures are ambiguous, unclear, and lack meaning.
   a. Many clinical pharmacy services are not routinely nor consistently measured across different organizations.
   b. Some vendor products request pharmacy departments to report clinical workload in terms of 15-minute increments. This is likely not measured accurately in any department, which leads to inaccurate reporting.
6. Normalizations are not applied consistently across hospitals, and often are not meaningful.
   a. Some pharmacy departments may purchase high-cost drugs, such as volatile anesthetic gases, contrast media, intravenous immune globulin, albumin and hemophilia factor products. The pharmacy departments in peer organizations may not. If this is not properly factored into peer group comparisons, it can make the department purchasing these products inaccurately appear to be a poor cost performer.
7. Reporting of pharmaceutical manufacturer rebates and expired drug credits are not applied consistently across hospitals.
   a. If a pharmacy department does not have these expense reductions credited against drug expense, then it may inaccurately appear to be a poor cost performer.

Table 12.2. Weaknesses of Commercial Vendor External Productivity Monitoring Systems *(Continued)*

8. Disproportionate share (340(b)) contract participation is not readily flagged in vendor systems.
   a. Non-340(b) participants should not compare themselves to 340(b) participants in terms of drug cost performance.
9. Vendor-reported labor- and cost-productivity ratios and suggested key performance indicators are flawed and often used inappropriately within organizations.
   a. Many reported include metrics in terms of patient days and doses dispensed, which can negatively affect performance versus more accurate indicators of patients discharged and medication orders processed.

Table 12.3. Examples of Frequently Used Pharmacy Productivity Ratios[1]

Cost-Based Productivity Ratios

- Total pharmacy cost per adjusted discharge*
- Drug cost per adjusted discharge*
- Labor cost per adjusted discharge
- Total pharmacy cost per adjusted patient day
- Drug cost per adjusted patient day
- Labor cost per adjusted patient day
- Total pharmacy cost per 100 orders processed
- Drug cost per 100 orders processed
- Labor cost per 100 orders processed

Labor Productivity Ratios

- Hours worked per adjusted discharge*
- Hours paid per adjusted discharge
- Hours worked per patient day
- Hours paid per adjusted patient day
- Hours worked per adjusted patient day
- Hours worked per 100 admissions
- Hours worked (paid) per 100 orders processed
- FTEs per order processed
- FTEs per occupied bed
- FTEs per dose billed
- FTEs per adjusted patient day

(Hours worked per 100 CMI-weighted revenue-adjusted patient days)
(Hours worked per 100 pharmacy intensity-weighted patient days)

1. Often, productivity ratios are weighted for acuity using a CMI-weighted index and adjusted using a pharmacy revenue factor adjustment when non-inpatient expenses are included in the inpatient department. Such weighting may occur for any productivity ratio. An example of these weightings is included for demonstration purposes in *italics* with the first labor productivity ratio in this table.
2. Preferred metrics are indicated by an asterisk (*).

then propose alternative groupings and the reasons behind them to administration. Come prepared with suggested substitute organizations and explain why these organizations may support a better comparison.

Moreover, select the key indicator metrics for comparing the pharmacy's performance to its peers. Select a few cost ratios and productivity ratios. If patient days are the key indicator ratio denominator, consider changing this to discharges (or admissions). Reporting labor or cost metrics by patient day may result in substantial declines or increases in performance, depending on how well the hospital manages the patient discharge process. If the hospital improves its performance in terms of reducing length of stay and thus patient days, the pharmacy's performance on ratios using patient days in the denominator could gradually worsen over time, solely because the hospital has improved in managing patient discharges. Also, most drug expense and the pharmacist labor requirement are associated with the front half of a patient's admission to the hospital, thus reporting metrics per discharge (or admission) rather than per patient day is simply the right thing to do. If doses charged (or dispensed) are reported in the ratio denominator, consider changing this to medication orders processed. Reporting doses charged (or dispensed) certainly does not measure the full range of pharmacy service activities. Comparing one's organization against a ratio based on doses dispensed is flawed because there are considerable differences in labor requirements for pure unit dose dispensing operations versus organizations that stock commercially available manufacturer-size products in automated dispensing systems. Such ratios are also easily altered by different computer systems that count doses differently. The same could be said for orders as well.

Report inpatient expenses separate from all other ambulatory expenses whenever it is possible, and work to avoid using a revenue adjustment factor in the performance metric altogether. When inpatient and ambulatory costs are combined into one department and revenue adjustments are applied in performance metric calculations, organizations with higher ambulatory markups can be identified (in error) as better inpatient performers, and organizations with larger ambulatory drug costs can be labeled (in error) as poor inpatient performers solely based on their larger ambulatory drug expense. Insist on using a combination of labor productivity and cost-based productivity ratios when measuring performance against peers. Poor labor productivity performers often provide a much higher level of clinical pharmacy services than the better labor productivity performers. Pharmacists are so effective at controlling drug expense in a hospital that the worse labor productivity performers may be the best pharmacy total cost performers. Because drug costs represent up to 85 percent of a pharmacy department's total cost, pharmacy directors must point out to their administrators the labor versus drug cost leverage when evaluating operational benchmarking performance metrics.

Review key indicator scores against the 25th, 50th, and 75th percentiles of the peer group. Work to explain positive variances in terms of the exceptional service the pharmacy provides. Identify data elements, indicators, or service and operating differences that may explain negative variances in a positive light. For instance, if labor cost per discharge is higher than the peer average, perhaps this is because the organization provides a different range of services or a higher level of quality pharmacy service than the peer group. Or perhaps, based on discussions with the peer group pharmacy directors, the pharmacy leader can determine that other hospitals report their data differently, which explains the difference. It may be that the pharmacy's cost-based metrics are out-performing those of its peers. Use caution when addressing variance; never explain a variance in terms of quality unless data exist to support the argument.

Develop a department expert to whom ongoing management of the system is delegated. This allows the pharmacy director's time to be spent on strategic planning to improve reported results. Develop a routine (e.g., quarterly) results monitoring system. Make certain that the routine monitoring system includes data integrity checks. If a peer's reported performance appears too good to be true, it usually is. Call the pharmacy director in that organization and ask about the reasons behind their exceptional performance. If the results of the pharmacy are unfavorable compared to the peer group's results, work to rule out each limitation as a potential cause of the problem. Based on the results, determine at least one opportunity to improve the overall labor efficiency and total cost performance. Let administrators know that the pharmacy department plans to develop a specific plan to improve performance relative to the peer group.

If pharmacy labor productivity ratios are worse than desirable, see how nursing productivity ratios compare against peers. It may be possible that pharmacy staff in the organization do work that nurses perform in peer organizations. This will most likely be the case if the department provides a 100 percent unit dosing service, maintains the nurse medication administration record, provides patient medication history taking and medication reconciliation services, or provides patient medication teaching for inpatients. If administration expects the pharmacy department to benchmark at or below the 25th percentile in terms of labor productivity, explain how performing at this "low labor level" may negatively affect patient safety and external quality score compliance, and ultimately increase the total cost of care and seek examples and opportunities in the peer group reports. Make the argument that the best financial performance always follows the highest quality service.

Measuring Productivity Using Internal Benchmarks

Internal benchmarking provides a measure of self-comparison over time. It is preferable to external benchmarking in that it is more controllable and eliminates many of the flaws of external benchmarking comparisons. However, it does require both an upfront and ongoing internal commitment of resources to establish and maintain a system of measures and targets. Having internal productivity targets and positive productivity trends data against those targets is helpful when working with administrators to maintain or expand pharmacy labor resources (e.g., FTEs). Internal benchmarking avoids inaccurate comparisons with dissimilar organizations and allows for an accurate measure of staff activities and of changes in practice and workload volume. It provides a means to account for department resources necessary to provide best-practice clinical and distributive services within the department. Internal benchmarking will ultimately help the pharmacy department to explain budget variances and to request additional pharmacy FTEs because of documented workload increases or avoided drug costs resulting from the expansion of patient care services. Internal benchmarks can also be of greater value than external comparisons because the pharmacy director has more control over internal processes.

There is no preferred method in the literature for internal productivity monitoring; there are different ways of conducting it, and not all measures will be perfect. The key is to strive for numbers that are validated, accurate, and applied consistently over time to assess the state of the department in workload and demonstrated efficiency. A good internal productivity and monitoring system will enable a pharmacy director to demonstrate improved performance in operational efficiency over time through monitoring of workload and cost metrics, and will provide objective data by quantifying total pharmacy workload to demonstrate upward trends. Depending upon the institution and contributing factors, simple metrics or productivity ratios may suffice, and the complexity of patient acuity and revenue factor adjustments can be avoided. See Table 12.4 for suggested internal benchmarking metrics.

Methods of Work Measurement

To develop a data-rich internal benchmarking system, a functional knowledge of work measurement methods is required. Time and motion studies are one set of methods that may be useful in determining the resources necessary to complete a task.

A time standard, the mean time required to perform a task, can be developed by directly observing, self-reporting, work sampling, or borrowing from a similar organization.[3-5] A volume indicator, the mean frequency of a reported task, may be routinely obtained in an automated fashion from the pharmacy computer system or hospital admit/discharge/transfer and patient billing system. They may also need to be obtained through self-reporting for certain activities, such as documentation of pharmacist clinical interventions. Multiplying

Table 12.4. Suggested Internal Pharmacy Benchmarking Productivity Monitoring Ratios[1]

- Total cost/admission
- Drug cost/admission
- Labor cost/admission
- Labor expense/1000 doses billed
- Pharmacist worked hours/order[2]
- Technician worked hours/dose[3]
- Doses dispensed/admission
- Doses/admission
- Pharmacist:Technician skill mix ratio
- Pharmacy cost as a % of total hospital cost
- Inventory turns/year
- Clinical interventions/pharmacist shift worked

1. Avoid using patient days in the numerator; admissions is a better predictor of pharmacist workload and drug expense.
2. Orders usually drive pharmacist workload more than doses.
3. Doses usually drive technician workload more than orders.

a time standard for a task times the volume indicator for that task provides the total time required to perform that task.

A good method for establishing a time standard is to perform a series of direct observations of a task, determine the average time required to complete the task, and assign a standard deviation to the average measurement.[3–5] Once time standards and volume indicators have been established for the majority of tasks that drive workload, the total time requirement for each major activity can be determined. Then the total time required for each activity can be summed to determine approximate total workload time requirement and staffing requirement for the department. Before initiating time standard or volume indicator measurements, first clearly define the activities to be measured.

To perform a direct observation time study, an observer will not interfere with the worker being observed (to avoid the Hawthorne effect) but will record the start and end time of activities with a stopwatch and clipboard. Direct times studies are most appropriate for high-volume activities with a clearly defined start and stop time that are short in duration. In conducting a direct observation time study, the staff to be observed will require notification of involvement in the activities that are to be measured. It may help to notify observers when a task is about to begin. A team approach should be taken to define a list of staff activities with the realization that some activities may differ across patient care types. Direct time studies are often used because they are easily transferred into a simple metric in which the determined time standard (e.g., time required to enter a medication order) is multiplied by the volume indicator (e.g., number of medication orders) to generate the total staff time requirement for a specified activity over a period of time (e.g., total time required to enter medication orders), usually in total minutes or 100 WLUs.

The direct observation time study method has some disadvantages, including observer influence over the pace of activities, observer variability, the large number of observations required to generate statistically valid time standards, and time constraints resulting in a limited sample size. Include both clinical and distributive activities, then establish definitions and have the staff validate these definitions before performing time standard measurements.

A second time study method is self-reporting.[3–5] In contrast to direct time study, the self-reporting method relies on staff to document the amount of time required to perform an activity. Self-reporting studies are best conducted in situations of low to moderate activity volume with easily definable start and stop times with little variation in activity interpretability. In using this method, one must be aware of some common flaws associated with self-reporting. First, inaccurate reporting can occur if the staff do not understand the true task definition with subsequent confusion over the objective start and stop times. Second, there can be unintentional skewing of data in the staff's attempt to achieve what they perceive as the desired results, which explains why there may be 12 hours of work documented for an 8-hour shift. Third, it can be difficult to accurately self-report time requirements during periods of peak workload. For these reasons, avoid self-reporting whenever possible, taking into consideration the dependence upon available resources.

Direct observation and self-reporting may also be used to generate volume indicators in addition to time standards. However, many volume indicators may be produced directly from pharmacy and/or hospital reports, and pharmacy directors should strive for these reports.

Work sampling is another method to estimate the percent of time that staff spend on various activities.[4,5] Work sampling is an indirect method of establishing time requirements. It does not involve actual timing of individual activities but estimates the proportion of time spent in various activities. The premise is that a sample of instantaneous observations at random times has the same proportion of observations as the entire segment. The work sampling method of measurement is ideal for measuring the relative frequency of all tasks staff perform, and for measuring intermittent activities that are not closely structured in time, occur infrequently, and thus would require an inordinate amount of time to collect through direct observation. When conducting a work sampling study, the study coordinator predetermines a list of workload activities to measure and from these activities designs a data collection form to be distributed to pharmacy staff. Pharmacy staff members, the study participants, are provided with the data collection forms along with a study pager. A random time schedule is created, and pagers are synchronized with this schedule to notify pharmacy staff members of these randomly designated times for data collection. When the pager signals the study participant (i.e., the pharmacy staff member) that person simply puts a tick on the data collection form for the activity he or she is performing at that point in time. After all data collection forms have been returned, the study coordinator tallies the total number of ticks for the tasks listed on the data collection form. Next, the number of ticks for each task is divided into the total number of ticks for all tasks to generate the percentage of ticks made up by each task. The tick percentage is assumed to be equal to the percentage of employee time spent on that task. This percentage may be extrapolated to a time standard for each task, as in the following example.

Let us say that there are a total of 5,000 pharmacist hours in a week at a particular institution. During the sampling period, it was noted that 10 percent of the total number of ticks recorded fell under the category of "order entry." This would approximate that 500 hours per week (10 percent of 5,000 hours), and thus 71.43 hours per day were dedicated to order entry. Subsequently, the institution reports a volume indicator that, on average, staff enter 2,500 orders per day. In converting the 71.4 hours into 4,286 minutes and dividing by 2,500 orders per day, one can determine that, on average, each order entry requires 1.71 minutes (1 minute 43 seconds). This time standard for order entry of 1.71 minutes per order can then be used to multiply by the volume indicator (number of orders entered) to determine the WLUs associated with order entry.

Work sampling is a good technique to measure the impact that system change has on how staff spend their time (e.g., measuring a desired shift from distributive to clinical activities). This method is also useful to establish a productivity monitoring system that incorporates a large number of tasks that staff perform when resources required for direct observation are not available.

Conducting time standard-based work measurement through any method requires a degree of caution. Care must be taken when combining various activities such as order types (e.g., new, modified, and discontinued orders) in developing time standards for workload measurement. Work measurement theory would dictate that different order types (or different activities) be split into separate time standards to make the time standards statistically meaningful. The closer the standard deviation is to the mean, the more accurate the time standard. The most reliable time standards will have a standard deviation within 5–10 percent of the mean. The required number of observations depends on precision (i.e., standard deviation around the mean), but this may be in the hundreds for that task under a number of different conditions (e.g., weekends, weekdays, evenings, days, different staff members, etc). Assuming the standard deviation is low, a time standard is fairly accurate.

Time standards developed like this are valid for the place and in the conditions under which they are constructed. Extrapolating them to other departments with other workers, conditions, logistics, or facility considerations must be done carefully. However, there is often an administrative "need" to use a standard developed in one facility in other environments. This can be done, but recognize the flaws in this approach. Using a time standard for select activities (such as order entry, compounding, performing a medication history, etc.) from a different organization or even across different patient care areas within a hospital may not be accurate if used to determine precise staffing needs, but this approach may be good enough for establishing an internal productivity monitoring system in a pharmacy department. Before officially adopting borrowed time standards, a few direct observations of each task should be performed to confirm that the borrowed time standard is within 25 percent of the observed time requirement in the organization. It will be more valid if used consistently over time to approximate trends in total time requirements and relative resource needs over time (e.g., use the estimated time requirements as a compass to help gauge relative staffing needs over time, not as a thermometer to determine precise productivity ratios).

No system will be able to quantify all tasks with complete certainty. One must either accurately measure delays caused by fatigue and interruptions or recognize that some uncertainty exists (say 10–15 percent) for all tasks that are reported, and that down times and non-productive times will occur (such as bathroom breaks, walking between care areas, etc). When using time standards to determine staffing requirements, the pharmacy director should be aware that there may be a wide variation in activity time requirements based on patient type and interruptions such as phone calls, stopping to check doses, stopping to answer a drug information question, and so forth. A pharmacist who is interrupted while entering medication orders, for example, will have a lower order entry rate per hour than a pharmacist who is not interrupted throughout that hour. However, it would be inappropriate to draw conclusions about either pharmacist's productivity without factoring in clinical interventions and other various interruptions. Because of differing staffing models, developing a standard across various hospitals for an acceptable number of orders a pharmacist should enter per hour or per shift would be impossible. The number of medication orders per hour that can be processed also depends upon the computer system being used for order entry. Some systems are more robust or easier to use than others. Merely having a different computer system can render two pharmacy departments difficult to benchmark against each other.

In summary, whereas time standards represent mean time requirements, volume indicators represent mean frequency indicators (e.g., number of admissions/time period). Unlike time standards, volume indicators can often be obtained through automated pharmacy-dispensing software, hospital computer-generated statistical reports, or self-reporting.

Practical Suggestions for Getting Started

Although developing an internal benchmarking system may seem to be a daunting project, identification of just a few core activities generally influence most of the total staff workload

Table 12.5. Daily Activities for Internal Pharmacy Workload and Productivity Measurement

- Order entry of medication orders
- Patient care rounds participation
- Clinical pharmacist interventions
- Admission medication histories
- Dose adjustments
- Dose checking (first doses, cartfill, floor stock)
- Discharge medication counseling
- Drug allergy avoidance
- Review of new orders for clinical appropriateness
- Intravenous solution preparation and checking
- Medication profile reviews
- Education (staff, patients)
- Patient drug therapy monitoring
- Drug interaction avoidance
- Pharmacokinetic monitoring

(e.g., medication order volume, doses dispensed, patient admissions and discharges, etc). Table 12.5 lists some daily activities that have been used in internal productivity work measurement for pharmacists. It may be best to start with just a few pharmacist and technician activities to keep the project manageable and then to expand included activities over time.

Next, determine how to measure workload (volume and time requirement) for each task, and consider possible available resources for workload measurement, such as pharmacy students, pharmacy residents, or industrial engineering students. A temporary solution may include borrowing standards from other organizations or using a Delphi process, whereby time standards are developed by pharmacy staff representing an internal expert panel for consensus of agreed-upon values with the help of a facilitator. A classic Delphi process involves a facilitator presenting panel members with a series of specific questions: in this case time standard-based questions, in which responses are collected anonymously and then averaged. Based on the average response, the panel members are given the opportunity to change their answers, and a new average is subsequently developed. This process is repeated until a consensus response is agreed upon. A modified Delphi process mirrors the classic Delphi process in that an average consensus of a metric is determined. However, after that metric is determined, a small-scale direct observation study (e.g., 10–20 observations) is conducted on a small sample to internally verify the average consensus that was made by the expert panel. If the subset direct study confirms the expert panel consensus average, the metric, (e.g., time standard) is then considered validated. If the direct study disagrees with the consensus average, the modified Delphi process is repeated until consensus can be reached and validated by a small number of observations.

After determining the data collection and extraction method, review the plan with staff and get their endorsement of the numbers to be used. Incorporate a continuous feedback loop in the event that the data may unintentionally lead to a misrepresentation of true workload. After accepting the benchmarking methodology, develop a monthly reporting system with subsequent communication of total workload to the institution's fiscal department each month for incorporation into the pharmacy budgeting process. Use these workload statistics to demonstrate efficiencies gained over time and to assist in demonstrating increased workload to justify new staff requests.

Another useful strategy in creating an internal benchmarking or productivity monitoring system is to separate each functional area of the department. For example, consider a separate productivity monitoring system for the sterile products area, repackaging area, purchasing activities, and decentralized clinical services provided. For the department as a whole, attempt to streamline this process by having total workload from each smaller part of the department roll into one or two high-level numbers for each major cost center (e.g., the inpatient pharmacy cost center) so that administration sees one workload number for each pharmacy cost center, and perhaps one for the entire department. Consider using a combination of both broad and specific activities that have time standards and volume indicators determined to be associated as combined workload for central and decentral workload. An example of this is provided for a fictitious pharmacy department in Figure 12.1. In this example, some specific activities have dedicated time standards, whereas other, broader activities, such as an ICU Patient Day, have time standards that are representative of several smaller activities rolled into one.

Conclusion

Making effective use of external operational benchmarking and internal productivity monitoring is challenging. Vendor-developed benchmarking systems typically assess and monitor a limited scope of pharmacy practice; have methodological flaws, hidden errors, and inconsistencies in data collection and categorization; and require focus, effort, and resources to manage effectively. Commercial models generally do not include measures designed to determine the overall quality and cost effectiveness of pharmacy services being provided. Productivity targets set by external benchmarking vendors and consultants may also conflict with the pharmacy department's goal of expanding clinical services and implementing best practices.

Pharmacy directors must understand how benchmarking and productivity monitoring can be used to support current pharmacy operations, focus their efforts on efficiency and quality, and support the growth of pharmacy services. The key to successful benchmarking is to demonstrate the level of quality and positive outcomes that the hospital is achieving from its investment in pharmacy services. Ideally, data supporting the patient care role of the pharmacist are integrated into productivity monitoring systems. This integration should include correlating total hospital cost and quality outcomes with pharmacy benchmarking results to demonstrate the positive impact of pharmacy services on the total cost and

	Time Standard (hrs)	Actual FY02 Vol	100 WLU	Actual FY03 Vol	100 WLU	Actual FY04 Vol	100 WLU	Budget FY05 Vol	100 WLU
Non-Production									
Admissions	0.2517	19,337	2,920	20,249	3,058	20,617	3,113	21,060	3,180
ICU Days	0.9733	17,143	10,012	19,477	11,375	19,612	11,453	20,776	12,133
Non-ICU Days	0.4917	101,760	30,019	105,335	31,074	108,436	31,989	111,929	33,019
Total Doses Administered	0.0117	3,371,936	23,604	3,589,777	25,128	3,976,176	27,833	4,160,000	29,120
Total Medication Orders	0.0375	1,306,035	29,386	1,581,744	35,589	1,787,661	40,222	1,750,000	39,375
Patient Transfers	0.1750	26,627	2,796	31,924	3,352	32,656	3,429	32,030	3,363
IV Solution Doses	0.1290	71,465	5,531	79,059	6,119	79,703	6,169	79,000	6,115
IV Solution Orders	0.1290	179,115	13,864	202,782	15,695	246,880	19,109	241,000	18,653
PCA Syringes	0.3625	18,876	4,106	18,446	4,012	19,034	4,140	19,500	4,241
Outpatients on Inpatient Units	0.5333	4,369	1,398	5,418	1,734	6,326	2,024	5,980	1,914
Infusion Center Orders	0.4750	3,635	1,036	4,037	1,151	3,830	1,092	3,900	1,112
Non-Production Dept Total			124,670		138,287		150,573		152,225
Sterile Products Area Production									
Injections	0.0275	139,618		126,423		106,480		110,000	
Minibags	0.0385	46,437		40,828		38,984		39,500	
Oncology/IDS	0.1192	19,697		17,082		14,700		13,500	
Short Expiration	0.0459	12,243		17,348		20,511		22,000	
Stock Injections (less PCAs)	0.0091	203,268		232,424		295,834		305,000	
Stock Minibags	0.0100	15,193		16,816		13,505		12,000	
Frozen Minibags		0		11,168		8,816		10,000	
PCAs	0.0532	11,235		13,010		12,697		12,000	
Flush Syringes	0.0091					0			
Allergy Preps	0.2000	4,142		5,867		6,336		6,700	
Plain IVs (including night workload)	0.0064	41,126		42,176		37,230		34,600	
Additive IVs (less CII IVs)	0.0532	43,338		61,746		65,806		69,500	
Schedule II (CII) IVs	0.0850	7,438		5,436		6,337		7,100	
Cardioplegia Solutions	0.2857					282		1,456	
TNAs	0.2310	6,586		6,684		7,176		7,000	
IV Solutions Labeled and Prepared	0.0850	98,488	5,023	103,922	5,300	109,373	5,578	100,600	5,131
Minibags/Syringes Prepared	0.0467	452,765	12,677	486,402	13,619	517,863	14,500	537,800	15,058
TNAs & Cardioplegias	0.2617	6,586	1,034	6,684	1,049	7,458	1,171	8,456	1,328
SPA Dept Total			18,734	597,008	19,969	634,694	21,249	646,856	21,517
Repack/Manf Production									
Emergency Boxes & Trays	0.1500	801		1,154		1,319		1,200	
Tabs/Caps	0.0030	453,212		495,666		589,347		600,000	
Manufacturing Items	0.0500	4,139		5,248		4,844		4,000	
Extemp Compounded Items	0.4117	179		834		1,129		1,200	
Misc Barcode Labeling	0.0096	25,151		54,612		54,661		58,000	
Prepacks	0.0700	1,385		1,668		2,612		2,000	
Orals (vials, oral syr, inhal, stock)	0.0240	133,825		146,668		187,571		185,000	
Robot Packaging	0.0048	737,454		917,743		971,053		1,000,000	
Mail-Outs	0.0333	7,667				0		0	
Suppositories	0.0500	2,700		2,820		2,394		3,000	
Units Packaged	0.0033	1,366,513	2,733	1,626,413	3,253	1,814,930	3,630	1,854,400	3,709
Stockroom									
Loan Borrow X-Action	0.2500	257		238		243		250	
Total Lines Keyed (Custmr-Custmr)	0.0053	142,113		131,384		151,201		141,000	
Total Lines Picked	0.0125	130,464		133,852		131,649		141,000	
Special Orders	0.3333	1,422		1,895		2,685		2,800	
Spec Rqst Stklist	0.0500	43,840		30,024		17,447		17,000	
Purchase Orders	0.3333	4,985		5,599		5,532		5,800	
279 Orders	0.1667	329		428		692		630	
PO Line Items Keyed	0.0433	36,284		42,494		43,978		46,000	
Total Line Items Picked & Keyed	0.0250	166,748	2,501	176,346	2,645	175,627	2,634	187,000	2805
Total Workload									
100 Workload Units			148,639		162,899		177,518		180,255
Total Staff Hours			247731		271498		295863		300425
Total FTEs required			119.102		130.528		142.242		144.435

Figure 12.1. Fictitious Pharmacy Department Workload Budget

outcomes of patient care. A well-designed internal productivity system assists in document-ing improvements in efficiency over time, directing pharmacist or technician resources, and obtaining additional resources when necessary.

References

1. Goetzel RZ, Guindon AM, Turshen IJ et al. Health and productivity management: Establishing key performance measures, benchmarks and best practices. *J Occup Envir Med.* 2001; 43(1): 493–504.

2. Bhavnani SM. Benchmarking in health-system pharmacy: Current research and practical applications. *Am J Health Syst Pharm.* 2000; 57 Suppl 2: S13–20.

3. Iglar AM, Osland CS, Ploetz PA et al. Time and cost requirements for decentralized pharmacist activities. *Am J Hosp Pharm.*1990; 47: 572–578.

4. Roberts MJ. Work measurement. In: Brown TR, Smith MC, eds. *Handbook of Insti-tutional Pharmacy Practice: Administration and Management.* 2nd ed.; 90–110.

5. Hepler CD. Work analysis and time study. In: Brown TR, Smith MC, eds. *Handbook of Institutional Pharmacy Practice: Administration and Management.* 2nd ed.; 71–89.

6. Medicare Prospective Payment System, American Hospital Directory. http://www.ahd.com/pps.html (accessed 2 June 2008).

7. Kaplan RS: When Benchmarks Don't Work. Harvard Business School Working Knowledge. http://hbswk.hbs.edu/tools/print_item.jhtml?id=5158&t=finance (accessed 16 January 2006).

8. Knoer SJ, Could RJ, Folker T. Evaluating a benchmarking database and identifying cost reduction opportunities by diagnosis-related group. *Am J Health Syst Pharm.* 1999; 56(11): 1102–1107.

9. Murphy JE. Using benchmarking data to evaluate and support pharmacy programs in health systems. *Am J Health Syst Pharm.* 2000; 57 Suppl 2: S28–31.

10. McAllister JC. Collaborating with re-engineering consultants: maintaining resources in the future. *Am J Health Syst Pharm.*1995; 52: 2676–80.

11. Summerfield MR, Go HI, Lamy PP et al. Determining staffing requirements in insti-tutional pharmacy. *Am J Hosp Pharm.* 1978: 35; 1487–1495.

12. Robinson NL, Stump LS. Benchmarking the allocation of pharmacists' time. *Am J Health Syst Pharm.* 1999; 56(6): 516–518.

13. Wong D, Lass G, Frandsen J. *Benchmarking data from Hospital Pharmacy Data Quarterly.* 1999: 2 (2); xx.

14. Krizner K. Benchmarking helps attain the delicate balance between cost and quality. *Managed Healthcare Executive.* 2003; 13(9): 36–38.

15. Camp RC, Tweeet AG. Benchmarking applied to health care. *Jt Comm J Qual Improv.* 1999; 20: 229–38.

16. Witt MJ. Improving group practice performance with benchmarking. *Healthcare Financial Management.* 2001; 55(2): 67–70.

Strategic Financial Planning

Michael R. McDaniel

Introduction

In pharmacy school, we don't get a particularly large dose of business training. To be truthful, we get modest or even no business training at all. However, as we progress in our careers, many of us find ourselves in positions of leadership that demand business skills. You do not have to occupy a formal management position to need these tools, but many directors and other managers must acquire these skills in order to succeed.

Strategic financial planning calls for a deliberate approach to determine your future actions as a department and as a leadership team. This approach is summarized in the diagram shown.

One definition of the word *strategic,* focusing on the root *strategy*, is "an elaborate and systematic plan of action." Strategic financial planning is just that. It is elaborate in that it attempts to take into account everything needed to achieve all desired goals, and it is systematic because one step must often be taken before another step presents itself. Years may go by before the final "bricks" are in place, which demonstrates the need to be systematic.

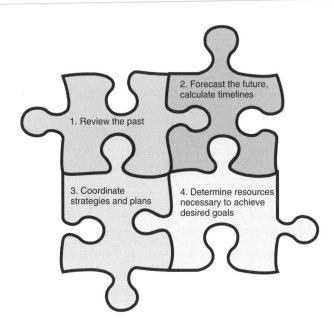

A plan of action denotes where a department is in its journey and prevents the manager from taking avoidable detours or leaving out necessary steps.

The steps delineated in the diagram are explained as follows:

1. Review the past: An old quotation says that those who forget the past are often doomed to repeat it. Simply put it's hard to go in a particular direction if you don't know where you are or how you got there.

2. Forecast the future, calculate timelines: Where do you want to be? Where does your organization want to be? How long will it take to get there?

3. Coordinate strategies and plans: It is important for your department to be working in conjunction with the rest of the organization. What you do and when you do it can be completed independently, but it should not be done haphazardly. Your plans may only address the pharmacy but should still point in the same direction and timeframe as the organization's plans.

4. Determine resources necessary to achieve desired goals. Meeting your goals or your organization's goals will probably require more resources—or different resources—than you currently possess. The essence of strategic financial planning is this: *"In order to do what needs to be done, what will need to be added?"* (i.e., what is the cost, and why is it worth the cost?)

This chapter will focus on the concept of strategic financial planning as used in a department of pharmacy and will follow the outline below:

*   Know your department
*   Know your facility
*   Know your organization's strategic goals and plan
*   Develop departmental operational goals
*   Develop the pharmacy strategic financial plan
*   Put it all together

Know Your Department

A deep and thorough knowledge of your department is the foundation of any planning process. There are several questions to answer before setting off on our strategic financial planning project: Where are we at from the perspective of

*   Space
*   Personnel
*   Processes
*   Practice

Space

The questions regarding space are basic. Do you have enough? Do you have too much? Is the space well used? Does your layout facilitate work or impede it? Is your space well located to serve the needs of your patients and customers? Why are these issues important in a planning chapter? Because space is normally an extremely scarce and highly sought-after commodity in hospitals and is often the most expensive barrier to overcome. If any aspect of space is a concern or barrier to achieving operational goals, then it needs to be addressed in your strategic financial plan.

Personnel

In the current era of pharmacy, personnel looms large on many directors' radar screens. Do you have enough people, both pharmacists and technicians, to do the job? Do you have the positions budgeted? Do you have the positions filled? If you do not have enough positions budgeted, how do you go about getting more positions funded? If you have adequate positions budgeted but too many vacancies, what needs to occur to fill these positions? Will more incentives, better salaries, a retention bonus, or an improved marketing budget help? Whatever the issue in the area of personnel, odds are that these issues are impeding your department's progress toward its current or future operational goals and should be addressed in your strategic financial plan.

Processes

Perhaps the most difficult aspect of developing your plans is knowing who to approach with the various issues in your department to and determining what needs to be done, where. The approach recommended in this chapter will be a "core processes" approach. We will divide the department into four core processes:

1.   Product procurement, storage, retrieval, and preparation
2.   Drug distribution
3.   Order management
4.   Clinical involvement

Although these four core processes do not describe every process used in a modern department of pharmacy, they provide a framework for the director to achieve two key goals:

1.   To have a rational, operations-based process to systematically identify department strengths and weaknesses, process by process.
2.   To have a structure for clearly outlining needs within the strategic financial plan that will enhance understanding by the non-pharmacists who will make decisions based on your plan.

Each of these core processes is unique and as such contributes to your operational plans and goals. There is also an opportunity within the plan to explain the consequences of not making necessary investments in each of the core processes.

Product Procurement, Storage, Retrieval, and Preparation

The first core process includes everything that a pharmacy department does to buy drugs, receive them, store them, retrieve them, and perform any necessary manipulations in order for them to be dispensed from the pharmacy. There are several different processes within this core process:

- The act of purchasing
  - Identifying proper contracts.
  - Assuring proper quantities of product to keep on hand.
  - Determining which products and dosage forms to keep on hand.
  - Making sure the prices paid are appropriate.
- The act of receiving and storing
  - Making sure the right product was received.
  - Making sure the product is in date.
  - Determining where it needs to be stored.
- The act of retrieving
  - Determining where the product is stored and how much is needed.
- The act of preparation
  - Indentifying what type of preparation is needed for each product; some require little or no preparation, whereas fluids such as TPN or sterile admixtures require significant preparation.
  - Compounding non-sterile products.

For these processes to occur, it is necessary to have the proper resources, including people, equipment, facilities, and so forth.

Drug Distribution

Once a dose has been pulled from storage and prepared, it is ready to be transferred to the appropriate patient care location. There are many ways to perform the intricate dance of distribution, and hospitals may use different models for different locations, including the following:

- Ward stock (hopefully extinct by now)
- Cart exchange—Either manual or robot assisted
- Automated dispensing cabinets located in patient care areas (such as Pyxis or Omnicell)
- Hybrid systems—part cart exchange and part automated dispensing cabinets

As you work through the planning process, it is important to understand the current state of drug distribution and the targeted ideal state. It is likely that personnel or capital resources will be required to move you from where you are to where you want to be. Either way, securing the necessary personnel and capital will need to be a part of your planning.

Order Management

The core process of order management is essentially everything the pharmacy does to understand, translate, perfect, and prepare the physician's order for fulfillment. Order entry, or order review, usually comprises a large part of this process. The computer system (and the functional systems and processes that it supports) is central to this process. There are also variations on this theme:

- Manual or computerized pharmacy review
- If computerized, stand-alone/interfaced or integrated pharmacy system
- If integrated,
  - Pharmacist order entry
  - Technician order entry
  - Nursing order entry
  - Physician order entry
  - A mix of the above

The pharmacy manager needs to understand the following about this process:

- Are orders written by prescribers or directly entered into the system?
- If directly entered, by whom?
- If written, how are the orders transmitted to the pharmacist?
  - Courier system
  - Pneumatic tube system
  - Scanning system
- How does order clarification work?

Although the order management process may sound simple, it takes a large amount of pharmacist time. Pharmacist time is expensive, and its use is well documented. Order management is certainly an area that pharmacy planners will address at some point. Components that should be under consideration may include:

- Pharmacist manpower needs
- Opportunities to structure the ordering process, including treatment guidelines and standardized order sets
- Technician and other non-pharmacist roles in the order management process
- Clinical information system upgrades
- Clinical information system replacement
- Order transmission technology
- Automated order clarification and review processes

Clinical Involvement

The process of clinical involvement encompasses everything a pharmacy department does outside of order management that affects patient care. Some, but certainly not all, of what can be considered to comprise clinical involvement include the following:

- Renal dosing services
- Pharmacokinetics services
- Nutrition support services
- IV to PO conversion processes
- Adverse drug event/adverse drug reaction detection
- Drug therapy management
- Duration of therapy review
- Medication reconciliation services
- And many others

Many non-pharmacists, and especially non-physicians, are unfamiliar with these services. To acquire the resources necessary to perform these valuable services, documentation and education is needed. The expansion or maintenance of these services must be addressed in any pharmacy department planning. A focus on patient care outcomes, the financial, patient care and quality aspects of these services is also in order.

Personnel Considerations

Once you have a firm grasp on the nature of the core processes, you will be able to address the needs of the department regarding one of the most valuable and hard to get (and sometimes keep) resources—people. Knowing the demands of your core processes allows you to document and articulate your needs regarding personnel. Knowing the skill sets and full-time equivalents (FTEs) required to make everything work well is the single-most important measurement you will make. The mix of people needed to run your pharmacy department is also critical. The complex set of skills and the challenges of documenting the needs for each future skill set require thoughtful assessment. Some of the skill sets that your pharmacy department may need include:

- Management
  - Director or chief pharmacy officer (CPO): typically only one, although health systems and larger, more diverse integrated delivery networks may require a more complex leadership model
  - Operations manager—or assistant or associate director (the number needed may vary)
  - Supervisors—technician or pharmacist or neither (the amount needed may vary)
  - Pharmacists

- Generalists
- Drug information and drug policy or medication safety officer
- Clinical staff
  - Specialists
  - Subspecialists
- Technicians
  - Staff technician
  - Advanced-skill technician
    - IV lab
    - Chemotherapy
    - Clinical support
  - Professional non-pharmacist
    - Nurse pharmacist extender
    - Business manager
  - Business Manager
    - Billing and compliance staff
    - Buyer
  - Informatics and automation support staff
    - Information technology pharmacist
    - Information technology support staff
    - Automation support staff

Knowing what you need to fill the gaps is important, but being able to predict your needs and adequately articulate why that need exists is vital. The ability to articulate your staff needs within the framework of your core processes will become apparent very quickly. Staff demands can increase or decrease, and changes might increase the demand for technicians while decreasing the demands for pharmacists, or vice versa. The ability to communicate effectively about the current state of the processes and personnel and how changes in the processes will affect the demand for personnel is an integral part of the strategic planning process, which is the precursor to the strategic financial planning process.

Space

We have covered processes and people, now we go to space, "the final frontier." If you have sufficient space in your pharmacy you are blessed. Many departments lack an adequate amount of space, and space is possibly the most expensive limitation to overcome. The capital costs for new space per square foot can be significant. Even the cost for renovating existing space can stress a facility's capital budget.

Why is space important? If you have too much space and use it poorly, it can make for inefficient core processes and wasted steps for your staff. However, if you lack an adequate amount of space, you will find your processes may be inefficient, and additional steps may be necessary. The most relevant question is, Will the space accommodate my future needs? If not, how will my space needs change and when?

Space changes often require a significant amount of lead time to accomplish because of the amount of planning required, the duration and nature of construction and other renovations, and the heavy capital costs often incurred. You will need to be able to address the following:

- What space is needed
- Why it is needed
- When it is needed
- What are the consequences of getting the required space and at the right time

Space can be the forgotten variable at times. Changes in your processes can either increase or decrease your need for space. Either way, a failure to evaluate your space needs in your strategic financial plan can be fatal to your plan, or at the very least cause serious delays.

Equipment

For many, equipment is the first thing that comes to mind when they hear the words *strategic, financial,* or *plan.* For many directors of pharmacy, the need for equipment first introduces them to the capital budget process. However, most of the time this type of financial planning falls more properly under the concept of tactical planning, because it is episodic in nature and often deals with just one piece of equipment and the resources necessary to support it. Equipment purchases often require application of planning and financial justification in several of the topics we have already discussed.

- What process needs the equipment?
- How will the equipment affect human resource needs? Will more staff, less staff, or a different skill mix be needed?
- Is there room for the equipment, or will the new equipment free up space?
- How much will the equipment cost? What will the support or maintenance costs be?
- Can the piece of equipment stand alone, or will it need other equipment to achieve its operational goals?

Our brief discussion of equipment completes our overview on knowing your department. In summary, we have discussed the major components that every pharmacy leader needs to be conversant with to convince hospital leadership that he or she is in firm command of the operational aspects of the pharmacy department.

Know Your Facility

The pharmacy department does not stand alone. It operates as part of the greater whole, the hospital or system. To be a convincing advocate for pharmacy needs, you must be aware of the overall environment within which the organization operates. This can be difficult because the department head group, of which the director of pharmacy is a member, is not always included in the communication process about the overall health and environment of the organization, or may lack sufficient detailed information to determine ways the pharmacy department can help.

If the organization has performed a SWOT (strengths, weaknesses, opportunities, and threats) analysis, getting access to this report or discussing it with the appropriate individual in leadership can be very valuable. (SWOT analysis is a useful tool for departments and processes as well.) The reason this information can be useful for the pharmacy is that it enables the department to evaluate how it

- Enhances a strength or could enhance a strength
- Contributes to or could eliminate a weakness
- Enables the hospital to capitalize on an opportunity
- Helps the hospital to deal with a threat

There are other sources of information regarding your organization:

- Interdepartmental meetings
- Department head meetings
- Memorandums
- Budget planning and progress meetings
- Intra-hospital publications
- Open communication with your administrator or other members of senior leadership
- Others

To position the department of pharmacy in the best position to support the goals of the organization, you must know where the organization is regarding its performance toward those same goals. Thus it is important to be conversant in those goals and the overall environment that the organization finds itself in.

Once this context is understood, it becomes easier to analyze the challenges the organization is facing and then to locate the opportunities the pharmacy department has to meet those challenges. Some examples of organizational environmental challenges that open opportunities for the pharmacy department follow:

- Core measures involving the use of medications. Many quality performance measures involve the use of medications. The pharmacy department can improve the organization's performance in many of these measures. Describing a plan to reallocate departmental resources to improve performance in some or all of these measures will result in a grateful organization. If the pharmacy department lacks the resources to address these issues right away, then the strategic organizational plan can describe the resources required, the costs, and the benefits of acquiring those resources.

- TJC RFI (The Joint Commission's requirements for improvements) involving the medication management standards or some other area that the pharmacy can influence.

- Performance issues within the medication administration or drug therapy processes that the pharmacy department can influence via an interdepartmental effort.

- The organization may need to enhance its visibility within the community it serves by opening up satellite ambulatory services. The pharmacy may help enhance the use of these satellite locations by offering a community pharmacy service co-located with the satellite services.

- Budgetary issues, such as drug expenses or overall cost of care per discharge, may allow for a larger role for the pharmacy than it currently has in the area of drug therapy management. Presenting the case for clinical capability expansion is certainly within the realm of strategic financial planning.

The Organizational Strategic Plan

As we close in the process of actually creating and maintaining a departmental strategic plan, we arrive at the necessary step of identifying the organization's strategic plans. Almost everything the department of pharmacy does should tie into, or relate to, a component of the organization's strategic plan. The degree to which an individual organization performs strategic planning can vary widely, from extremely sophisticated to nonexistent.

If your organization has a strategic plan, then you must address it within the boundaries of the pharmacy's strategic financial planning. Organizational plans often cover several different areas. Whatever those areas are, the pharmacy leadership team is responsible for evaluating how the pharmacy can assist the organization in achieving these strategic plans.

An example of an organization's strategic plan is described below.

Strategic Plan

- Quality: Achieve benchmark or higher measures in all TJC and CMS (Centers for Medicare and Medicaid) standards.

- Employee engagement: Improve employee engagement as measured by an X percent increase in overall engagement scores.

- Growth: Enhance capacity/efficiency such that the time a bed is requested to the time placed in bed is under two hours, and adjusted discharges are increased by 7.8 percent.

- Physician relations/referrals: Cultivate mutually beneficial relationships with physicians, resulting in an overall physician satisfaction score of X percent.

- Image: Become consumer-driven as evidenced by an X percent increase in patient satisfaction score.
- Safety: Maximize employee and patient safety through process improvement or through implementation of appropriate automation initiatives.

Knowing the organization's strategic plan is not the same as understanding it. It is important to understand these goals and the timelines surrounding these goals. Without understanding it will be difficult, if not impossible, to effectively work toward doing what you can to help the organization achieve its goals.

A department will often need to do some planning of its own to support the hospital's strategic plan. Resources may need to be realigned, altered, or added to, to make progress possible. This is why the preceding steps have emphasized knowing the pharmacy and its capabilities intimately.

The Pharmacy Strategic Financial Planning Process

We have finally arrived at the beginning of our goal: starting the department's strategic financial planning process. Now we know where each of our processes stand in regard to our overall goals. We have an idea of our manpower needs, our space needs, and how the pharmacy stands to contribute to the organization's strategic plans and goals. All that is left is placing this information into a single coherent document that accomplishes the following:

- Emphasizes the overriding goal of the pharmacy is to support the mission and strategic plan of the hospital or organization
- Is structured in a logical fashion
- Ties each need to a goal
- Ties each departmental goal to a corresponding organizational goal (if applicable)
- Has a logical and achievable timeline
- Discusses the pros and cons of each proposal
- Discusses the costs of achieving the goal, as well as the costs of not pursuing the goal
- Enhances the ability of non-pharmacists to understand it by being written with as little jargon as possible
- Is designed to be updated as needed

A typical departmental strategic financial plan will cover a span of several years. Few departments and organization have the resources or budget to pursue a large number of projects at the same time or possess the ability to absorb too much change too fast. Some components of a strategic financial plan will also be required before others in order to build a foundation for subsequent components.

Using the preceding model of an organization's strategic plan, let us develop our pharmacy's strategic financial plan.

Preamble

It is the mission of the Hypothetical Hospital Department of Pharmacy Services to work in conjunction with the hospital to deliver the best patient care services possible. In particular, the goal of the department of pharmacy is to lead superior drug therapy management for every patient while at the same time promoting the safest possible approach to the supply and usage of medications. A further goal of the pharmacy department is to evaluate possible ways to achieve superior drug therapy management and medication safety while at the same time working to contain the overall cost of patient treatment. It is recognized that cost effective care, assisted by the pharmacy department, will make available needed resources that can improve patient care, treatment outcomes, and safety in areas not directly affected by the pharmacy.

Background

The work of the department of pharmacy is encompassed within four core strategic processes:

1. Drug procurement, storage, retrieval, and preparation: This is best described as everything the pharmacy does to make sure the proper medications, purchased from reliable sources at the best price, are available when needed and in the proper formulation for timely and safe administration to the patient.

2. Drug distribution: The significant process of moving 7,000,000 patient-ready drug doses from the pharmacy to the point of acquisition by nurses for administration to the patient each year.

3. Order management: The department's pharmacists are responsible for reviewing each of the 1.7 million medication orders generated annually to assure that each order is safe; is in the proper dose, dosage form, and frequency of dosing; does not conflict with other medications, lab values, or procedures; and is in compliance with all formulary requirements and protocols.

4. Clinical involvement: Every patient will be provided the clinical capabilities that fall within the province of the clinical pharmacy services, namely:

   a. Renal dose adjustments for patients with impaired renal clearances

   b. ADR (adverse drug reaction) monitoring based on the use of specific trigger drugs

   c. IV to PO conversions to limit patient exposure to the more risky injectable dosage forms

   d. Clinical monitoring to assure the use of ASA, ACEI, and ARBs for patients with AMI or heart failure

   e. Monitoring the use of anticoagulants

   f. And others

The pharmacy department leadership monitors each of the above core processes to assess continually the department's achievement of the goals of each core process and the resources necessary to maintain the appropriate level of goal achievement.

Departmental Alignment with Hospital Strategic Plan

Strategic Goal	Departmental Current State	Departmental Future State
Achieve benchmark or higher measures in all JCAHO and CMS standards.	Departmental clinical workload is heavy and has increased significantly over the past three years. Pharmacists are capable of significantly increasing core measure scores in the area of DVT prophylaxis, use of ASA in AMI, and others.	Increase clinical pharmacist resources to accommodate current clinical and patient safety initiatives and to allow for pharmacy leadership in the area of DVT prophylaxis and the use of ASA in AMI.
Improve employee engagement as measured by an X percent increase in overall engagement scores.	Pharmacy experienced a 17 percent increase in employee engagement in the last engagement survey. Two problematic areas, however, are the decrease in the number of 5 scores in "I get to do what I do best" and in "I have the equipment and supplies to do my job."	Pharmacist small group discussions reveals an increase in frustration in being able to achieve their clinical goals daily because of the overall increase in clinical and order review workload. The proposed increase in pharmacist staffing will improve the department's performance on this strategic goal as well.
Enhance capacity/efficiency such that the time bed requested to the time placed in bed is under two hours and adjusted discharges are increased by 7.8 percent.	Nursing and physician satisfaction with pharmacy performance remains high.	The improved clinical pharmacist staffing already mentioned will have an incremental contribution to this strategic goal as well. Physician satisfaction with the organization is affected by the level of clinical contributions provided by our clinical staff. We have several clinical areas of contribution requested by our physicians that we have been unable to satisfy at our current staffing/workload level.
Cultivate mutually beneficial relationships with physicians resulting in an overall physician satisfaction score of X percent.	Pharmacists work very closely with our medical staff in a wide range of areas. Expansion of our services is requested by our medical staff in almost every medical department.	Again the expansion of our clinical pharmacist resources will enable the appropriate involvement on the patient care team as desired by our medical staff. This would be expected to have a positive incremental impact on our physician satisfaction scores.

Strategic Goal	Departmental Current State	Departmental Future State
Become consumer-driven as evidenced by an X percent increase in patient satisfaction score.	Most patients and their families are unaware of the availability of pharmacists to consult on questions they may have about their drug therapy. Pharmacist workload and a large number of patients renders it impossible for our pharmacists to consult with every patient. However, whenever we do, the patient or the family is extremely grateful.	This is another area where an expansion of our clinical resources will render an incremental improvement in the organization's achievement of the strategic goal. The more patients that the pharmacy can interact with, the more overall positive scores we will see.
Maximize employee and patient safety through process improvement or through implementation of appropriate automation initiatives.	CPOE, bedside bar-coding are currently not installed but are planned. Clinical rules exist but need considerable expansion.	Informatics complexity within the pharmacy, or in areas directly affecting the pharmacy, is growing and will continue to grow. The department's informatics resources are small and will be completely consumed by the current clinical information system initiative and existing automation support and database maintenance. Additional resources need to be added and training initiated before we tackle CPOE or bedside bar-coding.

Once this task is accomplished, we can see our primary needs. It appears that our essential needs are resources in the form of more of the right kind of employees. Hospitals view labor expense as something to be examined closely. It will be beneficial in our strategic financial plan to show how these additional employees work to help the organization achieve its goals.

Strategic Financial Planning Tools to Consider

Although examining and aligning your department goals with that of the overall organization is important, it may not reveal internal issues that need to be addressed or medication process issues not pointed to by the hospital strategic plan.

SWOT Analysis: Strengths, Weaknesses, Opportunities, Threats

For our particular example, we would want to map each of these concepts.

Strengths

- Clinically capable staff
- Well regarded by medical staff
- Well regarded by nursing staff
- Large number of clinical programs
- Low turnover

Weaknesses

- More clinical opportunities than man-hours to achieve them
- Difficulty in recruiting new staff
- Lingering image of heavy workload environment
- Space in main pharmacy is marginal. No more room exists for automation installation, and work counter space needs expansion

Opportunities

- Medical staff demanding more involvement in pharmacy-based consults
- Other departments requesting placement of pharmacists (ED)
- Counter-detailing opportunities are unlimited

Threats

- Increased activity by local pharmaceutical sales representatives
- Dramatic workload growth

A SWOT analysis is useful in demonstrating that a thorough overview of the environment in which the department is operating has been conducted. It is often useful in identifying surprising aspects of the environment that have not been previously identified.

In this example, we have identified another issue for our strategic financial plan—space!

Gap Analysis

Another tool that can be useful is a gap analysis, which is used to point out the difference between where a particular department or process is versus where it should be. The value of a gap analysis is to demonstrate the thoroughness of examination for the issue. Some simple examples of gap analysis include the following:

- The number of daily admissions versus the number of medication reconciliations performed
- The potential number of IV to PO conversions versus the total number performed
- The number of clinical services possible versus the number of clinical services offered

This analysis can be simple or complex. The situation should dictate how detailed the analysis needs to be.

For our example, we will consider the need to package 6,000 doses per month, but our manual process and technician staffing only supports 3,000 doses per month. To close this gap, we need either

- An additional technician FTE to staff the packager for two shifts five days per week
- A robotic automatic packager to facilitate packaging on demand and prepare the department for the future demand of bed-side barcoding.

Other Tools

Many other tools can be used for ideas on what to include in your strategic financial plan. Some of the other tools include the following:

- Brainstorming
- Soliciting ideas from your staff
- Stealing ideas from other departments
- Stealing ideas from other hospital pharmacies (attendance at national meetings is a great way to find out what best practices are evolving in your profession)

Pharmacy Strategic Financial Plan: Main Body

Year One

Proposal

Add two floor pharmacists and one clinical specialist to current pharmacy staffing.

Rationale

Current workload is heavy for both our clinical staff pharmacists and our clinical specialists. This workload prevents us from expanding our services into new areas. Additional staff will enable the following organizational goals to be advanced:

- Achieve benchmark or higher measures in all TJC and CMS standards.
- Improve employee engagement as measured by an X percent increase in overall engagement scores.
- Enhance capacity/efficiency such that the time bed requested to the time placed in bed is under two hours and adjusted discharges are increased by 7.8 percent.
- Cultivate mutually beneficial relationships with physicians, resulting in an overall physician satisfaction score of X percent.
- Become consumer driven, as evidenced by an X percent increase in patient satisfaction scores.
- Maximize employee and patient safety by process improvement or implementation of appropriate automation initiatives.

Each of these goals will be furthered by the proposed staff expansion. Pharmacists play a key role in helping organizations to achieve higher levels of compliance with many aspects of the medication standards. Improved capacity for clinical involvement and projects will raise the department's response on the engagement question: "I get to do what I do best at work." Facility throughput will be enhanced by the decreased order turnaround time and by the raised involvement with medication therapy management provided by the new pharmacists, enabling an incremental gain on enhanced capacity and efficiency.

Physician demand for pharmacist services will be facilitated by this staff expansion as well. We will focus on one specific area for pharmacist involvement this fiscal year (increased capacity for anticoagulation management). With these three additional positions, our ability to perform more patient encounters and teaching episodes will enhance the patients' familiarity with the pharmacy, and their satisfaction will potentially be enhanced.

Certainly, three additional pharmacists to expand our clinical involvement and programs will have a measurable impact on patient safety initiatives.

Financial Analysis

Each pharmacist's starting salary plus benefits: $125,000 × 3 = $375,000 less the established return on investment for pharmacists of 150 percent (base salary $100,000) $450,000 yields a net gain of $75,000.

Proposal

Pharmacy space is severely limited. The capital cost for an entirely new pharmacy is extremely high. The pharmacy department has a back wall that is unusable because of electrical cabinets. Engineering has determined that space exists in nearby equipment rooms to relocate these electrical cabinets along the entire 30 feet of the back wall. Our proposal is to move these cabinets, clearing the length of the wall and allowing for a more efficient use of the back of the pharmacy. Approximately 200 functional square feet will result from this.

Although this upgrade is not as optimal as a new pharmacy, it does allow for a reconfiguring of the main pharmacy to use space more efficiently.

Financial Analysis

Remodeling costs will be $189,000. This equates to $945/sq ft., a high cost but substantially less than moving the entire department to a new location that would have to be built from the ground up.

Year Two

Proposal

Continue the expansion of pharmacy staff as indicated by current departmental workload and desired clinical program and project expansion.

The goal is the same as year one: two clinical staff pharmacists and one clinical specialist. We will focus this year on enhancing our ability to provide in-depth clinical services into the late afternoon and evening. Our order review data shows that, although our mid-morning peak is still intact, we have an emerging pattern of a second medication order peak lasting from 2 p.m. through 4 p.m. It is anticipated that this trend will continue and that this staff will be necessary to accommodate the order workload and the clinical opportunities that typically accompany a large number of medication orders. Discharge counseling consults are expected to grow, and these resources will enable the department to cope with this growth.

Financial Analysis

Each pharmacist starting salary plus benefits is $125,000 × 3 = $375,000 less the established return on investment for pharmacists of 150 percent (base salary $100,000) $450,000 yields a net gain of $75,000.

Proposal

Integrate an automated unit-dose packager with our central pharmacy carousel team to streamline the packaging of our non-unit dosed oral solids into the carousel unit-based cabinet replenishment process. The current packager system is completely manual and offers several opportunities for errors. An integrated packager with bar-code identification offers a safer packaging process with fewer opportunities for error. Our current packaging process is falling behind our packaging volumes. A purchase at this time would position the pharmacy department for the future bed-side bar-coding initiative.

Financial Analysis

Purchase price $250,000 plus annual support expense of $10,000. Offset expenses include one technician FTE redeployed and one technician FTE avoided, a net annual savings of $62,500. Annual packaging savings (purchasing a select number of products in bulk at a net savings), $5,000. The payback period based on dollar savings (not NPV, net present value) is 3.7 years (not including annual support).

Years 3–5 would follow the same model.

Summary

Strategic financial planning performed at the departmental level can provide both the department and the organization with a direction otherwise lacking in a fiscal year-by-fiscal year approach. The multiyear approach to a plan helps hospital senior leadership comprehend the impact of delays or of elimination of components of the pharmacy strategic plan. The financial component of the multiyear approach allows for cash flow modeling to be conducted as well as relative value analysis (i.e. which of several departments' budgetary requests promises to best fulfill the organization's financial and strategic goals). Linking the departmental strategic financial plan to the organization's strategic plan shows that the pharmacy department is supportive of the organization's goals and has taken proactive steps to achieve the maximum level of departmental support.

Financial Planning and Assessment for Pharmacy Education and Research Programs

Alan H. Mutnick
Peter K. Wong

Introduction

We first came across the term *intellectual capital* in a book by Thomas A. Stewart. The author defines *intellectual capital* as "intellectual materials, knowledge, information, intellectual property, experiences that can be put in use to create wealth."[1]

This definition can remind us of what we do each day in pharmacy. The pharmacy department is composed of a team of competent and experienced clinicians. Together the team provides pharmaceutical care to patients. The collective knowledge and wisdom ensures that patients receive cost-effective care while avoiding any potential adverse drug events. It is difficult to estimate the wealth of the intellectual capital, because it is not stated on the corporate balance sheet or any company's financial statements. Some companies may state the number of employees in their annual report. However, this report does not list the experience, wisdom, education, or any other factor that comprises the human intellectual capital (HIC) of the company. The HIC is difficult to describe because no uniform measurements and comparators exist. The company's assets and liabilities statement does not recognize the HIC; therefore, managers and executives possess no measure to understand how to preserve, build, deploy, or grow such assets. Moreover, most of the employees are employed at will. Consequently, employers and employees are free to choose whom they work for, how they work for the company, where they want to work, and when they want to work. Mismanagement of these HIC assets will lead to a brain drain, and the company will lose its competitive edge.

In many business schools, subjects such as financial management, human resource management, and organizational behaviors are a part of the current curriculum. Seldom is HIC management discussed. In this chapter, we will demonstrate and discuss the costs and benefits of growing and deploying the HIC in pharmacy. The development of pharmacy employees will not only have a positive return on investment in patient care, but it can also result in a positive cash flow to the department providing residency and pharmacy student training. Furthermore, such training efforts can also serve as fertile ground for staff recruitment and the advancement of the pharmacy profession. In short, to remain successful, the pharmacy profession must grow and preserve its human intellectual capital. At the end of the chapter, we will suggest several measurements for human intellectual capital. Although these measurements have not been widely adopted, it is useful to articulate them to the health system administrators on a regular basis.

Management of Pharmacy Wealth

Pharmacy has traditionally been a product-oriented department in many health systems. The advent of clinical pharmacy and the pharmaceutical care model have changed the nature of the department. Not only do pharmacies provide drug products, they also dispense care in the form of knowledge and information. With health care's growing focus on cost containment, pharmaceutical care has gradually played a greater role in the selection of appropriate drug therapy and the monitoring of patient outcomes. Seasoned, knowledgeable, and experienced clinicians are difficult to recruit and retain. The management of human intellectual capital is vital to the success of the pharmacy department.

With the demand for new skills required in the appropriate delivery of pharmaceutical care, many pharmacy departments have developed programs to assist the management of these resources. Programs such as staff development and training of residents and pharmacy students are growing. When these new programs are presented to the institution's chief financial officer (CFO), the pharmacy director will often be asked whether these programs can be financially self-sustaining and whether these programs have any return on investment. We hope this chapter will answer some of these questions and prepare pharmacy administrators to defend our position.

Funding Sources for Residency Programs

Recent review of Policy 0005 by the American Society of Health System Pharmacists (ASHP) Council on Educational Affairs and the ASHP Board of Directors found that the policy was appropriate for assuring that pharmacists engaged in direct patient care "require the development of clinical judgment, which can be acquired only through experience and reflection on that experience." The policy goes on to state that pharmacy departments should "establish as a goal that pharmacists who provide direct patient care should have completed an ASHP-accredited residency or have attained comparable skills through practice experience."[2]

An earlier review of ASHP Policy 9911, also carried out by the Council on Educational Affairs and also deemed still appropriate, included the following statements: "To continue efforts to increase the number of pharmacy residency training programs and positions available; further, To expand efforts to make pharmacy students aware early in their education of the career choices available to them and the importance health-system employers attach to the completion of a residency."[3] This approach to setting policy and the sustained growth in patient care-based education and on residency training mirrors the value placed on the programs in our discussion.

In a portion of her recent Harvey A. K. Whitney Award presentation, Sara White described the early foundations created by Whitney. She reiterated how Whitney's implementation of a formalized internship program trained future hospital practitioners and formed the stepping-stone to today's formal accreditation process for assuring uniform quality to the post-graduate residency programs in our constantly changing health care system.[4]

During the earliest of times in the evolutionary process of the American Society of Health-System Pharmacists, professional training and minimum standards for hospital pharmacy practice have been a core strength of the association's persona. More recently, the expansion of residency training programs and the need for amending accreditation standards to meet the needs of a changing health-care system have been the more contemporary core strengths in the association's charge.[5]

Similar to colleagues involved in medical training, the need to establish and grow post-graduate programs whose purpose is to provide out-of-classroom experiences, which enable pharmacists to attain the necessary advanced practice skills and knowledge to meet the needs of today's diverse patient populations. The act of training hospital pharmacists in the management of pharmacy services in hospitals has changed substantially since its inception, but the vision for hospital pharmacist training created by Harvey Whitney during his pioneering efforts at the University of Michigan more than 70 years ago is still paramount to the future success of health systems pharmacy.

As vital as residency training is in developing clinical maturity in pharmacy practitioners, the residency training program requires resources—both in manpower and in dollars—if they are to continue being able to address the growing needs placed on them by society.

Before the late 1990s, little information was published in pharmacy-related journals on the methods used to fund pharmacy residency programs. However, with the landmark publication in the *American Journal of Health System Pharmacy* by Linda Cortese Annecchini and Donald Letendre, this changed because of the findings shared from a questionnaire focusing on various aspects of pharmacy residency programs. The response rate was exceptional (93 percent), reflecting the interest in the survey topic, and the respondents represented more than 300 residency program preceptors representing 774 resident positions.

A major finding from the survey was that fewer than 50 percent of pharmacy programs eligible for reimbursement sought and received graduate medical education (GME) pass-through funds. Additional findings included that hospitals or health systems were responsible for funding more than 60 percent of residency positions alone, 8 percent of residency positions jointly funded with a pharmacy college, 9 percent jointly funded by the Department of Veterans Affairs, and 7 percent funded as a Veterans Administration prime initiative. Colleges of pharmacy funded 4 percent of respondents' residency positions, and no mention was made of residency positions funded by industry.[6]

A subsequent article by D. E. Miller and T. W. Woller attempted to increase the level of visibility for the graduate medical education pass-through funding process by better acquainting pharmacy managers with pass-through funding as a way to reimburse health systems for pharmacy residents. Miller and Woller, in a basic, stepwise approach, were able to illustrate the manner in which a pharmacy manager could develop a business plan, which would then be used in demonstrating the financial basis for obtaining pass-through funding for pharmacy residency programs.[7] Formal training of health-care professionals to improve the quality of care provided to the patients being served is an approved activity that can be paid for thorough pass-through reimbursement.

Paramount to the preparation of a formal business plan is the need to identify direct educational costs associated with residency training (i.e., salary, benefits, photocopying expenses, teaching time for residency training, professional dues and subscriptions), indirect educational costs (i.e., office space, equipment depreciation, housekeeping), and the hospital's Medicare patient load. Additionally, value to the hospital might center on the contributions that residents might have during their program when they provide online staffing functions as part of the department's operations activities. One example might include a department's requirement that its residents provide collateral operations staffing every other weekend for 16 hours (Saturday and Sunday, 8 hours each shift). Five residents providing such activities over the course of 11 months of a residency program would translate to just under 2,000 hours of collateral coverage. At an average salary of $80,000 per newly hired pharmacist, that would represent a staffing savings of about $77,000. One pharmacist FTE could be spent in another non-operations function because of the staffing contributions provided by the pharmacy residents.

Most academic medical centers that provide services to Medicare patients have created a group of financial reimbursement specialists who work with respective residency program directors to identify the direct and indirect costs of residency training and Medicare patient load to create a more complete business plan for hospital administration. An annual report is then created by the reimbursement specialists, which includes the medical center's educational expenses, direct, indirect, and Medicare caseload, to prepare the overall reimbursements as part of the pass-through funding process.

It is apparent from the August 1, 2003, decision by the Centers for Medicare & Medicaid Services (CMS) that the level of visibility for residency funding through the Medicare pass-through has dramatically improved over the last decade. As evidenced by the letters of support to CMS by thousands of ASHP members along with members of other organizations, preservation of funding for first-year pharmacy-practice residency programs was achieved and represented a fundamental misunderstanding of pharmacy education by officials at CMS.[8] Today's health system pharmacy departments are much more aware of the contributions of Medicare's pass-through funding opportunities, and current goals as recently described by Stein, center on the ongoing needs for similar funding for the specialized or post-graduate year 2 (PGY2) residency programs, which currently are not being funded.[9]

As optimistic as the CMS acknowledgment might appear, it is clear that today's health systems pharmacy leaders still have their work cut out for them in ensuring a strong financial future for residency training. A recent survey of U.S. academic medical centers conducted by J. Hoffman et al hoped to identify the most important and challenging issues involved in pharmacy training. Using a 5-point Likert scale to assess levels of importance and challenge, respectively, for the survey prompt, "Maintaining financial resources to continue current programs at the size currently offered," mean scores of 4.3 and 3.1 were reported. The only concerns that had a greater mean level of importance were the "recruitment of residents" (4.8), "completing residency research" (4.5), and "complying with the evaluation and documentation requirements" (4.4).[10]

From the initial survey carried out by Cortese Annecchini and Letendre, it was apparent that the majority of funding opportunities for residency programs were derived primarily by the specific hospital or health system, and that is probably the area that prompts the greatest concern for today's pharmacy managers.[11]

What will happen to such revenue streams as dollars become tighter within these hospitals, and what can pharmacy leaders do to mitigate the potential for reducing available dollars? Some would say that we should consider a greater level of interaction with our academic colleagues to increase teamwork in supporting residency training. Others would say that we should take advantage of the growing interest from the pharmaceutical industry to carry on such collaborative efforts. Still others would say that we must continue to demonstrate to health system administrators the beneficial effects that residency training has on staff retention and recruitment and patient outcomes. Each of these comments may present viable alternatives to avoid the reduction in residency training and perhaps even allow for occasional increases in programs, depending on potential revenue streams. However, they might also represent less than desired outcomes if each situation is not evaluated thoroughly.

Collaboration with Colleges/Schools of Pharmacy

We strongly believe that it would be in the best interests of our academic colleagues to increase efforts of collaboration for future residency programs, both within the health system and outside in the community setting. The increased numbers of colleges/schools of pharmacy and the growing demands of the out-of-classroom, real-world environment will continue to increase dependence on health system pharmacists to provide suitable environments for experiential training. As evidenced by the most recent standards approved by Accreditation Council for Pharmacy Education, Accreditation Standards and Guidelines for the Professional Program in Pharmacy Leading to the Doctor of Pharmacy Degree, a growing emphasis is placed on the quality of experiential training programs, the level of expertise placed on preceptors and experiential coordinators, and the need for suitable learning sites to afford students the opportunity to actively engage in patient care–related activities.[12]

The answer of how each college/school of pharmacy should adequately address the newly provided standards would appear to be a rather elementary one. Experienced preceptors who are willing and able to serve would be of great benefit, and the ability to support such goals might be best served through the financial support for residents who can fill such preceptor roles once they have completed their residency training. An alternative method, which had been used in the past, might use a dedicated faculty member to serve the health system as a practitioner/educator. Unfortunately, unlike many current faculty role models who possess other non-hospital-based priorities, which might be viewed more as visitors to the health system rather then preceptors, this type of faculty member would need to become more completely entrenched in the health system to serve as an appropriate residency preceptor.

Certain aspects of the academic model currently existing among faculty involved in PharmD students' education during experiential training might not be beneficial for residency training. One aspect of the model involves the faculty member serving more in a patient care-consultant role, primarily in attendance at the institution as a preceptor for students rather than as an active practitioner. Residency training requires a greater degree of mentorship from such preceptors, and, if the faculty members were not able to relate effectively to the overall practice model and departmental mission within the health system, it would not prove beneficial to the resident.

One can merely speculate as to the posture taken by the academic community but would hope that those engaged in pharmacy academia would recognize that the long-term future of the profession and its ability to meet the growing needs being placed on it by society will be better served through a collaborative effort. If the health systems are not able to train patient care-focused practitioners adequately, the future students passing through experiential training sites might not obtain the necessary expert training to make them future contributors to our profession. If viewed globally, the collaborative approach is a logical one.

Collaboration with the Pharmaceutical Industry

In his Harvey A. K. Whitney Award lecture, McAllister stated that we must more successfully engage the pharmaceutical industry and develop our common purpose.[13] Many subscribe to this message and for years now have done what they can do to build better fundamental relationships, which work to benefit both pharmaceutical companies and pharmacy departments. However, there are others who have seen the impact that such relationships can have on the ability to maintain unbiased evaluations when serving as an active participant in clinical decision making activities. For the health systems pharmacist, this might become a difficult challenge when attending a meeting of the pharmacy and therapeutics committee and asked to provide a constructive evaluation on competitive drug products, with one product being from a collaborating pharmaceutical company.

Discussion of Medicare reform, drug importation, and government-established price controls has made the pharmaceutical industry the center of much debate within the health-care industry.[14] An ongoing process that is currently unfolding within many academic medical centers is a growing awareness of collaborative relationships with the pharmaceutical industry, and the concern that such relationships have on access, marketing, and formulary management. Marketing strategies used in today's competitive health-care environment have forced many institutions to begin clarifying their relationships with the pharmaceutical industry, and for several leading institutions such clarifications have resulted in a substantial reduction in the level of interactions among health-care providers and representatives from the pharmaceutical industry.

Conflicts of interest represent an expanding challenge for pharmacists as their therapeutic influence grows and therefore will require appropriate evaluation to minimize the potential appearance of such conflict.

Collaborative funding with the pharmaceutical industry for residency training can take several different forms and venues. However, when monies are given to health-care systems to fund residency positions, it would be naïve to think that the collaboration is merely the unilateral flow of monies from the pharmaceutical company to the hospital. It is that part of the collaborative relationship, which will be troubling for some residency directors as they ponder the successful outcome goal to be appreciated by the collaborating party, in this case the pharmaceutical company.

A recent letter by Young provided a chilling reminder of the issues for which pharmacists must be prepared to comply with the federal antikickback law.[15] In the brief letter, Young singles out the development of a legitimate educational or research program, which, if funding is tied in any way to the purchase of the pharmaceutical company's product, the parties are breaching the antikickback law. Grants to support residency training or research within the department or health-care system are permissible; however, caution must be exercised in the entire grant package to avoid legal issues that would certainly not help such a training program.

Demonstration of Resident Value within the Health System

During the last 20 years, the demonstration of the positive contributions of pharmacy services to the outcomes associated with patient care has been an area of growth in pharmacy literature. Throughout the peer-reviewed literature, articles continue to present positive findings based on expanded levels of pharmaceutical practices, which directly affect patient care.[16, 17, 18] The available literature can prove valuable to pharmacy leaders in need of evidence demonstrating the valuable contributions that contemporary pharmacy services have for health systems. (Refer to Appendix A for a list.)

Pharmacy managers planning on using the literature to obtain support from their respective administrators should provide an ongoing dialogue with the necessary evidence from the literature, along with ongoing highlights from the department that provide additional proof of such value. A one-time barrage of evidence, or timing an initial discussion during the annual budget process, might not be as effective a strategy as providing information as part of an evolving educational strategy.

An additional strategic goal might also include the identification of areas within the hospital in need of an expanded level of service that might benefit through the addition of a pharmacy resident as part of the hospital's annual performance improvement efforts. One such area, which might represent a critical issue for senior administrators, might be the involvement of pharmacy residents in improving the institution's medication reconciliation program, or any of the other national patient safety goals as developed by the JCAHO. The ability to dovetail a much-needed hospital initiative as a part of a given residency program's responsibility might be a small activity to become engaged in to implement a residency program.

One final strategy that might prove of benefit would be the potential impact of a residency program on the recruitment of future pharmacy practitioners for the health system. As would be demonstrated through the residency program, the value that a resident would have to the institution could be appreciated both as an addition to the staff during times of pharmacy shortage and the advanced level of practice at which the resident would be able to practice once completing a residency training program.

The strategic plan of the American College of Clinical Pharmacy states that "Formal, postgraduate residency training will become mandatory before one can enter practice."[19] The American Society of Health-Systems Pharmacists has a detailed 2015 Initiative, which demands that pharmacists be at the patient's bedside, directly involved in patient care, actively communicating with other members of the health-care team, and monitoring all pharmaceuticals to be assured that the patient is receiving necessary treatments for select outcomes-based disease states.

The profession has much to deal with, and many believe that only through the active support for post-graduate residency training will the profession have enough qualified practitioners to make the above-mentioned initiatives possible. As the health-care system continues to demonstrate its dynamic changes, and with the growing rise of consumerism across the country, today's pharmacy leaders will need to work carefully to make sure the staff engaged in practice within our facilities are able to function at a level worthy of a cautious, highly educated society. If we are able to carry out our mission appropriately, the consumer will reward our profession, but if we are not able to meet the challenge, we may have lost our opportunity, which may not resurface again.

Professional Obligation to Train Future Practitioners

The Accreditation Council for Pharmacy Education (ACPE) announced the release of the revised *Accreditation Standards and Guidelines for the Professional Program in Pharmacy Leading to the Doctor of Pharmacy Degree,* adopted by the ACPE Board of Directors on January 15, 2006. The new standards and guidelines (*"Standards 2007"*) were effective on July 1, 2007. The release of "Standards 2007" brings to a conclusion a three-year revision exercise, initiated in January 2003 with the decision by the ACPE Board to revise the accreditation standards for Doctor of Pharmacy degree programs.[20]

With the formal release of the document came a growing level of interest in several important aspects of the new standards. Many pharmacy educators and experiential education-focused faculty were concerned that the standards directly related to the out-of-classroom, experiential aspect of pharmacy coursework.

At the conclusion of the actual document is an Appendix C, referred to as "Additional Guidance on Pharmacy Practice Experiences."[21] Mentioned within Appendix C are direct descriptions of the qualities of experiential preceptors, which includes the following characteristics: (1) practice ethically and with compassion for patients, (2) accept personal responsibility for patient outcomes, (3) have professional training, experience, and competence commensurate with their position, (4) use clinical and scientific publications in clinical care decision making and evidence-based practice, (5) have a desire to educate others (patients, care givers, other health-care professionals, students, pharmacy residents), (6) have an aptitude to facilitate learning, (7) be able to document and assess student performance, (8) have a systematic, self-directed approach to their own continuing professional development, and (9) collaborate with other health-care professionals as a member of a team and be committed to their organization, professional societies, and the community.

Most academicians view the characteristics in a favorable manner but also recognize the need to increase the availability of qualified experiential preceptors outside of the university setting (adjunct faculty). Traditionally, experiential programs have used adjunctive academic appointments to place students into out-of-classroom experiences with non-college faculty. Some experiences have proved beneficial to students based on the dedication and commitment of the respective preceptor(s). Students have viewed other experiences as more of a convenience to meet the required activity with little commitment to the overall academic purpose for the student involved in the out-of-classroom experience.

The standards appear to be on a collision course with the current workforce demands placed on health-care providers, including pharmacists. As the number of new colleges/schools of pharmacy grow along with total experiential exposures, each of us within the health-care setting will be called upon to help the profession adequately educate future practitioners. This will benefit the profession and society by ensuring enough professionals practice at a high-enough level to safeguard the medication use system. Unfortunately, much concern has been expressed in the manner in which our colleges/schools of pharmacy will implement the changes in experiential training and whether currently practicing pharmacists will have the interest, motivation, and skill sets to accomplish the mission.[22]

In his Harvey A. K. Whitney Award lecture, McAllister more than encouraged pharmacists to collaborate with representatives from the pharmaceutical industry. He also added, "We need to create partnerships with our colleagues in academia and other practice settings to ensure future generations have the optimism, commitment, and stewardship to make our profession absolutely essential and its practitioners invaluable."[23] The authors believe that such a partnership will be in the best interests of the profession, and pharmacy leaders must do everything in their power to make these partnerships work.

An area for such partnerships to occur was provided in a recent article by Trovato and Edwards. According to the authors, an important place to start the partnership would be for pharmacists in various practice settings and colleges/schools of pharmacy to begin sharing similar missions and visions.[24] Additional issues that will need to be addressed include the balance between patient care and service for the pharmacists within the health system. An additional discussion point might include the role that clinical pharmacy faculty will play in the partnerships, if they are to become stakeholders in the future, and what balance will exist between patient care, service, and research—fundamental missions consistent with the academic model.

Confucius made the following comment, which might apply directly to those not yet overwhelmed with the idea of actively participating in the partnership described above. It is a good place to start when beginning to put a preceptor team in place:

> Tell me and I will forget
> Show me and I might remember
> Involve me, and I will understand

The quote can be applied to many of the reasons behind experiential learning as a critical part of pharmacy education. The experiential programs in the United States place pharmacy students in various pharmacy work environments with mentors or preceptors, who are responsible for demonstrating up-to-date practice activities for the pharmacy students.

A promotional piece identified on the Web site of the Delta Synergy Group included a statement that "our ability to retain what we have learned increases markedly with interaction." Additionally, they add that from data they have researched, "We retain 90% of what we do, 30% of what we see, 20% of what we hear, and 10% of what we read." The authors are not suggesting that each potential pharmacy preceptor needs to attend a session with the Delta Synergy Group in Canada. It would seem logical to assume, however, that potential preceptors, in particular those not yet convinced of the need to collaborate with academic

Table 14.1. The Value of Mentoring for the Mentor

A mentee can help the mentor establish a legacy
A mentee can provide the mentor a role in the molding of successors
A mentee can provide an extension of the mentor's power base
A mentee can reinforce a mentor's professional identity
A mentee passes on personal knowledge that will help the mentor stay up-to-date in the field
A mentee can provide assistance with the mentor's projects
A mentee can bring to the mentor a sense of achievement or accomplishment
A mentee can help the mentor acquire new technical knowledge

colleagues, that experiential opportunities will likely pay large professional dividends to pharmacy, as mentors provide more students with a hands-on, involved experience during the initial years of their professional development.

The American Society of Health-System Pharmacists supports the need for practitioners to support the educational needs of students and have expressed their goal "to encourage practitioner input in pharmacy education," and "to encourage pharmacists and pharmacy leaders to recognize that part of their professional responsibility is the development of new pharmacy practitioners."[25] For most pharmacy practitioners within the health system, such future partnerships, if adequately developed, will be a welcome sight, as most would agree that out-of classroom exposures will maximize the skills, professional maturity, and commitment of the next generation of pharmacists. Paramount to this partnership will be the need to provide the necessary skill sets, motivation, and experience to those who have not been preceptors in the past. We have recently seen within our profession a growing interest in the concept of mentoring as a way to grow the profession.

Much has been written about the concept of mentoring and its value to both the mentor and the mentee (Table 14.1 and 14.2). However, the manner in which the partnership develops is of great importance in ensuring a collaborative spirit that will be mutually rewarding for both the college/school of pharmacy and those engaged as preceptors within the health system.

Table 14.2. The Value of Mentoring for the Mentee

A mentor provides a fund of knowledge that expands a mentee's information base and points the
    mentee to new resources
A mentor can target the skills needed for successful career development
A mentor provides individual recognition and encouragement
A mentor gives honest criticism and informal feedback and keeps the mentee on track
A mentor can demonstrate an increased awareness of formal and informal rules and builds a mentee
    who is perceptive
A mentor can advocate for the mentee (promotion, salary, resources, and appointments)
A mentor can protect a mentee during stressful times
A mentor may, if willing and competent, give advice on balancing career and personal tasks

Traditionally, the use of clinical pharmacy faculty to serve as experiential preceptors in health systems has been the norm. In many schools, the clinical faculty has been supplemented by on-site preceptors who carry out many of the purposes of an experiential preceptor. One criticism from both students and these types of preceptors has been a result of their level of patient care, which on occasion will disrupt experiential schedules. However, if we are to begin training pharmacy students to recognize the real-world situations involved in pharmacy practice, such disruptions because of patient care needs will serve as an excellent source of commitment and gratification for our students.

Various models have been used, and newer innovative models still need to be developed to solidify the partnerships necessary between our schools and the respective practice sites. The notion of regionalizing experiential training has been used at other institutions, and serving in more of a liaison role with a school allows for greater flexibility in timing of rotations while assuring the students' real-life experiences will shape their professional future in a positive way. The model does not come without costs, both to the school and the hospital site. Resources are needed to assure adequate training of preceptors, and the liaison must be able to schedule an acceptable level of precepting that will encourage staff participation rather then discourage it. However, several key ingredients will be required by the schools and health systems if the models are to be valuable in lieu of the new accreditation standards:

- Funds necessary to support the manpower resources used by the onsite pharmacy department in carrying out a quality level of experiential training
- Suitable office space for students to use to carry out much of their non-patient care activities (article reviews, literature searches, case report write ups)
- Availability, where indicated, for dedicated college clinical faculty serving as preceptors with a commitment to patient care and the mission of the department of pharmacy
- A real-time evaluation instrument, which adequately addresses student, preceptor, and hospital site performance, and which will be used as part of the review process for student and preceptor (at the end of each learning unit) and for the hospital and college/school (at the end of each annual contract year)
- Mutual respect between the school and health system in the education of future pharmacy practitioners

Staff Development and Training

The 2001 Institute of Medicine report *Crossing the Quality Chasm: A New Health System for the 21st Century* stated that safety and quality problems are occurring among our highly trained care providers.[26] It is not that our health-care professionals are not committed to their jobs. In fact, they are trying to produce quality care and to protect patients from harm. However, our learning system does not support them adequately once they leave the academic environment and enter into practice.[27]

When the transition to the practice environment is suboptimal, the outcome is frustration. Despite the intensive training provided within the Doctor of Pharmacy curriculum, it does not guarantee the right experience for the right job in the right practice setting. Even when the student possesses the right training and the right job, he or she may not fit into the practice environment. The "fit" for the practice environment normally refers to the team. Therefore, team building is also an important task for the pharmacy department manager and/or director to perform. Achieving a team's peak performance is the dream of a committed manager. However, excellence does not come easily, and it requires much development. The team and all of its needs must be viewed as an investment in intellectual capital, and the use of effective teamwork and crew resource management training is critical in high-risk areas. An effective manager will also understand how team members can be motivated to achieve the greatness to which he or she aspires.

Think back to the first day of your new job and how you were oriented to the environment, the people, and the department policies and procedures. Traditionally, the pharmacy staff orientation or facility orientation is far from adequate. Normally it lasts one or two days and is loaded with information. Members of the organization come in and out, speaking on many different subjects. By the end of the orientation, most of the new employees are brain dead. Most orientation sessions are not suitable for an adult learning style. Information may be presented with the best of intentions, but most of the information provided was not retained at all. Consequently, a new pharmacist on the job may be less confident, and, when compounded with high workload and work pressure, mistakes are bound to happen.

On the other end of the spectrum are experienced pharmacists who are being introduced to new programs and new initiatives without training and education. Consider a pharmacist in an anticoagulant management service as one example. If all pharmacists in the designated pharmacy department are not trained in the same manner and are not properly instructed before providing the service, the pharmacists may not adequately carry out the job required or may perform or monitor a given patient's anticoagulant therapy incorrectly. The unwanted consequences create significant patient safety concerns. Mistakes cost the institution more resources. If harm is caused by improper care delivered to the patient, the institution will likely be liable for damages incurred because of the services provided. Many examples like this are routine occurrences at every provider level—from physicians to nurses to pharmacists to housekeepers—in today's health-care systems.

To minimize the waste in hospital resources from scenarios similar to the above, we must focus on the level of staff training and development. To yield a significant return on investment in staff training and development, we must make sure that training is conducted properly. Otherwise, it becomes another mandatory activity to prevent its reoccurrence. We will discuss the business case for necessary staff development and training later in the chapter.

One might argue, "Why do we need staff development when most pharmacists are required to complete continuing education on a regular basis to keep a license active?" Many pharmaceutical companies provide dinner meetings as a method to present information on new products or as part of annual or semiannual professional association gathering. It would appear that pharmacists have more than enough learning opportunities and should be familiar enough with new information to apply it on-the-job. However, many of these learning opportunities are random, fragmented, and not focused on key elements of the pharmacists' day-to-day activities. In many cases, the subject matter does not build on current levels of practice, and consequently connecting the dots with the organizational objectives becomes a challenge.

An additional point for consideration is that all pharmacists do not learn at the same pace and do not retain the same degree of information received. Moreover, even if every pharmacist within a single pharmacy department attended the same continuing education program, there is no guarantee that each program provides a competency demonstration requirement based on the hospital's practice environment. At best, most continuing education programs require some form of a posttest. When the pharmacists encounter a subsequent patient situation, there is no guarantee that the information obtained from the program will apply to the patient's situation, and even so patient care variations exist. Patient care variations may not be bad, but they can make the care provided by the department inconsistent, which will create performance gaps.

Consider learning a specific subject in college in which lectures are given routinely, and each new lecture builds on the previous lecture. There are homework or practice sessions out of the classroom, and students are tested at a regular interval to ensure that an expected level of knowledge is instilled. The earned knowledge, coupled with the practice opportunities, becomes the intellectual property of the individual. The application of this intellectual capital drives the quality of pharmacy care.

Now contrast the classroom experience with learning associated with continuing education. Even the most self-disciplined pharmacist, who religiously attends continuing education programs, cannot be guaranteed of the ability to apply the information obtained from the respective educational offering. Furthermore, most participants forget the majority of the information once they leave the presentation.

Unlike the continuing education program, staff development and training is structured in a way that achieves specific goals of the pharmacy department or a person's specific career goals. Staff development must be planned for, well coordinated, and should be based on the departmental or personal goals. One of many ways to plan for the pharmacy department's staff development and training program is to begin with the organizational goals and objectives. Table 14.3 depicts the organizational goals of the ABC Hospital for the current year.

Once the pharmacy director receives the organizational goals, he or she must review what the pharmacy department can contribute to the organization's goals. The pharmacy

Table 14.3. Organizational Goals of ABC Hospital for the Current Year

1. Achieve 90th percentile of the benchmark score with similar size and services hospitals on the publicly reported quality core measures for heart failure, heart attack, pneumonia, and surgical care improvement prevention.
2. Improve patient safety by reducing adverse events by 10 percent.
3. Reduce resource consumption for surgical patients by 5 percent of total costs.
4. Reduce the average length of stay for psychiatric patients by one day compared to the previous year baseline performance.
5. Achieve outpatient revenue growth to 35 percent of total organizational revenues.

Table 14.4. Pharmacy Department Practice Ideas to Support the Organizational Goals of ABC Hospital for the Current Year

1. Achieve the publicly reported quality core measures for heart failure, heart attack, pneumonia, and surgical care improvement prevention of 90th percentile.
   * Improve the use of angiotensin inhibitors for both heart attack and heart failure patients at patient discharge.
   * Improve the use and documentation of flu and pneumococcal vaccines for pneumonia patients.
   * Make sure antibiotics are used appropriately for pneumonia patients and in surgical prophylaxis.
2. Improve patient safety by reducing adverse events.
   * Streamline drug therapy for poly-pharmacy patients.
   * Implement anticoagulation service to reduce adverse drug events.
3. Reduce resource consumption for surgical patients by 5 percent.
   * Improve prophylactic antibiotic usage and maximize their discontinuation within 24 hours for surgical procedures.
   * Maximize the conversion of IV therapy to PO therapy.
4. Reduce the average length of stay for psychiatric patients by one day.
   * Streamline the psychiatric patient's medications.
5. Achieve the outpatient revenues growth by 5 percent.
   * Implement outpatient medication therapy management.

director will then meet with his or her management team to brainstorm ideas to support the organizational goals. Table 14.4 provides a list of how the pharmacy department could support the organizational goals. After ideas are generated, the pharmacy management team can prioritize the suggestions. The prioritization should be based on an idea's quality impact to the patient care and the financial impact to the institution. Once the ideas have been prioritized, they become the goals of the pharmacy department. Table 14.5 depicts an example of the pharmacy department goals for the current year.

Based on the goals established, the pharmacy department will begin developing training modules and will formalize implementation procedures for the pharmacy staff. The department will also begin measuring a baseline level for each of these initiatives.

Table 14.5. ABC Hospital Pharmacy Department Goals for Current Year

1. Establish an outpatient anticoagulation clinic to increase pharmacy revenues by 1 percent of annual pharmacy revenues.
2. Implement inpatient anticoagulation services to reduce adverse events documented by anticoagulation by 50 percent.
3. Implement appropriate antibiotic review program to ensure antibiotics are used appropriately 100 percent.
4. Implement an IV therapy to PO therapy switch program.

As illustrated above, the staff development program for the purpose of this discussion employs goals 1 and 2. The staff development objectives will provide the knowledge and skill for staff to monitor anticoagulation therapy while also providing outpatient anticoagulation services.

The next step in the process is to assess the learning style of the staff members. If this is the first staff development program, direct discussions with the staff will help design a program that will be most beneficial to all participants. Some staff may learn better through books, some may receive better instructions through multimedia, whereas others may be better learners through active involvement in the learning activity. Nevertheless, the style of learning for adults is important.

Traditional classroom style learning is outdated and not suitable to staff development because we cannot put the department's workload on hold to allow the staff to attend the necessary classes. More likely, the staff development program will take the shape of self-learning modules and case studies with demonstrated competency and directly supervised practice for an initial set of patients being cared for. Of all these activities, the staff demonstrated competency to provide vital care, and the care provision should be consistent among all pharmacists within the department. Once the completion of the training modules is completed, each pharmacist should also be coached by the pharmacy experts. In many instances, the person who supervises the trainees is the clinical coordinator or other type of clinical practitioner.

This type of staff development does not come without associated costs and requires an extensive work force. However, the outcomes are significantly better than with continuing education. Pharmacists will become more satisfied with their jobs, productivity will increase, and patient care will improve. As the program grows, the pharmacy director may be able to justify more staff based on the reduction in adverse events or increases in outpatient anticoagulation service revenues.[28] The program, if planned appropriately, should yield a significant return on investment.

Staff Development in Form of Personal Career Development

Staff development can also be used as a form of career development—either voluntary or involuntary. The involuntary form of career development is used when a staff member shows deficiencies in his or her performance. A structured development plan will be created between the staff member and the department manager (on behalf of the department) to improve performance. A timeframe, 90–180 days, is often deemed necessary to correct the deficiencies. The plan should include measurable goals and performance metrics to assess the success of the program. Failure to meet all the requirements stated in the plan will lead to disciplinary actions or relief from current duties. It may sound unpleasant, but this type of corrective staff development is essential for the pharmacy department to provide consistent quality patient care.

To facilitate this type of staff development, the pharmacy leader must communicate his or her vision of the department, the performance expectation, and the measurements of performance. The review of performance should take place at routine intervals, such as 90 days, for all employees in the pharmacy department. Positive feedback and improvement opportunities should be discussed with each employee. If necessary, the above-mentioned staff development plan should be put in place. This is a powerful way of developing the staff. However, this evaluation must be consistent to avoid employee grievances and frustration. The measurements being used within the evaluation have to be fair and attainable.

Another type of staff development is for the career growth of particular individuals within the department. This person may aspire to move up within the department or organization or to become specialized in a designated area(s) of practice. Formal education may be required, such as the Master of Business Administration or other specialized education programs. In some organizations, a formal mentoring program, which can be found in many progressive organizations, may be available for managers or peak performers who wish to advance. A person who is interested in being mentored will make his or her intention known to the department head or the organization's human resource (HR) department. The HR department, through a formal matching process, might assign a mentor to an individual for a period. Some organizations may require a personality inventory test before assigning a mentor. The results of the personality inventory test will match the personal traits of the mentor with those of the individual being mentored. The individual and the mentor will meet to discuss subjects related to the organization. The individual may spend time shadowing the mentor for a designated period, perhaps a day, a week, or longer. The individual can also ask for advice from the mentor.

Organizations use many methods to identify candidates to succeed the organization's key leaders. The purpose of succession planning is to guarantee that the organizational values are propagated and the legacy continues. Once these individuals are identified, they will go through many skills assessments (e.g., leadership skills, managing finance, project management, etc.). Results from these assessments will be used in the future development of these key leaders. Over the course of several years, these individuals will develop their skills through various organization-sponsored activities. If their performance is not derailed, these individuals will be given first consideration for advancement in the future. This type of staff development is called talent management.

Staff development is essential for the future growth of the pharmacy department. It provides the necessary knowledge for the staff to render quality pharmaceutical services. The alignment of organizational goals with the staff development program is the backbone for staff development and can yield significant results. The pharmacy profession must develop staff. The 2001 Institute of Medicine Report *Crossing the Quality Chasm: A New Health System for the 21st Century* identified that health professionals are not adequately prepared to meet the needs and expectations of the nation's patient population.[29, 30, 31, 32] Americans are becoming more diverse, are expecting more from the practitioners, and are more knowledgeable because of the Internet. The old model of patient-provider relationship will not meet future needs. Recognizing the need to overhaul health professional education, a recent Health Professions Education Summit was held on June 17–18, 2002. Five areas were identified that are related to the training of staff and educating health professionals in the future:

- Provide patient-centered care: identify, respect, and care about patients' differences, values, preferences, and expressed needs.

- Work in interdisciplinary teams: cooperate, collaborate, communicate, and integrate care in teams to ensure that care is continuous and reliable.

- Employ evidence-based practice: integrate best research with clinical expertise and patient values for optimum care.

- Apply quality improvement: identify errors and hazards in care, make improvement as needed.

- Use informatics: communicate, manage knowledge, mitigate error, and support decision-using technology.[33]

Although it is unclear how the formal, academic education will change to incorporate these areas, the practice environment, like the pharmacy department, must embrace these concepts and begin to develop training programs for future students, residents, and staff. If we use quality improvement as a subject, many pharmacists have never been formally trained on all the improvement principles and lead a performance improvement project. Training related to these areas cannot be neglected. Training is the building block for the future of health-care.

Business Case

Today's health-care facilities are facing many challenges, including rising health-care costs, shortage of qualified health-care professionals, cost containment, cost reduction, aging facilities, and increasing public expectation on quality care, to name a few. These challenges have created tremendous pressure for facility administrators to balance the budget while attaining a reasonable margin for future growth of the facility. Therefore, the facility administrators must be selective in investing precious resources. Training and education have been perceived as luxuries that are not essential to the operations. Some administrators still have the notion that they are hiring the most capable and the best people, so they do not believe in training. As cost pressures begin to mount, the first thing cut from the operating budget is the staff training and development programs. This belief is also strengthened by the lack of demonstrated results from the training and development program, such as travel and meetings. For a mid-sized hospital (200–300 beds), the pharmacy department may budget $10,000 for the travel, meetings, and staff development. However, outcome measurements, which adequately demonstrate the value staff members obtain by such funding, have not traditionally been reported to administrators. Therefore, when finances get tight, this line item will be the first cut. Yet residency training programs, student teaching, and staff development and training are vital to our future success in providing quality care to our patients. We have demonstrated the importance of training pharmacy residents, students, and staff members. Several recommendations can make the business case for these training and development programs:

1. Link the staff training and development with specific outcomes. Use the case presented in this chapter. The pharmacy director can measure the adverse events related

to over-anticoagulation and under-anticoagulation and quantify the total costs of no anticoagulation services (benefits assessment) and the costs to provide the services (cost assessment). The net benefits can be calculated by subtracting the costs from the benefits.

2. Measure cost-effectiveness of the department services. Every program in the department should be evaluated for cost-effectiveness on a regular basis. For example, what are the total costs to review medication orders and to enter them into the computer system? How effective is the service? Can we identify any waste (time, people, information, distance, motion, inventory, etc)? By eliminating the waste, the program will become more cost-effective. If the pharmacy director measures the cost and effect of all programs, the pharmacy management team is better able to justify the existence of each program and to provide a ranking of each program based on its cost-effective ratio. The programs with low-ranking numbers must improve or otherwise cease to operate.

3. Profile human intellectual capital (HIC). There are several nontraditional metrics that we can use to evaluate human intellectual capital. Unlike traditional human resources measures, HIC measures quantify the human capital assets of the pharmacy department. We need both sets of measurements to manage human capital.

Traditional Human Resource Measures	Recommended Human Intellectual Capital Measures
• Turnover rates • Vacancy rates • Employee satisfaction • Payroll dollars • Absenteeism • Costs of replacement	• Return on investment of each program • Individual pharmacy employee contribution margin • Total number of years of progressive pharmacy experience of the department • Cost-effectiveness ratio of each pharmacy program including distribution functions • Number of adverse events that can be avoided with pharmacist interventions • Pharmacist's impact on publicly reported quality measures

With the measurements from both columns, pharmacy management can articulate the value proposition for the pharmacy services being provided. If a pharmacy program is not having an appropriate impact on patient care, the pharmacy director should eliminate the program before being asked to do so. For example, during the 1980s, aminoglycosides uses were high, and many dosing regimens were irrational. Many pharmacy departments implemented pharmacokinetics dosing programs as a way for the pharmacy department to better coordinate the cost-effective use of aminoglycosides. With the arrival of newer antibiotics in many hospitals, the use of aminoglycosides has been reduced, and the pharmacokinetic dosing services are not having the impact today that they had previously. The pharmacy director must decide whether a pharmacokinetic service for aminoglycosides is still warranted.

The pharmacy profession cannot afford not to train their staff. If we fail to train staff properly, we fail our patients through our inability to provide cost-effective quality care.

Conclusion

The literature is filled with various attempts to define the term *profession*, and as evidenced by the various sections of the current chapter, the attainment of knowledge and the ongoing effort to obtain additional knowledge to carry out professional activities is an important issue for the pharmacy. According to the *Encyclopedia of Education,* the five criteria necessary for a profession include: (1) Performance of an essential social function, (2) The requirement of a lengthy period of training and experience, (3) The respective practitioners are service oriented, (4) There is the official recognition of the professional status by the government, and (5) The profession has standards of competence.[34]

The British ethicist Paul Rowbottom also suggested six characteristics for the recognition of a profession: (1) a body of knowledge, (2) which has practical applications (technology); (3) exclusive competence—that is, the knowledge and technology are too complicated to be employed by the laity; (4) the profession must develop and transmit its own knowledge; (5) practitioners accept a service ethic; and (6) the profession controls the entry of its members.[35]

The authors have provided in this chapter a series of challenges, suggestions, and warnings regarding a key characteristic found in most respectable definitions of a *profession.* The education of future practitioners, the sharing of knowledge with current practitioners, the transfer of knowledge, the implementation of new skill sets as the occasion rises, and the ability to provide ongoing opportunities for career development have been described as a function of today's practitioners' roles in residency training, student teaching, and staff development. To provide an environment worthy of such activities, today's pharmacy management team must demonstrate the value for such efforts to non-pharmacy leaders, who will require outcomes assessments to allow the performance of such activities.

Pharmacy as a profession will continue to change as the dynamic health-care environment continues to change. Such change requires the ongoing need to adapt our practices to meet the needs of a society, which will expect more and tolerate less. We must continue to invest in our future through the education of our students in the best manner possible. We must continue to identify future leaders to provide them with opportunities through residency training, staff development, and ongoing educational opportunities, which will provide successors in our practice sites. We must look to those within our own institutions for the continued commitment to professional growth that will ensure our next generation of pharmacists a viable, willing, and acceptable place for them to practice.

We have come a long way from the early days in which Whitney worked to create a post-education formal training program for pharmacists. We now must work to see that the level of practice that we expose our future practitioners to represents the level of expectation which our society so badly needs and expects.

Appendix A: List of Recent Publications Describing Benefits of Clinical Pharmacy Practice to Patient Care

1. Kaboli PJ, Hoth AB, Mcclimon BJ et al. Clinical pharmacists and inpatient medical care: a systematic review. *Ann Intern Med.* 2006; 166: 955–64.

2. Schumock GT, Butler MG, Meek PD et al. Evidence of the economic benefit of clinical pharmacy services: 1996–2000. *Pharmacotherapy.* 2003; 23(1): 113–132.

3. Bond CA, Raehl CL, Franke T. Clinical pharmacy services and hospital mortality rates. *Pharmacotherapy.* 1999; 16: 556–67.

4. Lada P, Delgado G. Documentation of pharmacists' interventions in an emergency department and associated cost avoidance. *Am. J. Health Syst. Pharm.* 2007; 64: 63–68.

5. Mutnick A, Sterba K, Peroutka J et al. Cost savings and avoidance from clinical interventions. *Am. J. Health Syst. Pharm.* 1997; 54: 392–396.

6. Scrivens JJ Jr, Magalian P, and Crozier GA. Cost-effective clinical pharmacy services in a veterans administration drop-in clinic. *Am. J. Health Syst. Pharm.* 1983; 40: 1952–53.

7. Chuang LC, Suttan JD, Henderson JP. Impact of the clinical pharmacist on cost saving and cost avoidance in drug therapy in an intensive care unit. *Hosp Pharm.* 1994; 29: 215–21.

8. Bjornson DC, Hiner WO, Potyk RP et al. Effect of pharmacists on health care outcomes in hospitalized patients. *Am J Hosp Pharm.* 1993; 50: 1875–84.

9. Boyko WL, Yurkowski PJ, Ivey MF et al. Pharmacist influence on economic and morbidity outcomes in a tertiary care teaching hospital. *Am J Health-Syst Pharm.* 1997; 54: 1591–5

10. Leape LL, Cullen DJ, Clapp MD et al. Pharmacist participation on physician rounds and adverse drug events in the intensive care unit. *JAMA.* 1999; 282: 267–70.

References

1. Stewart TA. Intellectual capital: the new wealth of organization. New York: Bantam Doubleday Dell Publishing Group, Inc; 1997.

2. ASHP Council on Educational Affairs. http://www.ashp.org/s_ashp/bin.asp?CID=6& DID=4010&DOC=FILE.PDF (accessed on 2007 February 13).

3. ASHP Council on Educational Affairs.<http://www.ashp.org/s_ashp/bin.asp?CID=6& DID=4010&DOC=FILE.PDF (accessed on February 13, 2007).

4. White SJ. Leadership: successful alchemy. *AJHP.* 2006; 63: 1497–503.

5. ASHP Web site. http://www.ashp.org/s_ashp/docs/files/AboutASHP_EarlyYears.pdf (accessed on 2007 February 17).

6. Cortese Annecchini LM, Letendre DE. Funding of pharmacy residency program—1996. *Am J Health-Syst Pharm.* 1998; 55: 1618–9.

7. Miller DE, Woller TW. Understanding reimbursement for pharmacy residents. *Am J Health Syst Pharm.* 1998; 55: 1620–3.

8. News item: One-year hospital pharmacy residencies retain eligibility for special Medicare payment. *Am J Health-Syst Pharm.* 2003; 60: 1933.

9. Stein GC. Battle for funding of pharmacy residency programs. *Am J Health-Syst Pharm.* 2005; 62: 1019.

10. Hoffman JM, Thomley S, Vermeulen L et al. Pharmacy residency training in academic medical centers. *Am J Health Syst Pharm.* 2004; 61: 2528–33.

11. Cortese Annecchini LM, Letendre DE. Funding of pharmacy residency program—1996. *Am J Health-Syst Pharm.* 1998; 55: 1618–9.

12. Accreditation Council For Pharmacy Education. http://www.acpe-accredit.org/pdf/ACPE_Revised_PharmD_Standards_Adopted_Jan152006.pdf (accessed on 2007 February 17).

13. McAllister JC III. What will be your legacy? *Am J Health-Syst Pharm.* 2003; 60: 1625–30.

14. Christel Farthing-Papineau E, Sutton Peak A._Pharmacists' perceptions of the pharmaceutical industry. *Am J. Health-Syst Pharm.* 2005; 62: 2401–9.

15. Young D. Pharmacists should heed antikickback law, experts advise. *Am J Health-Syst Pharm.* 2004; 61: 878–880.

16. Kaboli PJ, Hoth AB, McClimon BJ et al. Clinical pharmacists and inpatient medical care: a systematic review. *Ann Intern Med.* 2006; 166: 955–64.

17. Schumock GT, Butler MG, Meek PD et al. Evidence of the economic benefit of clinical pharmacy services: 1996–2000. *Pharmacotherapy.* 2003; 23(1): 113–132.

18. Bond CA, Raehl CL. Clinical and economic outcomes of pharmacist-managed aminoglycoside or vancomycin therapy. *Am J Health-Syst Pharm.* 2005; 62: 1596–605.

19. American College of Clinical Pharmacy. The strategy plan of the American College of Clinical Pharmacy. ACCP Report 2002; 21(10): S1–7.

20. Accreditation Council For Pharmacy Education. http://www.acpe-accredit.org/pdf/ACPE_Revised_PharmD_Standards_Adopted_Jan152006.DOC (accessed on 2007 February 18).

21. Accreditation Council For Pharmacy Education. http://www.acpe-accredit.org/pdf/ACPE_Revised_PharmD_Standards_Adopted_Jan152006.DOC (accessed on 2007 February 18).

22. Trovato JA, Edwards JM. Education and training of pharmacy students. *Am J Health-Syst Pharm.* 2004; 61: 1956–7.

23. McAllister JC III. What will be your legacy? *Am J Health-Syst Pharm.* 2003; 60: 1625–30.

24. Trovato JA, Edwards JM. Education and training of pharmacy students. *Am J Health-Syst Pharm.* 2004; 61: 1956–7.

25. ASHP Council on Educational Affairs. Education and Traning—Positions. http://www.ashp.org/s_ashp/bin.asp?CID=6&DID=4010&DOC=FILE.PDF (accessed on 2007 February 13).

26. Institute of Medicine. Crossing the quality chasm: a new health system for the 21st century. Washington DC: The National Academies Press; 2001.

27. Greiner AC, Knebel E, eds. Health professions education: a bridge to quality. Institute of Medicine Report: Quality Chasm Series. Washington DC: The National Academies Press; 2003.

28. McDaniel MR, DeJong DJ. Justifying pharmacy staffing by presenting pharmacists as investments through return-on-investment analysis. *AJHP.* 1999; 56: 2230–2234.

29. Cantillon P, Jones R. Does continuing medical education in general practice make a difference? *British Medical Journal.* 1999; 7193: 1276–79.

30. Davis D, OBrien MA, Freemantle N et al. Impact of formal continuing medical education: Do conferences, workshops, rounds, and other traditional continuing education activities change physician behavior or health outcomes? *JAMA.* 1999; 282(9): 867–74.

31. Halpern J. The measurement of quality of care in the veteran health administration. *Medical Care.* 1996; 34(3): 55–68.

32. Pew Health Professions Commission. Critical challenges: revitalizing the health professions for the twenty-first century. San Francisco, CA: UCSF Center for the Health Professions; 1995.

33. Greiner AC, Knebel E, Eds. Health Professions Education: A Bridge to Quality. Washington DC: National Academies Press; 2003, 45–46.

34. Encyclopedia of Education. NY: Macmillan, 1971. p. 432. *Ref. LB15.E47. vol. 3.*

35. Paul Rowbottom in Curtis, Erik K. Defining a profession. *Journal of Arizona Dental Association.* June 2000; 14(12): 5.

Outsourcing Pharmacy Services

Doug Wong

Introduction

Outsourcing the pharmacy department can be one of the most critical decisions a member of hospital administration will make. That decision will certainly have an impact on many aspects of patient care and ultimately patient safety and outcomes. With the explosion of new oncology and biotechnology drugs in the past decade, pharmacy has rapidly become an area of focus for hospital leadership. Outsourcing this clinical area is a decision that should be made through a well-informed process that allows senior leadership to evaluate the benefits and risks of an outsourced relationship and its potential long-term and short-term impact on the quality and efficiency of the pharmacy department. In this chapter we will explore outsourcing of various pharmacy tasks as well as outsourcing of all pharmacy operations. We will review current services and contractual options that are available through outsourced providers, and we will consider how to evaluate the risks and benefits associated with certain contractual arrangements.

Defining Pharmacy Outsourcing

ASHP's Guidelines on Outsourcing Pharmaceutical Services defines *outsourcing* as "a formal arrangement by which a health system contracts with an outside company to obtain selected pharmaceutical services or comprehensive management of the organization's pharmacy."[1]

Functional Outsourcing

Nuclear Radiopharmaceuticals

Radiopharmaceuticals are one of the most commonly outsourced functional areas in pharmacy with close to 90 percent of all radiopharmaceutical doses originating from a radiopharmaceutical outsourced provider. Rigorous environmental standards of practice often make it economically impractical for each facility to provide an appropriate environment. Prior to dispensing these drugs, pharmacists must also be licensed in their state of practice, be classified as an authorized user on a radioactive materials license, and have a minimum of 700 hours total of didactic and clinical experience in the use of radiopharmaceuticals. Because of these challenges, several outsourced providers can deliver a team of specially trained personnel, familiar with the U.S. Department of

Transportation (US DOT) regulations surrounding safe preparation and transport of radioactive materials, ensuring compliance with the US DOT specification 7A testing requirements.

Intravenous (IV) Compounding

IV compounding is another functional area of pharmacy that is occasionally outsourced. These providers typically deliver a range of products, including standard compounded IV admixtures with single or multiple additives, specialty and neonatal parenteral nutrition, cardioplegia solutions, sterile talc, dialysis solutions, and antibiotics. They are delivered in a patient-specific form. Outsourcing this functional area allows the pharmacy to redirect their professional staff to patient-related activities, while reducing drug waste and inventory needs. The cost of this service must be weighed against the potential safety and economic impact of the redirection of staff time.

Clinical Services

Outsourcing of clinical services may be one of the last areas that a pharmacy would consider outsourcing. The patient care aspect of pharmaceutical care is an area in which the profession of pharmacy is continuously expanding. However, several outsourced providers are gaining traction in this area. It appears that this phenomenon is driven by two unique needs: a lack of access to clinical pharmacy personnel in some areas, and specialization. These providers work collaboratively with health systems to manage drug usage, enhance patient safety, and influence the overall cost of care. Often with smaller hospitals, the clinical pharmacist will be available on a part-time basis to complete a host of activities related to the Pharmacy and Therapeutics (P&T) Committee and required activities for compliance with the Joint Commission on Accreditation of Health System Organizations. In addition to these activities, the clinical pharmacist will typically educate the existing professional staff and coordinate a drug-monitoring and intervention program through the current staff. Activities can include the following:

Clinical Activities

Intervention Activities	**Documentation**
IV to oral conversion	Intervention activity
Renal dosage adjustment	ADE, DUE, and DSE reporting
Culture and sensitivity report analysis	Credentialing
Monitoring Activities	**Miscellaneous**
Adverse drug events (ADE)	Physician rounding
Drug usage evaluation (DUE)	Newsletter generation
Disease state evaluation (DSE)	Drug information services
Cost Containment	P&T Committee meeting preparation
Formulary development and management	
Dosing guidelines and protocols	

Packaging Services

In recent history there has been tremendous pressure applied to health-care organizations (HCOs) from third-party payers to increase patient safety using barcode technology. This has been a challenge for many pharmacies, where many doses do not come from the pharmaceutical manufacturer with a barcode at the dose level, and the pharmacy lacks the infrastructure and technology to label these doses. Subsequently, numerous HCOs have turned to vendors for solutions. These vendors provide solutions that range from onsite software packaging and labeling systems to offsite production of low unit of measure machine-readable barcodes in a variety of formats. Numerous vendors provide ready pouches for dispensing robots and packaging machines that can package runs on 300–500 different formulary items on demand. Offsite products are packaged in a cGMP (current good manufacturing practice) environment according to strict FDA guidelines. Offsite production by vendors is typically only for products with high volume, because FDA guidelines require a shorter expiration date on these items.

After Hours Order Entry

A growing area of interest in the outsourcing market is the provision of after-hours order entry service. The shortage in pharmacists in the marketplace and the evolution of technology has driven a critical need supported by vendors. These vendors can provide support during times of pharmacist shortage on day or evening shifts and full coverage during hours when the pharmacy is closed, including thorough medication review to comply with *JCAHO* medication management standards. Support is typically driven through a remote site that accesses the pharmacy information system through an encrypted Internet connection. This link can provide remote pharmacists with the ability to access patient medication profiles, allergies, laboratory data, and medical history.

Clinically trained licensed pharmacists review each order for appropriateness and can enter them into the order entry system. This review is essential for safety, quality care, accurate billing, implementation of electronic MAR (medication administration record), automated profile systems, and bar coding.

The American Hospital Association and the American Society of Health System Pharmacists support 24-hour pharmacy services as a best practice. Remote order entry allows orders to be checked by licensed pharmacists every time.

Market Drivers

Health-care organizations may elect to outsource for a variety of reasons. These include addressing regulatory challenges, filling staffing and leadership vacancies, controlling the rising cost of pharmacotherapy, and advancing operational, technological, or clinical initiatives. The most urgent driver is typically lack of compliance in a completed or pending regulatory survey, whereas the most common drivers are staffing and leadership shortages—in addition to the need to control rapidly rising pharmaceutical expenditures.

Organizational and Operational

Staffing Turnover

According the ASHP 2007 national survey of pharmacy practice, the estimated vacancy rate was 6.4 percent of FTE pharmacists and was 4.1 percent of FTE pharmacy technicians nationally.[2] The overall turnover rate for pharmacists was 7.7 percent and 13.6 percent for technicians. For a large pharmacy department with 100 employees, that means working 7 people short on average and recruiting and integrating over 20 new employees into the department in a year's period. The 2006 survey commented that it took approximately 6 months to hire a pharmacist and 1.8 months to hire a technician.[3]

Knowledge of pharmacist job turnover—including its prevalence, the types of employees leaving, and how turnover occurs—is important because the supply of pharmacists is limited and because job turnover is costly to health-care organizations. Organizations lose the efficiency of the person leaving (the "leaver") and incur costs associated with hiring temporary employees and recruiting and training new employees. Also, employees who remain have to work harder to make up for the leaver. The cost of replacing an employee has been estimated to be up to four times the employee's annual salary.[4]

Cost Containment Challenges

- Aging population: More than 75 million people over 55 years old by 2010. By 2030 the U.S. Census Bureau projects more than 25 percent of U.S. population will be 65 years old or greater.

- Use of multiple drugs to treat a single disease.

- Total prescription spend was $252 billion in 2005, growing at 5–8 percent annually. Biotechnology drugs were growing at 17 percent with generics growing at 20 percent.[5]

- Federal forecasters predict that U.S. health-care spending will double by 2016 to $4.1 trillion per year. That's one-fifth of the nation's gross domestic product (GDP). Health spending in 2006 was projected at $2.1 trillion, or 16 percent of the GDP. "There is a relatively modest and stable projection for 2006 to 2016, with an average growth rate of 6.9 percent," John Poisal, deputy director of the National Health Statistics Group at the Centers for Medicare and Medicaid Services (CMS), said during a Tuesday teleconference. He noted that with projected growth rates falling slightly in 2006 and 2007, "that would result in five consecutive years of slowing growth."[6]

- U.S. prescription drug spending should reach $497.5 billion by 2016, more than double the expected level for 2006. Prescription drug spending will grow at an average annual rate of 8.6 percent until 2016. The cost of hospital care is expected to climb to more than $1.2 trillion by 2016, versus $651.8 billion expected for 2006. The growth rate for hospital spending is expected to slow, from 7.9 percent in 2005 to 6.6 percent in 2006.[7]

Key Benefits and Risks

An experienced outsourcing vendor can provide a number of benefits. An optimally managed pharmacy department can have a positive impact on nursing, the medical staff, and most importantly the patient. Additionally, time spent by hospital leadership on pharmacy-related issues can decrease dramatically. Finally, the health system can experience many positive financial benefits with strong pharmacy leadership and management.

Their expertise can drive operational efficiency, improve distribution performance, and enhance pharmacy workflow. Management companies also have the personnel and expertise to make changes efficiently without interrupting services. The management company can assist the hospital by staffing hard-to-fill positions, thus allowing the organization to reach optimal staffing levels for achieving productivity targets. Management companies also have the expertise to reduce and maintain the cost of pharmacy services. They shift the cost of employees, benefits, and liabilities to themselves. They also increase the hospital's financial operating margin by purchasing drugs at reduced prices because of volume discounting, improving billing accuracy, reducing drug diversion and pilferage, improving the drug formulary system, and implementing drug inventory management procedures that have been tested. They can also improve the level of pharmaceutical care provided to patients and the support provided to medical and nursing staff. The pharmacy management company can also resolve regulatory and accreditation problems relating to pharmacy services and ensure continuing compliance with legal and accreditation rules and regulations.

Contract Negotiations

Term and Termination

Most pharmacy management agreements require the health system to commit to a one- to three-year term. This allows the outsourcing company adequate time to influence pharmacy operations, invest in change management, and recoup their investment for an appropriate return. The pharmacy leader must pay careful attention to the termination clauses in these agreements. Termination for cause usually requires a breach and cure period, whereas termination without cause by the health system can result in penalty fees and the prohibition to hire the current leadership if they are employed by the outsourcing company. It is important to negotiate appropriate terms for hiring these personnel should the health system elect to end the outsourcing contract.

Exclusions

Buyer beware! Exclusions are the most critical area for any HCO to consider when entering into a comprehensive capitated, outsourced relationship. Under a capitated relationship, vendors will not accept risk for certain high-cost existing and future formulary items. This is reasonable on their part; however, the structure of the contract as it relates to exclusions, price increases, and risk sharing becomes critical to determining the financial success of the contractual relationship for both the vendor and the HCO.

Evaluating Providers

Understanding the selected vendor's capabilities, history, and resources will enable the pharmacy leader to make an informed decision about this critical partner. Below is a list of preliminary questions that should be asked of the vendor during the request for proposal (RFP) process and during the final interview and negotiation process.

How long have they been in business?

How many HCOs are they currently serving?

What is their average contract tenure?

What is their average annual contract renewal rate?

How many clients have chosen to terminate their agreements in the past three years, and may those clients be contacted to understand their reasons?

What is their performance record on regulatory surveys (Board of Pharmacy, JCAHO, CMS, FDA, etc.)?

What human resources does the vendor have in new operations? Who will be responsible for the initiation of the contractual relationship?

Who will the director of pharmacy report to at the vendor? Request the résumé of this person.

References

1. American Society of Health System Pharmacists. ASHP Guidelines on outsourcing pharmaceutical services. *Am J Health-Syst Pharm.* 1998; 55: 1611–7.
2. Pedersen CA, Schneider PJ, Scheckelhoff DJ. ASHP national survey of pharmacy practice in hospital settings: Prescribing and transcribing—2007. *Am. J. Health Syst. Pharm.,* May 2008; 65: 827–843.
3. Pedersen CA, Schneider PJ, Scheckelhoff DJ. ASHP national survey of pharmacy practice in hospital settings: Dispensing and administration—2005. *Am. J. Health Syst. Pharm.,* Feb 2006; 63: 327–345.
4. Mott DA. Pharmacist Job Turnover, Length of Service, and Reasons for Leaving, 1983–1997. *Am J Health-Syst Pharm.* 2000; 57: 975–984.
5. Hoffman JM, Shah ND, Vermeulen LC, et al. Projecting Future Drug Expenditures— 2007. *Am J Health-Syst Pharm.* 2007; 64: 298–314.
6. Gardner A. U.S. Health-Care Costs to Top $4 Trillion by 2016. http://www.washingtonpost.com/wp-dyn/content/article/2007/02/21/AR2007022100524.html (accessed 2007 February 21).
7. Borger C, Smith S, Truffer C et al. Health Spending Projections Through 2015: Changes On The Horizon. *Health Affairs.* 2006; 2: 25: w61–w73 doi: 10.1377/hlthaff.25.w61.

Building the Financial Plan for a New Pharmacy Service

Paul W. Bush

Introduction

Expansion of pharmacy services requires dedication of resources, equipment, or facilities. Whether it is a new service, additional space, equipment, personnel or a renovation, developing a written business plan will communicate the proposal, secure funding, guide the initiative, and keep it on track.

Health-care organizations use a standardized approach to allocating resources. The organization's annual planning cycle usually includes a segment dedicated to receiving requests for major new programs, projects, and equipment. These requests are categorized by type and size of the investment and then reviewed by health system leadership and budget review committees.

A key to success in acquiring new resources is the ability to communicate the value of the proposal clearly to the organization. This is accomplished through the development of a business plan. The business plan is a document with a standard format and structure that clearly explains the what, why, when, who, and how of the project. It is a comprehensive explanation of the opportunity, the people involved, the money required to implement the plan, where the resources will come from, and what financial results the opportunity is likely to produce.[1]

This chapter describes the process for developing, writing, and presenting a business plan.

The Business Plan Process

There are six basic steps to the business plan process:

1. Conceptualizing the initiative
2. Researching the feasibility and details of the concept
3. Evaluating and refining the concept based on data obtained
4. Outlining the plan
5. Preparing the business plan document
6. Presenting the plan

Conceptualizing the Initiative

Health care and the profession of pharmacy continue to evolve in the pursuit of improving the public health. The many unmet health-care needs and the extremely high cost of treating disease, linked with the important role medications play in improving patient outcomes, results in many opportunities for new pharmacy programs and services. Developing a business plan for a new pharmacy service begins with a thorough understanding of current services and their adequacy to meet the needs of the patient and the organization. New or expanded services fill the gaps in existing services, improve access, or add new services. A needs assessment conducted during the planning process may result in identification of multiple opportunities for the department. Through the planning process, the pharmacy department will identify and then prioritize the most important opportunities to address. Typical initiatives identified through the planning process may include addition of pharmacist staff to participate in the medication reconciliation process, expansion of repackaging capabilities to support a bar-coded medication administration program, or the opening of a new ambulatory pharmacy. Each initiative begins as a concept that may result in a business plan and eventually provide a new service.

Researching the Feasibility and Details of the Concept

Developing a business plan is more of a business research project than a writing assignment.[2] A successfully prepared business plan will contain extensive background information and have a clear and comprehensive description of the program or service. A thorough review of published literature describing similar programs or services should be conducted. In many cases, recent programs may not be well documented in the literature, so communication among hospital pharmacy leaders and site visits to learn about the program may be an alternative. Another source of information on programs and services and their value are white papers or best practice guidelines published by national health-care organizations, such as the Joint Commission, the Health Care Advisory Board, American Society of Health-System Pharmacists, American Pharmaceutical Association, or the American College of Clinical Pharmacy.

Evaluating and Refining the Concept Based on Data Obtained

Once the research and data collection process is underway, the information gained should be used as a basis for evaluating the feasibility of the concept. The concept should be reassessed and modified to ensure a good fit for the organization and the success of the initiative. A thorough evaluation at this stage of plan development is time and effort well invested, because concepts and proposals that do not show sufficient merit and return on investment will be deferred or eliminated and viable initiatives will be pursued.

Outlining the Business Plan

The business plan is composed of several sections addressing specific aspects of the plan and operation. Plans used for departments within health systems will not contain all components or the depth of detail included in the plan for a new stand-alone business. The readers of the plan will have an understanding of the health-care organization and current role of the pharmacy service. The plan for a new pharmacy service should include the following sections:

I.   Cover Page
II.   Table of Contents
III.   Executive Summary
IV.   Description of the Proposed Program or Service
V.   Consistency with the Organization's Mission
VI.   Market Analysis
VII.   Marketing Plan
VIII. Facility and Equipment
IX.   Management and Organization
X.   Financial Summary
XI.   Evaluation

Preparing the Business Plan Document

I.   Cover Page

The first page of the business plan is the cover page. This page should include the following information: name of the plan, month and year the plan was prepared, and name and contact information of the preparers.

Example:

Business Plan
For
Medical Center North Pharmacy

Plan prepared February 2008

Paul W. Jones, Pharm.D.
Director of Pharmacy Services
Department of Pharmacy Services

Logo

II. Table of Contents

The table of contents provides an overview and easy access to reports contents.

III. Executive Summary

The executive summary is the most important section of the business plan. It must be clear, succinct, and written with adequate enthusiasm to compel readers to review the entire document. It is brief, 1–3 pages in length, and written in narrative style, drawing information from each section of the business plan. The summary should be written after the entire plan is complete. It should demonstrate that the plan makes sense, is thoughtfully and thoroughly researched and written, can be accomplished by the pharmacy team, meets an organizational need, and is financially viable. An example of an executive summary is included in Appendix A, the Medical Center North Pharmacy Business Plan.

IV. Description of Program and Services

The first major section of the plan provides an overview of the program or service proposed. For example, if the pharmacy manager proposes to open a new ambulatory pharmacy, this section should include a description of the location, scope of services provided, benefits, staff involved, differentiating factors, and rationale, and reference other organizations that have similar pharmacies. If this is the first ambulatory pharmacy for the health system, information describing the prevalence of ambulatory pharmacy services in other similar organizations and rationale for a health system providing this service should be included.

Background information describing the anticipated start date, financial and volume trends, and previous program history should also be included in this section of the plan.

V. Consistency with Mission

This section of the business plan explains how the proposed program serves to support the mission, philosophy, and strategic objectives of the health system. Aligning departmental programs and services with the health system is a necessary attribute and provides greater potential for approval, and subsequent program success. Given the finite nature of financial resources, a major consideration in new program development is cost of the program and return on investment. This, and other positive impacts on organizational performance, should be stated clearly. If there are ethical issues to address, they should be discussed in this section of the plan. Finally, the role the program may play in meeting the needs of the community or special needs of specific providers or patients should be addressed.

VI. Market Analysis

When deciding to propose the new program, the pharmacy leader operates under the premise that the new program will provide a service for which there is a need. Communication of this identified need is a key objective of a business plan. The business plan should clearly identify the market (i.e., group of customers with a set of common characteristics who want to buy the service) for the services of the new program. This is the section of the plan where the market, barriers to market entry, and projected trends are discussed. Included should be a description of how the market research was done and with what resources.

A statement should define the customer profile or target population of customers who may want to buy the services (or products). The demographics of the market, the primary and secondary geographic areas served, the referral sources, the historical and projected market size, and the potential market growth rates should be discussed. Key service characteristics, including level of service and quality measures planned, should be described. The economics of the market should be included if applicable to the service provided, by including a discussion of price sensitivity and current and future reimbursement. If there is substantial competition in the market for the proposed service, the plan should address it candidly, directly, and in detail.

Disclosure of possible barriers to market entry and how they will be addressed should be included in this section. Barriers to discuss may include licensure, professional, business, and other regulations, the potential antititrust implications, needed technology, pharmaceutical pricing, and availability of staff. A statement on how well the program can serve the proposed market in terms of resources, strengths, and weaknesses will reinforce the proposal.

Investment in the business plan will be dependent upon continued success in future years. A business plan should include a discussion of the market trend over the ensuing five years. Include the clinical, technological, reimbursement, and site aspects. As an example, new technology may bring new products or services into the marketplace that may affect the new program positively or negatively.

VII. Marketing Plan

A good marketing plan is essential to business development and success.[3] The plan to inform potential customers of the new service and ongoing marketing efforts should be described in the business plan. The initial focus of the marketing plan will be to introduce the new service. The marketing plan for programs that provide services to various groups will include an overall strategy and may include tactics for each target group. Collateral materials and media should be described to provide additional insight on how the new service will be promoted. A schedule for introducing the new service and promoting it should be included, as well as a general plan for tracking results of the marketing effort.

VIII. Facility, Technology, and Equipment

Many new pharmacy services require additional facilities or modification of existing facilities. In the health system environment, securing space may be as challenging as obtaining the commitment of financial resources. The plan should indicate the planned location and availability, including the square footage and a description and schematic of the layout. The extent and plan for construction or renovation should be discussed. In addition to office fixtures and equipment, technology, such as computer software and hardware, point-of-care diagnostic instruments, or robotic dispensing devices, should be described. Refer to the appendix for an example of the scope and level of detail required.

IX. Management and Organization

Most new pharmacy programs or services will report directly to the leadership of the department of pharmacy services. A pharmacy department may have divisions in one or more legal entities of the health system (i.e., not-for-profit or for-profit, inpatient, ambulatory services, or home care divisions), and the type of new program or services may dictate in which legal entity it will reside. The business plan should clearly indicate the capabilities and expertise of the department's management team and how the new program will be overseen. The department organizational structure should be provided as a diagram with the new program and line of authority highlighted. If the plan calls for new managers, pharmacists, or support staff, availability of staff and the timing of adding them to the payroll should be discussed. A staffing plan should be developed and included in this section of the business plan. Contractual relationships, such as contracted staffing or repackaging agreements, should be described. The impact that the new program will have on other programs and services within the department and outside the department should be discussed.

An implementation plan with a timetable indicating key milestones should be developed and provided in this section of the business plan. The overall size and complexity of the project will influence the scope of the implementation plan.

X. Financial Summary

This section of the business plan summarizes the financial information provided in appended tables, spreadsheets, and graphs. Guidelines to consider in preparing the financial forms include: be conservative, be candid, use standard formats and financial terms, be consistent, and seek the advice of the financial services staff. The actual expenses and revenues are of primary interest, although costs avoided by implementation of the program may be included if clearly indicated.

The type of new program will dictate which forms to include. Health system-based proposals often include a start-up expense budget; staffing budget (based on the staffing plan); projected payer mix; a three-year pro forma income (profit and loss) statement showing volumes, expenses, and revenues; and assumptions. The narrative content of this section of the business plan should provide adequate detail such that review of the financial forms is optional.

XI. Evaluation

The performance of the new program or service that prompted development of the business plan should be monitored closely during the first year to make programmatic adjustments to ensure success. In developing the concept and business plan, many assumptions were necessary, and adjustments may need to be made. The business plan should include the performance indicators and frequency of monitoring. Suggested indicators include financial, clinical, market, and customer satisfaction. Successful performance of certain indicators may be critical for program success, and their performance should be closely monitored and may be chosen for a quarterly report to the director of pharmacy and administrator. The health-care organization's leaders may be supportive and willing to approve programs that include criteria for program success (and continuance).

Presenting the Plan

The plan should be a formal document that has been edited and proofread carefully by more than one person. Be sure that the language is clear and the graphs and charts enhance the message. Several texts devoted to developing business plans provide guidance on layout design and presentation.[4] Using both black and white and color in the document will improve the presentation. Binding the plan will give it a polished, complete look.

Many health-care organizations have new program budget review committees that convene to hear the presentation of new program requests. A well-prepared slide presentation based on the business plan is generally an expectation of an internal budget review committee. A copy of the business plan should be available to each member of the committee before the meeting. Meetings with key members of the committee or other organizational stakeholders such as members of the medical staff, nursing leadership, or specific program leadership should also be considered to build support and to receive input regarding the focus of the plan and presentation.

Conclusion

Many factors contribute to acceptance of new program business plans. The organization's availability of funds and current funding preferences and needs will be overriding factors. A well-done business plan is important—and in many organizations critical—to gaining approval for programs that require significant resources.

Appendix A
Sample Business Plan for an Ambulatory Clinic Pharmacy

References

1. Schumock GL, ed. How to develop a business plan for clinical pharmacy services: a guide for managers and clinicians. Kansas City, KS: American College of Clinical Pharmacy; 2001.
2. Abrams R, ed. The successful business plan: secrets and strategies. Palo Alto, CA: The Planning Shop; 2003: 13.
3. US Small Business Administration. How to write a business plan. www.sba.gov/idc/groups/public/documents/sba_homepage/pub_mp32.pdf (accessed July 29, 2008).
4. Abrams R, ed. The successful business plan: secrets and strategies. Palo Alto, CA: The Planning Shop; 2003.

Appendix: Sample Business Plan

Medical Center North Pharmacy Business Plan

Proposed on March 1, 2008
By Paul W. Bush

Medical University of South Carolina (MUSC)
Medical Center North Pharmacy
Table of Contents

Medical Center North Pharmacy
Executive Summary

Purpose of the Business Plan

This business plan was created to secure commitment and funding to open a multifunctional pharmacy operation in the Medical Center North Building to serve our patients and employees.

Background

The pharmacy will be located on the first floor of the Medical Center North located in North Charleston. It will be positioned adjacent to the entrance for easy recognition and accessibility. The pharmacy will dispense prescriptions, compound chemotherapy and intravenous admixtures, and provide pharmacotherapy services.

An outpatient pharmacy located in this medical center will augment the department's goal of providing optimal pharmaceutical care, increasing accessibility to pharmacy services, advancing pharmaceutical knowledge, and promoting enhanced patient outcomes. Achieving these goals supports the organization's MUSC Excellence pillar goals.

The Market

With pharmaceutical spending increasing at a rate of more than 8 percent in 2007, there is substantial growth in the industry, which will fuel sustained profit for this pharmacy. There are currently no other pharmacies in the area providing pharmacotherapy services or capable of compounding the chemotherapy our patients need. The Medical Center North Pharmacy will offer differentiated services that satisfy patient needs.

Organization

The pharmacy will have a pharmacy coordinator, who works in the pharmacy on a regular basis and who is responsible for operating the pharmacy on a daily basis. This coordinator will report to the manager of ambulatory pharmacy services, who directly reports to the MUSC director of pharmacy services. The initial staff necessary for the daily operations of this pharmacy includes two pharmacists and two technicians.

Finances

The initial cost to develop the facility and open the Medical Center North Pharmacy is $460,000. Based on five-year amortization of start-up expenses, the pharmacy will be profitable by the end of the first year. A conservative estimate of the return on this investment would be an annual profit of $275,000 beginning in year 2.

Conclusion

The addition of a MUSC ambulatory pharmacy at the Medical Center North will not only provide additional revenue for MUSC, but also, and more importantly, it will better serve our patients and our employees.

Medical Center North Pharmacy
Business Plan

Description of the Medical Center North Pharmacy

The Medical Center North is a new facility located on Highway 78 just off I-26 that provides residents convenient access to MUSC's comprehensive medical expertise and vast health-care resources. The Medical Center North Pharmacy will be located on the first floor of the Medical Center North facility, adjacent to the entrance and across from the waiting room. The pharmacy will provide outpatient prescriptions and over-the-counter medications for patients visiting this medical center, as well as MUSC employees, staff, and students; will provide pharmacotherapy services for patients seen by physicians of the medical center; and will provide compounded chemotherapy for the planned outpatient oncology clinic.

Establishing a pharmacy in the Medical Center North will provide MUSC patients who visit this facility a convenient location to fill their prescriptions. The pharmacy will also provide MUSC employees, staff, and students, who live in the North Charleston area, a local MUSC pharmacy where they can fill their medications. This location will use the Public Health Services 340B prescription pricing that is currently used by the other MUSC ambulatory pharmacies. The provision of pharmacotherapy services at this facility will also offer a convenient location for MUSC patients to meet with a pharmacist to have their medications managed. With the opening of an outpatient oncology clinic in the Medical Center North, a need for chemotherapy arises. The pharmacy in this center will be capable of compounding chemotherapy and other parenteral medications needed by the oncology clinic.

The Medical Center North Pharmacy will require a full-time coordinator and part-time pharmacist and two full-time technicians to fill prescription medications and over-the-counter requests and to compound chemotherapy infusions. In addition, an ambulatory clinical pharmacist specialist will provide pharmacotherapy services on specified days and for specified times. In the event that the demand for pharmacotherapy services requires a full-time pharmacist, the addition of another pharmacist to this facility will be considered.

The Medical Center North Pharmacy will differentiate itself from other area pharmacies through several services. It will establish a convenient location where MUSC patients can fill their outpatient prescriptions. It will also access MUSC's electronic documentation systems, which will allow pharmacists to double-check the strength, dosage form, and appropriateness of a prescription before dispensing. Through the network of MUSC ambulatory pharmacies, patients will have access to medications that are not commonly stocked in the retail chain pharmacies because of high inventory-carrying costs and low demand. There are currently no pharmacies in the area that offer pharmacotherapy services, and, with reimbursement of medication therapy management services for Medicare patients, our pharmacotherapy services can be extended to more disease state management through collaboration with MUSC physicians. Lastly, no outpatient pharmacies in the area support chemotherapy infusion services.

We will benchmark our services based on our other outpatient pharmacies and in comparison to other University HealthSystem Consortium member outpatient services to ensure that we are optimizing patient care while maximizing profits.

The anticipated opening of Medical Center North Pharmacy is November 1, 2008. Prescription drug expenditures are projected to increase at an annual rate of 8.0–8.4% between 2007 and 2015.[1] The usage of prescriptions has increased 71 percent from 1994 to 2005.[2] MUSC already has three outpatient pharmacies located on the downtown Charleston MUSC campus that have achieved prescription growth of more than 15 percent over the prior year and have generated a significant profit for the organization. The newest pharmacy is located on the first floor of the hospital and has been open for two years. In fiscal year 2007, the MUSC ambulatory pharmacies had a profit of $5.8 million. With experience in outpatient pharmacy services, the pharmacy services department is confident that the pharmacy at the Medical Center North facility will be a sound investment for the hospital.

Consistency with MUSC's Mission

The mission statement of the Department of Pharmacy Services is to work collaboratively with other health-care professionals to provide optimal pharmaceutical care to all patients, to advance pharmaceutical knowledge through educational and scholarly activities, and to promote positive patient outcomes. As part of the clinical services provided by Medical University Hospital Authority, the Medical Center North Pharmacy will provide optimal pharmaceutical care through outpatient dispensing and patient counseling during prescription pickup; provide advanced pharmaceutical knowledge through pharmacotherapy clinics and availability of pharmacists to answer physicians questions at the medical center; and provide a convenient clinic for patients to receive chemotherapy services, thus promoting enhanced patient outcomes.

In promoting MUSC Excellence, the Medical Center North Pharmacy will enhance the pharmacy goals involving the excellence pillars of service, quality, finance, people, and growth. The Medical Center North Pharmacy will enhance service by providing a convenient location for patients to fill prescriptions and to receive pharmacotherapy services and chemotherapy. It will enhance quality, using our electronic technology to ensure the proper medication, dose, and strength are combined with excellent patient counseling. It will enhance finance, by increasing pharmacy revenue through this additional pharmacy location. It will enhance people, by offering a variety of services that require talented and intelligent staff. It will enhance growth, by extending our pharmacy services to a new location in the North Charleston area.

Market Analysis

Our target markets are MUSC patients visiting the Medical Center North and MUSC employees, staff, and students who live in the area. With significant growth occurring in Charleston County in the north area, this area possesses the ability to have a large demand for pharmaceutical services. As of 2000, the North Charleston population accounted for about 39 percent of the total Charleston County population. North Charleston experienced the second largest growth in the county, with a rate of 12 percent between 1999 and 2000, second only to the city of Charleston.[3] In addition to the North Charleston population; the Medical Center North Pharmacy will also serve patients traveling from outside areas, including Goose Creek, Summerville, and St. George. Having a pharmacy to serve those patients visiting the Medical Center North will be beneficial, because they will not have to travel downtown to obtain specialty prescriptions or pharmacotherapy services.

With the aging baby boomer population nationwide, the growth of pharmaceutical spending will remain constant. Ninety-one percent of patients 65 years old and older incurred a drug expense in 2003.[2] Twelve percent of the total population in Charleston County is over the age of 64 years.[3] This population represents a significant target market in our area and a significant revenue generator.

MUSC is the second largest employer in Charleston. We currently employ 7,550 people, second only to the Navy.[3] We would need to consult our human resources department to determine the exact percentage of our employees living in the North Charleston area. The pharmacy would offer services to those employees and students living in the North Charleston area.

Drug expenditures are predicted to increase 5–7 percent in outpatient settings in the year 2008 and increase 14–16 percent in drug expenditures in clinics.[4] Reimbursement continues to be a significant factor in sustaining a profit in outpatient pharmacies. With the advent of Medicare Part D, a larger amount of the United States population over the age of 65 is now insured for pharmaceutical coverage. The medication therapy management services program established by CMS will also reimburse our pharmacotherapy clinic. Figure 16.1 illustrates the breakdown of ambulatory patients by payer type.

Although there are several benefits to opening this pharmacy, several barriers also exist. There are already several established retail pharmacies in the North Charleston area that our potential customers frequent. We would have to secure our potential customers' interest in using our services. By offering fast and convenient service, we have an advantage over

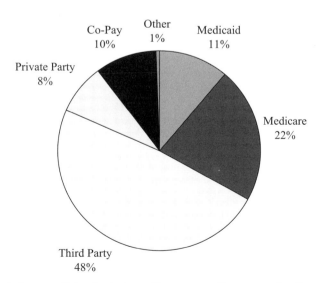

Figure 16.1. Breakdown of Ambulatory Pharmacy Revenue by Payer

the larger retail chains. Through use of our integrated electronic clinical record, we provide superior pharmaceutical counseling to our patients because of our knowledge of their current medication usage and current disease states. Another barrier to entry into the market is obtaining the staff needed for this operation. The pharmacist would need to be qualified in compounding chemotherapy and intravenous admixtures needed by the clinics. We would also have to restructure our current pharmacotherapy clinical pharmacists' schedules so that they could travel to this area to provide a service to these customers. As demand increases, we may hire a full-time pharmacotherapy specialist to work at this clinic. With a shortage of pharmacists and pharmacy technicians, we would have to offer a competitive salary and benefits to recruit for these positions.

In summary, there is a substantial need in the North Charleston area to justify pharmacy services in the Medical Center North and to sustain a profit. With excellent patient counseling, pharmacotherapy services, convenient location for employees and patients, and chemotherapy compounding services, this pharmacy would offer numerous unique and differentiated services to the North Charleston area.

Marketing Plan

With over 7,500 employees at MUSC, 700 hospital beds, 31,274 annual inpatient admissions, and greater than 940,000 outpatient clinic visits annually, there is an established market for outpatient prescription services. To introduce our new services to employees, pharmacy services will inform staff by electronic mail, the MUSC and pharmacy services Web page, and the MUSC newspaper, the *Catalyst*. To introduce our clinic physicians to the pharmacy services provided, pharmacy services will personally contact every practice in the Medical Center North facility and describe our services. Contact will be extended using electronic mail, flyers, and personal meetings. To introduce our patients to our services, a banner will be hung at the entrance to the building, flyers will be placed in every physician's office waiting room and at the downtown facilities, and information will be on the MUSC Web site and media services. We will also publicize through local newspapers and radio stations.

We will track our marketing plan results by measuring prescription volume and by collecting customer and employee surveys. Should we not generate the desired prescription volume anticipated, we will increase our radio and newspaper advertisements, increase our pamphlets and flyers available to patients, and use our current MUSC pharmacy staff, social workers, and administrators to increase our verbal communication concerning this pharmacy with patients.

Facility and Equipment

This new pharmacy will consist of areas that include prescription drop-off and pickup counters, patient consultation area, prescription order-entry and filling stations, medication storage, limited over-the-counter medication sales, offices for pharmacy coordinator, two pharmacotherapy exam rooms, staff break room, staff bathroom, and an admixture and anteroom for chemotherapy preparation and intravenous admixtures. See Figure 16.2 for the schematic layout of the clinic floor plan and proposed location of the pharmacy. See Appendix A for a list of fixtures and equipment needed.

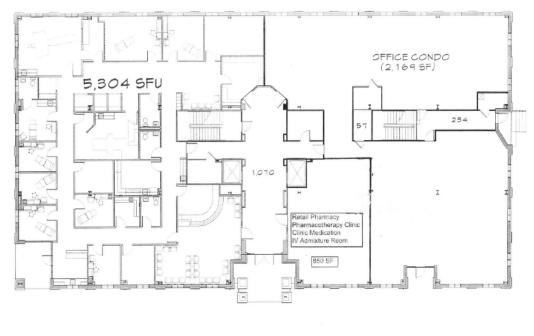

Figure 16.2. Floor Plan

Management and Organization

The Medical Center North Pharmacy will report to the manager of ambulatory pharmacy services, who is responsible for all of the organization's ambulatory pharmacy operations. The organizational structure is illustrated in Figure 16.3. The pharmacy will be supported by the department's administrative staff and an extensive support services staff of procurement, billing and reimbursement, prescription assistance, drug information, and informatics specialists.

The proposed initial staffing plan specifies 3.69 full-time equivalent employees and is illustrated in Appendix B. Initially, the pharmacy will require a pharmacist coordinator and a second part-time pharmacist. The pharmacy will also require two full-time technicians to assist the pharmacist in the pharmacy operations. In addition to staff who will be responsible for the retail and compounding activities of the pharmacy, one of the ambulatory care specialists from the MUSC campus will be assigned to provide pharmacotherapy services two half-days per week. As demand for the pharmacotherapy services increases to the point of needing a full-time clinical specialist at this facility, this position will be requested.

The pharmacy will be open weekdays and a half-day on Saturday. The hours of operation are to be determined based on prescription volume, physician offices hours, and outpatient infusion and oncology clinic chemotherapy needs.

After receiving approval to proceed, a detailed floor plan and construction schedule will be developed. Assuming funding for the project in July 2008, construction and setup of the

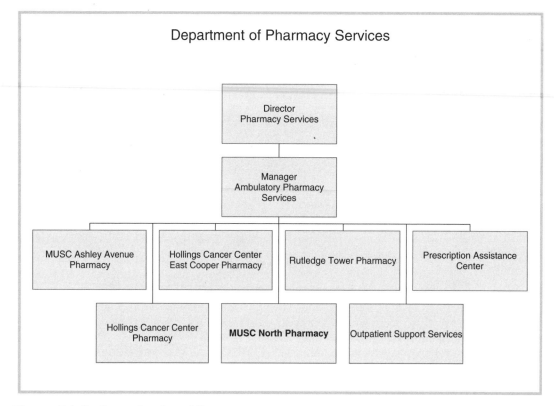

Figure 16.3. Organizational Structure

pharmacy will take approximately four months. The planned opening date of pharmacy would be November 1.

Financial Summary

The initial expenses to develop the site and outfit the pharmacy are estimates based on experience gained in establishing the organization's other ambulatory pharmacies. As illustrated in Appendix C, the major start-up expenses include design and construction costs, fixtures, equipment, software licensing fees, and the opening inventory.

A three-year pro forma income and expense statement is illustrated in Appendix D. Prescription volumes have been conservatively estimated at an average of 70 prescriptions per day for the first year with increases in years 2 and 3. The cost of pharmaceuticals and expected revenue are estimated using an average prescription price of $70 and cost of goods of 70 percent. Over-the-counter medications and convenience and food items will also contribute to the pharmacy revenue.

It is anticipated that chemotherapy will be administered at this site by the medical oncology practice. Pharmacy staff will prepare and deliver the chemotherapy and other medications using inventory provided by the oncology practice. The pharmacy will be reimbursed for the pharmacist and technicians' expense, supplies, and overhead for the equipment used. Although this is represented in the pro forma as an allocated expense, the specifics of the agreement will likely be set up as a fee-based service and described in a service agreement.

The focus of the pharmacotherapy service will initially be patients referred for management of anticoagulation, for which there is a significant demand. Patient visits and reimbursement have been estimated based on experience at the department's other two clinics.

Based on five-year amortization of start-up expenses, the pharmacy will be profitable by the end of the first year. A conservative estimate of the return on this investment would be an annual profit of $275,000 in year 3.

Evaluation

The progress and success of this new pharmacy will be monitored on a quarterly basis through financial, quality, and patient/customer satisfaction ratings. Clinic patient satisfaction will be monitored using the Press Ganey satisfaction survey. Quality control of admixture services will be monitored using the same methods employed in the medical center and cancer center pharmacies. Patient satisfaction with prescription services will be continuously monitored using the Web-based survey methodology employed by the other health system pharmacies.

A consolidated quarterly evaluation report will be prepared by the pharmacy coordinator for review by the department manager and director.

References

1. Borger C, Smith S, Truffer C et al. Health spending projections through 2015: changes on the horizon. *Health Aff.* 2006; 25: W61–73.
2. Kaiser Family Foundation. Prescription Drug Trends. June 2006. www.kff.org (accessed 2008 July 29).
3. Charleston Chamber of Commerce. www.charlestonchamber.net (accessed 2008 July 29).
4. Hoffman J, Shah N, Vermeulen L et al. Projecting future drug expenditures–2007. *Am J Health-Syst Pharm.* 2007; 64: 298–314.

Appendix A. Equipment and Fixtures

Retail Pharmacy Services

Drop-off and pickup counter

Medication storage shelves

Prescription order-entry workstation

Prescription filling station

Access to the QS/1's RxCare Plus pharmacy software

Admixture and Anteroom

Compounding Aseptic Isolator

Compounding Aseptic Containment Isolator

Shelving and medication storage

Computer workstation

Access to Horizon Meds Manager pharmacy software

Pharmacotherapy Counseling/Exam Rooms

Counseling stations

Computer workstation

Point-of-care diagnostic equipment (i-STAT)

Access to PMSI's Practice Partner software

Office/Meeting Room

Office furniture

Computer workstation

Appendix B. Staffing Plan

	S	M	T	W	Th	F	S	S	M	T	W	Th	F	S	FTE	PTO Factor	Total FTE
Coordinator		1	1	1								1	1		0.5	1	0.50
Pharmacists	0	0		0	0	1	1	1	0	1		1	1		0	0	1	0.7	1.1	0.77
Technicians		2		2	2	2	2			2		2	2	2	2		2	1.1	2.20
Clinical Specialist	0	0.5	0	0.5	0	0	0	0	0.5	0	0.5	0	0	0	0.2	1.1	0.22
TOTAL																	3.69

Appendix C. Start-up Expenses

Building Upfit	$300,000
Fixtures	$ 50,000
Software license fees	$ 9,000
Inventory	$ 80,000
Refrigerator	$ 1,200
Computer terminals	$ 3,200
Print server	$ 300
Label printer	$ 300
Laser printer	$ 1,500
Telephone—Multiline (2)	$ 830
Telephone installation	$ 460
Fax Machine/Copier	$ 500
Biological Safety Cabinet (2)	$ 12,000
References/textbooks	$ 500
License and permits	$ 500
Total	$459,290

Appendix D. Three-Year Pro forma Income and Expense Statement

	Year 1	Year 2	Year 3
Prescriptions	19,500	25,000	26,000
Clinic visits	1872	2080	2080
Prescription sales price	$ 70.00	$ 73.50	$ 77.18
Cost of goods sold	70%	70%	70%
EXPENSES			
Salary and wages			
Clinical Specialist (0.2 FTE)	$ 20,000	$ 20,600	$ 21,218
Pharmacist (1.3 FTE)	$ 124,000	$ 127,720	$ 131,552
Technician (2.2 FTE)	$ 64,065	$ 65,987	$ 67,967
Employee Benefits	$ 58,258	$ 60,006	$ 61,806
Salary Allocation to Chemotherapy Infusion	$ (63,033)	$ (64,923)	$ (66,871)
Rent (@$24/square foot)	$ 24,400	$ 24,400	$ 24,400
Software Maintenance	$ 1,500	$ 1,545	$ 1,591
Depreciation and amortization	$ 76,660	$ 76,660	$ 76,660
Utilities	$ 1,800	$ 1,854	$ 1,910
Telephone	$ 3,000	$ 3,090	$ 3,183
Office Supplies	$ 1,200	$ 1,200	$ 1,200
Marketing and advertising	$ 2,400	$ 2,400	$ 2,400
Pharmaceuticals	$ 955,500	$ 1,286,250	$ 1,404,585
OTC Drugs	$ 10,530	$ 15,000	$ 15,000
Medical Supplies	$ 1,200	$ 1,200	$ 1,200
Office Supplies	$ 1,200	$ 1,200	$ 1,200
TOTAL EXPENSES	**$ 1,282,681**	**$ 1,624,188**	**$1,749,000**
REVENUE			
Prescription	$ 1,365,000	$ 1,837,500	$ 2,006,550
OTC Sales	$ 15,000	$ 20,000	$ 20,000
Clinic	$ 56,160	$ 62,400	$ 62,400
TOTAL REVENUE	**$ 1,380,000**	**$ 1,857,500**	**$ 2,026,550**
NET INCOME	**$ 97,319**	**$ 233,312**	**$ 277,550**

Entrepreneurial Opportunities—Beyond Traditional Hospital Pharmacy

Billy Woodward
Sharon Enright

Introduction

Since the 1980s the Medicare cost control strategy, known as the Prospective Payment System, based on diagnosis related groups (DRGs), has created a systematic shift in care from the acute care environment into various ambulatory care settings, including clinics, skilled nursing facilities/long-term care, and home care. With this transition, there has been a growing financial pressure in the inpatient environment, including pharmacy. This pressure has resulted in a succession of fiscal crises as hospitals struggle to deal with a sea of change in payment strategies and tactics. Actions and programs to meet this challenge have included layoffs, budget cutbacks, and various administrative pressures to control costs and to seek new sources of revenue. These efforts often involve waves of consulting engagements designed to help the organization get ahead of the curve of reimbursement change.

As with any challenge, opportunities appear where we least expect them. If progressive managers and professionals are open to change and possess an entrepreneurial spirit, pharmacy can benefit from an unusual opportunity, because drugs and drug therapy are a universal patient requirement throughout the continuum of care. To be an effective financial manager, it is imperative that pharmacy leadership recognize opportunities beyond acute care and become capable of expanding into such practice settings with clinical, operational, and financial success equal to their acute care practice. This chapter is intended to describe such opportunities and discuss some of the unique financial challenges that may be anticipated as one ventures beyond the traditional hospital pharmacy setting.

Every busy pharmacy manager may understandably wonder, "Why expand beyond the daily, endless demands of the typical hospital pharmacy environment? I have more than I can do now, why dilute my efforts in areas outside my core acute care practice?" These are understandable and valid questions, with at least four acceptable answers.

The first answer is simply because it is the right thing to do for patient care. Today's complex health-care system often makes navigating patient transitions from outpatient to inpatient and back to ambulatory settings difficult, frustrating, fragmented, and less than satisfying for the patient and family. Beyond the frustrations associated with this system, it is fraught with the potential for serious error and mismanagement. A pharmacy department that develops the necessary services across the continuum can do much to bridge this gap, improve patient care services, and avoid critical medical and drug therapy errors.

The second answer for taking on such ventures is based upon the reality of today's hospital financial landscape, in which all opportunities that are consistent with the mission of the organization must be exploited. Highly integrated pharmacy departments, such as Scott & White in Texas, have demonstrated this point over the past two decades with expansion into ambulatory clinics, retail, and mail-order pharmacies, managed care pharmacy, home infusion pharmacy, and even a pharmacy benefits management company.[1] As a result of this entrepreneurial expansion, gross pharmacy revenues were four or five times the hospital's historic levels, with net pharmacy revenues equivalent to almost one-fourth of the net revenue of the entire health system.[2] Such revenues proved to be essential both to the success of the health system and to the fiscal credibility of the pharmacy and its leadership.

A third and less obvious answer is that expanding pharmacy practice and related business ventures beyond the hospital setting typically has a dramatic positive and elevating impact on the position of the pharmacy and its leadership within the overall organization. For example, the Scott & White Department of Pharmacy experienced this impact as their expansion positioned the department at the corporate level, where pharmacy leadership was responsible to the administration of all three corporate entities: the hospital, clinics, and health-care plan. Pharmacy leadership interacted with the boards of directors of all three and was able to affect clinical and financial outcomes more expansively than most other hospital departments. The overall pharmacy financial scope grew more than fourfold from the original hospital level, and the number of staff grew from less than 50 to over 250 in 15 years.[3] Because of this scope of responsibility, the influence, financial viability, and effectiveness of pharmacy was elevated within the institution. This was important, not as an ego trip for a few, but rather because it allowed the pharmacy leadership and staff to pursue many of their clinical and patient care goals that would have languished without adequate support.

A fourth answer is that a well-planned entrepreneurial strategy places the pharmacy in a positive building mode that is proactive, rather than supporting a financial status quo, sometimes evolving to a shrinking mode, often the case with today's hospital departments depending on acute care revenues alone. With today's shorter patient stays and increased acuity, there is no shortage of clinical and operational challenges for pharmacy. However, it also seems the hospital is struggling to survive on a shrinking island of reimbursement, in which clinical departments such as pharmacy are daily challenged to deliver optimal care with fewer resources. Expanding beyond traditional pharmacy practice also has the effect of putting pharmacy's financial strategy into a much broader and balanced portfolio of budgets and revenues, much like a diversified portfolio for one's personal investments, which improves the likelihood that in a given budget year, some areas may be growing and seeing improved bottom lines whereas others may be struggling with reduced reimbursement, and so on. The net result is a less crisis-driven, more stable pharmacy financial environment.

It is clear there is a much greater potential for long-term financial success and stability if such an entrepreneurial strategy is embraced with the same vigor as traditional hospital pharmacy services and related financial initiatives.

What's Different about Pharmacy Financial Management beyond the Hospital Setting?

In many ways, the financial management of a pharmacy service is much the same regardless of setting, patient requirements, and unique operational environments. Certainly the fundamentals of budgeting, supply chain management, and fiscal oversight are quite similar, because the basic elements for control, including costs of drugs, operational efficiencies, manpower costs, supplies, equipment, and overhead related to the services are much the same. Each of these elements requires budgeting, procurement, pricing, and inventory control, and management and oversight of all necessary resources. All of the previous chapters within this text, with some adaptation, can be applied in this setting and should be fundamental to any entrepreneurial strategy on the part of pharmacy leadership. There are, however, significant differences in each unique area that will require understanding, assessment, and strategic planning to assure success. Those considerations are described in the following paragraphs.

Competitive Environment and Financial Setting

The competitive environment and financial setting for the new service is an important area of difference. For example, the retail pharmacy environment presents a much different fiscal setting than a hospital. The type of drugs dispensed and managed are quite different, as are patient condition and related drug requirements, cognitive status, out-of-pocket expense issues, reimbursement and pricing strategies, and purchasing conditions. Dispensing typically involves a month's supply of an oral medication directly to the patient for home administration and self-management, which is dramatically different than preparing an intravenous injection for administration by a nurse to a patient in the hospital setting on a 24/7 basis. Certainly the basics of buying the drug, controlling the costs of manpower and related operations, supply chain, and billing concerns are quite similar, but the details and environment are much different. Understanding and adapting to those differences is critical to financial success in each area.

Reimbursement Environment and Approach

Another unique area that presents new challenges is the area of reimbursement for pharmacy services. Today's retail pharmacy adjudicates claims electronically online in real time in a matter of seconds in strict accordance with provider contract parameters, which include patient eligibility, drug coverage, days supply, patient co-pay, and payment schedule, including drugs and related fees. Although such a transaction can be a challenge, given the complexity of many of today's prescription drug plans and pharmacists often must spend far too much time getting the claim to process once the financial process is finished and payment is virtually assured. By contrast, in the hospital setting, each dose administered is billed from pharmacy, typically through the master patient billing system, posted to a cumulative account, and the net financial results of that transaction may not be known for weeks or months. Also in the acute care hospital environment, various reimbursement methodologies may apply, including capitated payment in the form of DRG payments for Medicare patients and discounted payments of billed services based upon managed care or third-party contract terms. This difference becomes complex in areas such as ambulatory clinics, in which reimbursement for drugs may be linked to special Medicare charge codes called J Codes. Reimbursement for home infusion drugs has come under intense scrutiny in recent years, and the challenge of billing appropriately and effectively has become a key to success or failure in this fiscal environment. Many hospital ventures into the ambulatory infusion business have been less than successful because of a failure to address the unique aspects of reimbursement in the ambulatory setting.

Regulatory Environment and Considerations

Another area of significant difference is the regulatory environment, which has financial implications for each pharmacy enterprise. Health care, and pharmacy in particular, has become increasingly subject to regulatory requirements because of the growing percentage of care paid for by various governmental agencies, including Medicare and Medicaid. Even those services not paid for directly by the government are subject to financially significant requirements because of the unique regulations imposed on insurance companies, managed care organizations, health-care entities, and health-care practitioners, including pharmacists. Often such regulation is linked also to reimbursement, so these two areas are often intertwined, although this is not always the case. Complying with regulations not only can affect reimbursement and thus directly affect financial success; it can also affect financial viability because of the level of resources, expertise, record keeping, and legal counsel required to be compliant. It is not unusual in many health-care ventures that regulatory compliance requires that significant manpower, expertise, and related expenditures must be allocated to meet that challenge yet somehow remain profitable. Although many of the regulations pertain to fiscal and reimbursement requirements, civil and even criminal legal penalties exist for infractions, even those that are not intentional. Fraud, waste, and abuse concerns have permeated every sector of health care, and, as a result, the corporate compliance departments in many hospitals have become the fastest-growing departments in the institution.

Operational Basics and Keys to Success

Within every pharmacy business area, there are some basic operational keys to success unique to the area that must be addressed to ensure financial success. These may include seemingly minor considerations, such as physical design detail, inventory savings tips for certain high-volume products, or a vital clause in a managed care contract, to major considerations, such as retail pricing strategy or ways to structure a business to qualify for own-use or 340(b) pricing. Thorough business research should identify many of the keys that could help ensure a faster ROI and ultimate financial success.

Each of these considerations will vary in different pharmacy financial pursuits and must always be researched, understood, and addressed if the entrepreneurial pharmacy leader expects success. Findings and judgments must be weighed to make them a vital part of the strategy and financial plans for that venture.

Research, Groundwork, and Developing a Business Plan

Any new business opportunity in pharmacy will require approval and funding to become a reality. Successful business proposals always start with thorough research and groundwork, which is then folded into a well-written business case that answers the essential financial questions necessary for approval. Too often, promising entrepreneurial concepts fall victim to a weak or nonexistent business case.

Research and Groundwork

Although resources, expertise, and infrastructure necessary to conduct effective research and planning for new business ventures is often lacking in the typical hospital pharmacy department, a thorough effort is critical to determine feasibility and the potential for success. The hospital environment and leadership are often risk adverse, so any departmental leader proposing an entrepreneurial venture will need to come to the table armed with sound research and an impressive business plan. Research fundamental to any venture should consider those variables unique to the proposed business and address the differences previously discussed here in an analytical thought process, including the following:

- Timing and administrative support: Many sound entrepreneurial opportunities fail to come to fulfillment because the pharmacy director does not do the advance development work with administration. This effort should be done discreetly with key leaders whose support will be critical for approval. It must precede the research and detailed groundwork and determine if the level of interest, understanding, finances and other resources are sufficient to warrant making this a strategic priority. In addition to the answers to these individual questions, there can also be a timing issue, in which a great idea cannot get traction simply because of other projects that are already underway. There is an art to this part of pharmacy leadership that must be learned, usually by failing several times and by misreading those signals, while learning to understand how key decision makers react to innovative ideas. Eventually, the successful pharmacy entrepreneur will learn to target the right people, to ask the right questions, to listen closely, and then to read the timing for moving forward with an idea. Some ideas require seeding long before expecting leadership to move forward decisively, and this seeding is part of the entrepreneurial strategy. Most successful entrepreneurs keep several ideas "on the back burner" by periodically mentioning them, assessing response, feeding information about successful examples, and sampling responses from leadership. At the right time, an idea will mature as a viable option, circumstances will change to make it more logical, and the thoughtful pharmacy leader then moves it to the "front burner" to make a proposal. This may sound a little ethereal for the pragmatic pharmacist, but its importance to success is often greater than all the business plans with glossy covers.

- Competitive environment analysis: This research includes an overview of the competitors, their nature, the number, and their advantages and vulnerabilities. This research also considers the overall size of the market in terms of gross dollars and net profits, clients and customers, and growth trends over the past three to ten years. Any external or internal trends that would affect the potential for success or failure should be includeed, as well as how this proposed venture would succeed in such an environment.

- Reimbursement analysis: This research considers the reimbursement issues unique to this business venture, outlining any advantages, leverage, or limitations to be considered. A realistic appraisal of how the reimbursement issues will affect the project and chances for success should be included. Strategies for maximizing any advantages and dealing with the challenges should be a part of this research and should become a fundamental component of the final business plan.

- Regulatory environment investigation: Research that considers the unique regulatory issues associated with this business must be thorough and is as important to success as any other financial factor in the project evaluation. An example in today's retail pharmacy marketplace would be the important role of Medicare Part D regulations and reimbursement and how they will affect the financial viability of any venture. In addition to the impact of provider contract reimbursement, regulatory environment investigation would also include the impact of Part D on Medicaid prescription volumes and market changes on the new plans and should be included in the business projections.

- Operational basics and keys to success: The basics of operating any pharmacy venture should be considered in light of this particular business environment. Included in such operational basics should be key financial metrics and factors:

  - Drugs and drug costs: Consideration of the types of drugs to be stocked and dispensed, any unique issues regarding their costs, cost of preparation and dispensing, wastage, handling, and inventory control. For example, in the case of opening a home infusion pharmacy, the costs per unit of the common antibiotic injections, anticipated wastage of partial vials, and expiration dates and unique shipping requirements would need to be considered and built into the plan when projecting such a venture.

  - Manpower supply and costs: Evaluation of the required services in the context of necessary manpower must be included in this research. Consideration of the manpower supply, costs, and demand issues unique to the venture is critical. For example, a hospital pharmacy seeking to open a retail pharmacy would need to consider the supply and competitive salary of pharmacists and technicians in the local and regional retail chain environment. It will also be important to consider the impact of expected higher retail pharmacist salaries on the salaries of existing pharmacists in the hospital setting. Once services expand beyond the traditional hospital setting, pharmacy leadership can expect wage and conditions parity issues to become a concern if not properly addressed across the department.

  - Operational issues and logistics: Location, space, facilities, and equipment are vital considerations in institutions in which space and location are among the most challenging and contentious issues. For retail pharmacy to be successful in the typical hospital environment, adequate space and a prime location for patient traffic is crucial. Hospitals and clinics typically move hundreds of patients with predictable prescription needs through their facility each day, and such movement, traffic, and visibility will determine where a proposed pharmacy should be located for success.

- Fiscal, structural, and political concerns: Any pharmacy venture beyond the traditional hospital functions will pose new concerns, including where the new venture should be within the organization's management structure, delineation of lines of authority and responsibility, and financial accountability for the new cost center. For example, whether a new ambulatory clinic is structured as a provider-based entity on the hospital's Medicare Cost Report will have significant implications for reimbursement and the use of PHS (Public Health Service) pricing in qualified hospitals. Where an infusion center is placed in the hospital's organizational structure will have consequences regarding revenue and reimbursement, in addition to the ability to purchase drugs for own-use purposes. New cost centers with significant revenues often create political and not-for-profit legal and financial questions when such issues are not considered before the project starts and revenues begin to flow. By their very nature, entrepreneurial ventures beyond the walls of the typical hospital pharmacy demand well-delineated structures and clear lines of authority and responsibility, and will encounter political stresses beyond traditional chain-of-command boundaries.

Developing and Presenting the Business Plan

Once the necessary research and groundwork for the proposed venture is complete, the development of an effective business plan becomes the next step before approval can be sought. The details of writing a business plan are covered in chapter 15, so we will not restate them here but encourage the reader to review these details in preparation for any entrepreneurial venture.

The business plan must be written in a format that reflects the philosophy and requirements of the institution. Although the basics of a sound business plan and financial projections are well documented in most business literature, the culture and approach of an individual organization may vary greatly from a standard plan described in the business literature. Some institutions have a formal and standardized approach with significant requirements for background information and detail, whereas others prefer to keep it short and simple, with additional details provided upon request. It is of paramount importance to understand leadership expectations and to tailor the report to meet these expectations. Many a good idea and sound business venture has met with rejection from having failed to properly assess this critical requirement.

Equally important is the understanding of expectations and approach for the presentation of the business plan. Spend the necessary time with institutional leadership to know their expectations and the preferred approach for presenting the business plan. Almost invariably, the formal presentation, particularly at the board level, allows inadequate time to address key concepts fully, so clear, concise visuals with a well-rehearsed script and a streamlined executive summary will be required. Being well prepared with backup materials, additional details, and a thorough knowledge of the proposal and the background research ensure the ability to anticipate any questions that might arise and will enhance the probability of success. The most common questions will focus on capital and manpower investment required upfront, projected return on investment (ROI), time until breakeven, and extended timeline for ROI. A rehearsal presentation to an astute financial leader—preferably a project champion who will be involved in the formal presentation group—before the actual presentation will assist with developing concise answers to these and other important questions.

Recruiting one or more champions for the plan who are at the level necessary to support the project, or possibly to copresent, will increase the chance for approval and success. In the typical hospital environment, this champion's support at the COO, CEO, CFO, and even board of directors' level is extremely valuable, because such a champion is equally well-informed and able to support the proposal within a peer group. Medical staff leadership who may have an interest in pharmacy ventures are also highly effective assets in addition to administrative and financial support from corporate leadership.

Financial Management Opportunities—Beyond the Hospital Pharmacy

To fully address the unique considerations a pharmacy leader may encounter in each of the pharmacy financial opportunities beyond the hospital setting requires a text of its own. For those who choose to pursue a specific area, some suggested references are included in this chapter. This chapter is intended to introduce the reader to such opportunities through a summary description that outlines the key considerations unique to each, including competitive environment and financial setting, reimbursement environment and approach, regulatory environment and considerations, operational basics, and keys to success. This background is presented from a pragmatic view, discussing the practical concerns, pitfalls, and keys to success a pharmacy leader might expect to encounter when pursuing pharmacy entrepreneurial opportunities in these areas.

Retail Pharmacy, Including Mail Service and Specialty Services

Introduction

For many years, the retail pharmacy services typically offered in most hospital settings have been limited to a small retail pharmacy, often referred to as the outpatient pharmacy. Typically located within the main hospital pharmacy, this outpatient pharmacy might offer a separate window, or, at best, a small space chosen more often for availability than for visibility and convenience for the patient. It is not unusual for the outpatient pharmacy to occupy a limited space in the existing pharmacy (typically in the basement, poorly located, and with little appeal for patients who have other options). All too often, the resulting prescription business is limited to discharge and emergency room prescriptions and employees and dependents of the health-care institution. With such limited potential for profit, these retail endeavors are frequently considered more of a "necessary distraction" than a viable revenue stream. The net result is often an outpatient pharmacy with limited hours, limited staffing (sometimes out of the main hospital pharmacy), limited space and resources, and with limited financial expectations or success. Hospital pharmacy leadership often considers these services an operational hassle, even a financial liability in times of economic stress on the hospital pharmacy budget. No wonder the retail pharmacy has commonly suffered from neglect in such an environment and with financial limitations.

A thoughtful pharmacy leader should reconsider this premise before accepting this status. Consider that today's hospital has typically seen great expansion beyond the walls of the acute care hospital into many ambulatory patient care services. Such services have been created to serve the growing needs of patients who are intentionally encouraged, usually for reimbursement reasons, to seek outpatient treatment and minimize inpatient stays and expenses. In almost every case, these patients have prescriptions that could be filled in combination with critical patient care services to assure continuity of care. The concept of offering retail and mail service pharmacies within the institutional setting is becoming a more common entrepreneurial consideration because of the potential for new revenue streams.

Competitive Environment and Financial Setting

The retail prescription business today has become highly competitive with large chain stores, grocery, and discount stores with pharmacies dominating the marketplace. The independent retail store owner has become much less common, with only about 22 percent of total prescriptions and 18.2% of prescription sales being filled in the corner drugstore or the mom-and-pop pharmacy.[4] Large regional mail-order pharmacies fill thousands of prescriptions daily and now account for about 7.2 percent of the total annual prescription volume in the United States, but over 19 percent of the prescription sales.[5]

Prescription pricing has been driven by highly competitive rates established by third-party payers, state Medicaid programs, and, beginning in 2006, Part D Medicare contracts. Unfortunately, the pressing daily demands of the online adjudication process for payment has driven and dominated the dispensing process in this setting, leaving little time for critical patient care clinical services.

In spite of this highly competitive and often frustrating climate for retail pharmacy, there is good news. Most patients show less concern for price shopping and more focus on convenience and availability of customer services because the price and patient co-pay are now most often determined by the third-party payer,. Thus, it is no accident that large chains seem to be expanding locations with large full-service, often 24-hour, facilities within close driving range of most populations in today's cities and suburban neighborhoods. Likewise, in this business environment a well-appointed convenient retail pharmacy located in a major health-care institution begins to make sense. If done properly, a convenient retail pharmacy can present a positive business case. Mail service pharmacy may also present opportunities for that population and setting in certain cases.

Reimbursement Environment and Approach

Today's retail prescription is reimbursed almost solely based upon contract payment terms set by the third-party payer and administered online. This is achieved through a real-time adjudication process administered through a pharmacy benefit management (PBM) company, which also sees that the providers are paid accordingly. When a patient presents a prescription to the retail pharmacy, the following steps in the financial process occur:

- From the prescription, the patient is identified, employee and patient identification is validated, with insurance coverage and benefit details identified.

- Prescribed drug and prescription details are entered into the pharmacy computer using common National Drug Codes (NDC), then through the electronic adjudication process the patient's coverage and plan is verified, including formulary status of the drug, days supply, and patient co-pay is calculated. If there are no clerical, business, professional, or patient care issues with the prescription, this process occurs in a matter of seconds. If the prescription fails to clear the electronic adjudication successfully, additional time-consuming manual steps are required to clarify any issue. This is one of today's greatest frustrations and productivity barriers in the retail pharmacy environment. Many pharmacists and technicians feel they spend more time managing insurance claims than providing vital clinical and patient care services.

- Assuming all the adjudication requirements are satisfied, the prescription is filled, the patient counseled, and the appropriate co-pay is collected. The patient is on their way.

- Behind the scenes, the electronic adjudication process has triggered the recording of a prescription drug event (PDE) that executes a payment process according to the contract terms. These financial transactions accumulate in a payment register for each provider with a payment ledger for each payer, all part of the financial function of the PBM. On a scheduled basis, this register is reviewed and cleared, and an electronic payment or paper check is forwarded to the pharmacy. Frequency of actual payment to the pharmacy is an important consideration when evaluating a contract.

A retail pharmacy located conveniently in a hospital can offer these same services by becoming a contract provider for all the major payers common to the area and patient population. Specialized retail pharmacy software is necessary to provide the adjudication capabilities necessary to handle the claims process and to track the payments and accounts receivable from the PBM payers. Many hospital pharmacy software systems include a retail package, but their range of capabilities should be thoroughly evaluated in comparison with stand-alone retail software. Any successful retail pharmacy business must have a fully functional retail pharmacy software package that effectively handles the adjudication and related business processes, which allows pharmacy leadership to maintain separate and full business accountability.

Reimbursement contracts are typically structured based upon pricing formulas, such as the following example:

Branded products: AWP–15% + $2.00 dispensing fee

Generic products: AWP–40% or MAC (max. allowable cost) + $2.00 disp. fee

See Figure 17.1 detailed notes regarding retail pricing formulas and related terminology.

Typical institutional own-use or group purchasing (GPO) pricing is discounted approximately 16–20 percent off of AWP (average wholesale price) with market share rebate and

Average wholesale price or AWP is the average list price for a product as listed in the *Red Book* reference. This list price has historically been used as the starting point for price formulas. Recent legislative efforts are beginning to change that with a move to ASP, or average selling price, for pricing drugs in clinics under Part B of Medicare. Current proposals are being considered to mandate the use of AMP or average manufacturers price for pricing Medicaid prescriptions. Both the ASP and AMP changes have the potential to change the net reimbursement to providers in a negative way.

Maximum allowable cost (MAC) is a standard cost price established by the payer (could be Medicaid or private payer MAC lists), which sets a standard price for products, primarily generics that see such a large variance in average wholesale price (AWP), and may be subject to misinterpretation and possibly misuse regarding justifiable cost reimbursement.

State Medicaid fees paid to retail pharmacies often vary based upon setting and certain criteria. Research as to the Medicaid reimbursement status of in-house institutional retail pharmacies is important, as in many states, such as Texas, the fees paid are less than the outside retail setting, and thus net impact must be included in the pro forma for the proposed retail venture.

Most contracts also state the formula followed by the wording "or usual and customary, whichever is less," which means that the provider pharmacy is obligated to pass on their usual price if it is lower than the contract formula. This prevents providers from collecting a price greater than their cash or walk-in price. Because of this language in most contracts, an unusually low "usual and customary" pricing matrix can result in reimbursement less than the contract formula. This factor needs to be considered when setting pricing methodologies and monitoring contracts and reimbursement expectations.

These formulas are often limited to 30-day fills, depending on the benefit plan. Refills for maintenance drugs for up to 90-day supplies may be authorized, sometimes for different co-pay amounts, depending upon the prescription benefit terms. Such refills also may be limited to mail service or in-house pharmacies. Mail service contracts are typically more aggressive, with fees as low as $.50 and discounts as high as 21 percent off of AWP.

Figure 17.1. Detailed Notes Regarding Retail Pricing Formulas and Related Terminology

competitive therapeutic classes offering additional discounts based upon performance. However, with aggressive retail reimbursement as much as 12 percent to 16 percent off of AWP for branded products, the net margins are reduced dramatically, and any business projections for retail pharmacy must consider all of this to ensure financial viability. Institutions that are able to garner highly competitive own-use pricing as defined by the Nonprofit Institutions Act[7] and use other price advantages, such as PHS or 340B pricing, which is the result of the Veterans Health Care Act of 1992,[8] may have a significant financial advantage when properly leveraged with a retail pharmacy located conveniently within the institution. As AWP is replaced by other cost and pricing benchmarks, these formulas will change; however, the tight relationship between the drug cost and reimbursement make a thorough review of cost and revenue a necessary part of the business planning process.

Regulatory Environment and Considerations

Retail pharmacies and pharmacists are primarily licensed and regulated by each state's board of pharmacy and are subject to significant variation from state to state. Thus state regulations for retail pharmacies must be thoroughly assessed before the venture considered reaches the business proposal stage, in which some key requirements may have potential financial impact. Variables in the regulations most commonly affecting the venture are requirements for ownership and licensure, type of licensure required based upon location within the institution and type of business, and operational requirements, such as minimum hours of service, signage, counseling, and staffing definitions.

Pharmacy mail services typically encounter additional board of pharmacy requirements that focus on handling out-of-state prescriptions. Pharmacies planning to provide mail service for patients outside the resident state often must seek licensure in those additional states and may encounter additional requirements regarding nonresident ownership, hard copies of prescriptions, telephone and fax orders, refill restrictions, special controlled substance requirements, and even delivery requirements and limitations. Any plans for mail service should include thorough research into these issues, so the financial impact may be included in the business plan.

Specific regulatory and record keeping requirements by the Drug Enforcement Administration (DEA) for handling controlled substances, and particularly record keeping in the retail setting versus hospital setting, should also be researched and incorporated into the plan.

Because the financial viability of retail operations will depend on the institution being able to purchase drugs at the best advantage, the question of using "own-use" drug pricing available through the hospital's group purchasing organization (GPO) or individual contracts is essential. Although always a concern, in recent years, legal opinions on this question seem to be more favorable toward allowing legitimate use within the institutional setting. To be sure that hospital legal counsel can support the venture, the question of using "own-use" pricing in the retail setting should be posed early, because he or she may choose to clarify this issue with the Federal Trade Commission (FTC). Having a letter from the FTC on file validating the answer based upon each hospital's retail structure and scope is ideal. Hospitals that qualify as disproportionate share hospitals (DSHs) may also qualify for the use of PHS or 340(b) pricing. If so, this pricing may be extended to certain outpatient drug purchases, including retail services, depending on the fact that the service and patients meet strict guidelines for such use. The potential for additional drug cost savings is substantial, if this can be incorporated into the retail strategy.

Any opportunity for new revenues in a not-for-profit setting, particularly retail ventures, always introduces the concern about the potential impact on the not-for-profit status of the institution. The venture will usually require the payment of taxes on the unrelated business income (UBI) but should not threaten the tax status of the organization. There are clear rules in this regard that need to be clarified by hospital counsel and restated somewhere in the background information for any new proposal.

Operational Basics to Consider and Keys to Success

There are numerous challenges that must be confronted to assure success in the retail pharmacy setting within a major institution. Here are a few of the more common ones to consider:

- **Understanding, monitoring, and reporting of key metrics to measure financial performance:** Every pharmacy must understand and monitor the basic business factors outlined throughout this text. However, in each area, key metrics are used to monitor that particular business. In the retail pharmacy setting, most metrics are based upon the common unit of a retail prescription dispensed, and include the following:

- Number of prescriptions filled (per hour, day, month, year)
- Brand versus generic prescriptions (numbers and percent of total)
- Cost versus revenue and net margin per prescription
- Cost per prescription broken down to manpower (salary + benefits), drugs, misc.
- Revenue per prescription broken down by payer type and individual payer

- **Finding location and space for the retail pharmacy:** Given the limitations of space in most institutions, this can be one of the most limiting challenges faced by a proposed new venture. Thoughtful consideration and planning to assure there will be adequate space in a visible location near the greatest patient flow must be a primary goal. Shared space within the existing pharmacy structure is rarely an effective answer, though often suggested by hospital leadership attempting to conserve vital space and to balance competing requests for space allocation. A retail opportunity with financial merit deserves appropriate space allocation to allow success.

- **Developing the retail initiative as a fully committed stand-alone business venture:** To be successful, the retail pharmacy strategy must be given the business acumen required for any successful business venture. It cannot be an afterthought or secondary consideration if leadership hopes to experience financial success. It must be approached both by pharmacy and hospital leadership as a retail business venture with its own unique requirements and not be combined by default with existing hospital departments with different agendas. Establishing the retail pharmacy as a separate cost and revenue center is essential for business clarity and accountability. This may even pose challenges as to where the retail center and infrastructure should reside within the organization, as opposed to the traditional hospital pharmacy structure. This should be reviewed, although thoughtfully and carefully, as a positive expansion of the scope of the pharmacy department within the organization, rather than trying to fit within the existing traditional infrastructure because it is comfortable or easier. Clear lines of authority and responsibility are essential to ultimate success.

- **Researching and accurately assessing the reimbursement climate for the retail pharmacy business against the institution's cost of drugs:** A thorough analysis of the reimbursement rates in the region is essential, including managed care contract rates and Medicare Part D and state Medicaid rates. A financial analysis should be performed, with the expected prescription benefit mix versus those rates, along with an accurate projection of institutional net drug costs, considering the potential own-use contracts and/or PHS pricing. An actual usage sample of typical prescription mix either using existing outpatient data and/or combining with managed care reports can provide an excellent picture of potential business. Close reading and understanding of provider contracts is important, particularly regarding the formulas that use AWP–X% versus MACs. AWP for generics is highly variable, and MAC lists range from standard to restrictive, including some branded and multisource branded products, so understanding these details is important to predict net margin on various provider contracts. Any expectations for handling indigent business, either no-pay or reduced payments, must be factored into the projections.

- **Recruiting knowledgeable and competent retail pharmacy expertise:** All too often retail pharmacy ventures in hospitals are relegated to existing pharmacy leadership and staff as another extension of the hospital pharmacy department. This is generally not a winning strategy, because the unique demands and expertise required in this area necessitate recruiting manpower with proven experience and financial success in retail pharmacy as a business. Because of the common differential in salaries in retail versus hospital pharmacy management and staff, the business plan must include this additional cost in contrast to hospital manpower market rates. Human resource departments in hospitals typically survey salaries in other hospital settings but fail to consider the very real competition from the retail pharmacy sector, particularly the aggressive chains that tend to absorb much of the local and regional manpower. Thus, it will be important to educate them on this market difference and to insist those salaries are included in the surveys and that the proposed staff is paid competitively.

- **Identifying and taking advantage of hospital leverage and other assets to attract prescription business:** The typical hospital setting has potential advantages and leverage, should they choose to venture into the retail pharmacy arena that may include the following:
  - Existing high volume and daily traffic of patients with prescription needs.
  - Ability to locate a retail pharmacy in a highly visible location near peak patient flow.
  - Name or brand recognition for the institution that represents a proven high-quality health-care provider.
  - Existing professional relationships with the prescribing physicians of patients, so that delivery of an efficient financial and clinical service is anticipated.
  - Access to "own-use" and in some cases PHS pricing, as well as institutional contracts and market share agreements, that when properly applied with physician support can offer significant net margins for the pharmacy.
  - Employee and dependent prescriptions that are paid for by the institution, which is at risk for those expenses, generating a cost of up to millions of dollars each year. A retail pharmacy or a mail service pharmacy can offer options for capturing a significant part of this volume, resulting in savings, new revenues, and enhanced patient convenience. Compliance with regulations in capturing this volume must be a key consideration. Clinical management of these patients may be combined with other pharmacy efforts so that overall care can be improved as well.
  - A well-conceived marketing plan for a retail pharmacy initiative is essential to be certain that all the potential business is realized. This is typically not a component of hospital pharmacy operations, so pharmacy leadership will need to give this as much priority as the clinical and financial operations plan.

One cannot assume that because the hospital builds it, they will come. Today's retail pharmacy market is driven by convenience, and any hospital venture must address that requirement first and then combine the inherent leverage of patient volume and access with advantageous pricing to assure ultimate success.

Mail Service Pharmacy—Additional Considerations

Although the term *mail-service pharmacy* often evokes a less professional image than the typical hospital pharmacy considers acceptable, pharmacy leaders should not automatically dismiss such an initiative in this environment. Some hospital pharmacies have incorporated mail service pharmacy into their retail strategy in a highly effective and professional manner. Scott & White Health System in Texas and the University of Wisconsin system have, in different ways, combined such services with their managed care and retail initiatives with great success, while managing to maintain a high level of professionalism.[9] Nearly every managed care prescription services proposal mandates a mail service provider, which may either be contracted or provided in-house. Expensive maintenance quantities of branded products have been effectively moved into this environment, where the institution is able to manage the patient and the prescription using highly competitive pricing through in-house contracts. Prices in this arena are often linked to market share rebates within therapeutic classes, but this approach keeps the savings and the clinical continuity within the pharmacy system.

The financial management of a mail service pharmacy represents a complex set of issues warranting detailed discussion, but to stimulate the reader's thought about key issues, the following points should be considered:

- Managed care contracts are typically the most aggressive in this provider sector, with AWP minus 20 percent or more plus fees as low as $0.50 for branded products being common.[10] These rates must be factored into this business; however much of this is offset by a higher percentage of mail-order business filling maintenance quantities of expensive branded products. Thus the average prescription price increases dramatically, so that in spite of lower reimbursement, there is still potential to drive significant net margins per prescription.

- Historical analysis has demonstrated that mail service represents around 7–8 percent of the total volume of any managed care plan, unless aggressive policies and co-pay incentives are built in to further drive this business. Thus reasonably managed, one can expect a similar percentage of total volume to come into the mail service pharmacy.

- Properly executing a mail service pharmacy requires more than moving prescription volume into a new or existing pharmacy. There are certain efficiencies in comparison to walk-in volume in that it is easier to dispense at a consistently efficient pace because there are no interruptions throughout the day as with walk-in patients. It is easier to push the volume primarily into the day shift, to consider a second shift for mail, and to staff Monday through Friday, in most cases until the volume reaches a certain level demanding weekend hours. This eases the pressure on manpower, hiring, and ability to recruit and retain competent help.

- There are also operational issues unique to this environment that must be considered. The packaging and mail function must be planned, including space, manpower, daily pickup details, and additional costs to assure financial success. On the front end, the critical requirement is an online system for electronic ordering through a Web site, combined with a call desk or service center receiving calls and service inquiries by phone. This front-end system is essential for smooth throughput into the pharmacy system for dispensing and delivery. Systems for handling physician calls, refills, clinical edits, and patient billing issues are all important considerations in mail service. Considerable planning needs to be included regarding policies for payment by mail, such as charging, credit and debit cards, and personal checks. With both members of most households working today, the ability to contact the patient can be a challenge. Above all, a mail service pharmacy's success is predicated on patient convenience and ease of use, highly efficient service and turnaround time, and using the batch process for dispensing to ensure cost efficiency.

- Location is typically not a concern when compared to walk-in retail pharmacies. This is a huge advantage in the typical institutional facility in which space and location are at a premium. However, the tendency to short-change the space allocation needed for efficient dispensing, packaging, and mailing processes is a common problem. Simply merge mail services into existing walk-in pharmacies to conserve space and manpower may be a temptation. Unfortunately, the net result usually creates havoc and inefficiencies for both sides of that pharmacy operation. Combination of services can be achieved, but only if the workflow, staffing, space allocations, and demands of each are duly considered within that facility.

- Mail service pharmacy requires the consideration of marketing approach and materials in a significantly different way than walk-in retail pharmacy ventures. An introduction packet to potential members, patients, and employees should instruct them how to access the pharmacy through the Internet. Phone service desk and Web site, designed in a manner that makes mail service use efficient is the key to success. With incentives built into the prescription benefit for the patient, including maintenance supply quantities and lower co-pays, it is possible to drive the percentage of mail service for a plan or employee group well beyond the typical 7–8 percent of total prescription volume for the plan. Some plans are able to selectively drive expensive specialty drugs to the mail service through mandated provider requirements, incentives for members, or penalties or noncoverage for using non-preferred providers.

It is important to consider the mail service pharmacy option as a potential financial opportunity. Although there are potential pitfalls in this extremely competitive business, there are also circumstances in which this option may actually be ideal. When considering the current managed care contract for mail for institution employees and dependents, it is important to recognize that mail is the one provider that typically has sole contractual authority. This means that business can be directed by contract to any mail service provider, including one developed by the institution. It is important to include mail service considerations in the retail research and analysis as another option the pharmacy and hospital leadership should consider as they plan an effective retail strategy.

Specialty Pharmacy—Other Considerations

Although there are significant distinctions between the specialty pharmacy and the retail pharmacy business, there are significant similarities. The consideration of a specialty pharmacy as a unique business is determined more by the type of product dispensed and the reimbursement mechanism than by the operational and financial basics of the pharmacy itself.

For example, the specialty pharmacy, like the retail pharmacy, stocks, prepares, and dispenses drugs to patients, primarily those in the home or other outpatient settings. The drugs are limited in number but tend to be expensive, frequently require administration by self-injection, and are often not routinely stocked in a neighborhood pharmacy. In some cases they require additional clinical expertise and high-touch monitoring and may require patient or family education to safely administer at home. In some cases, the distribution of such products may be limited to certain specialty pharmacies by the manufacturer either for logistics or legal reasons, or both. Such limitations have sometimes created a controversy with physicians, patients, payers, and provider pharmacies because of concerns about restricted access, controlled pricing, and continuity of care. Unique and expensive products such as blood coagulation factors, biotech drugs, growth hormone, interferon, disease-modifying anti-rheumatic drugs or DMARDs, and other expensive treatments for unique diseases all typically fall into the specialty pharmacy category.

The greatest difference from retail pharmacy in this sector is in the specialty drug reimbursement model. Drugs are generally paid for by insurance through specialty carve-outs from the medical insurance benefit rather than as part of the prescription drug rider. Often prescriptions must be approved through a prior authorization process by the plan medical director or pharmacist, are subject to different deductibles, co-pays, and capitation requirements. They may also be restricted to provision by approved providers. Reimbursement often includes a low percentage markup, because the base drug costs are so expensive, and fees may include the necessary handling and clinical management requirements. Such aggressive margin management, combined with the cost of inventory and clinical infrastructure, require close financial scrutiny and sound projections to justify this business venture.

Costs for these drugs are rising dramatically faster than the cost of other drugs, thus generating a considerable concern among both employers and health plans, as they track the escalating costs to their plans.[11] The current pipeline of drugs being researched for Food and Drug Administration (FDA) approval contains many additional agents, primarily the biotech drugs that will fall into this category. Payers and providers alike are struggling to determine how best to meet the needs of the patient while assuring the financial viability of their organization.[12]

Although existing arrangements and contracts for specialty pharmacy services are typically carved out and negotiated separately, this highly expensive and sometimes clinically demanding portfolio of drugs should not be ignored by the entrepreneurial pharmacy leader. The combination of high costs, high-touch patient care requirements, and the need for continuity, as well as the potential for negotiating pricing leverage on these products, should stimulate every pharmacy leader to consider providing these products and services through the expanded retail pharmacy services. Of particular interest should be the consideration to provide this service for employees and dependents to assure continuity of care and to take advantage of institutional pricing on these expensive products. This opportunity should entail the same detailed research, groundwork, and financial projections as other retail ventures to ensure that adding it to the pharmacy's portfolio is a sound clinical and financial decision.

Managed Care Pharmacy—Opportunities in Institutional Settings

Introduction

If asked about managed care pharmacy in their institution, most hospital pharmacists would answer they have few if any such issues, concerns, or opportunities. Despite this common misperception, when one looks more closely at most every institution, there are managed care pharmacy issues, some of which may offer entrepreneurial opportunities with financial returns far greater than those pursued in more familiar areas. It is not unusual for an institution to own or contract with one or more health maintenance or preferred provider organizations of which the hospital staff has little knowledge or understanding, yet that provide valuable managed care services to a patient population. Almost every hospital has some form of self-insured health-care plan for employees and dependents that also includes a prescription drug benefit or drug rider. Often this prescription plan represents 10 percent or more of employee health costs, which translates to millions of dollars annually.[13] Prescription plan costs are rising at a percentage dramatically higher than the rest of employee expenditures, and the responsibility for this typically rests with the employee benefits division of human resources, which has little detailed knowledge of the issues. The benefit is usually coordinated through a prescription benefits manager (PBM) who answers to the benefits manager in human resources, but neither have much connection with the pharmacy, overall drug policies for the organization, or the organization's formulary. Often the formulary and related policies, directed by this PBM, may differ substantially, or even be in direct conflict with the goals and policies of the P&T committee and medical staff of the institution. No wonder a physician may become frustrated when contacted about discrepancies that result with a request to change from hospital formulary preferences.

Most hospital pharmacy staff and leadership have some managed care challenges and related opportunities in their institutions. This area of hospital activity represents an opportunity for a progressive pharmacy leader to become involved and to develop a new entrepreneurial pharmacy service. This section of the chapter is intended to briefly outline the most common managed care issues pertinent to this environment and then to describe the financial variables, as well as some challenges and opportunities.

The Competitive Environment and Financial Goal Setting

By definition, *managed care* is a highly competitive arena in which the primary strategy is to offer a comprehensive bundle of health-care services for a set fee over a specific amount of time, using principles of health management and financial control. Managed care is a risk-based business and a form of insurance. Thus it is regulated by each state board of insurance, as well as by a growing number of national regulations and mandates, partly because of negative experiences or perceptions of managed care in the last two decades. The plan or plan sponsor, in this case the hospital organization, is ultimately responsible for the delivery of contracted services for the specified contracted amount. In contrast to the typical hospital business venture, this risk-based business can be brutal and unforgiving. Deliberate and thoughtful financial analyses are essential to avoid the pitfalls of assuming such risk without fully understanding and projecting the related costs. For example, in the 1980s, even huge managed care organizations with years of experience rushed in to the senior marketplace to offer medical plans, including the drug benefit, at no additional cost. In some cases, that decision became a major factor in the demise of the plan, when the prescription drug bills began accumulating for this resource-intensive patient population.

The prescription drug benefit has become a vital part of overall managed care coverage, with the plan responsible for defining the benefits, including formulary coverage, co-pays, deductibles, and caps according to the specifications of the employer, who is picking up most of the expenditures. The prescription drug benefit portion is often defined by the plan and priced on a per member per month (PMPM) basis. Then a prescription benefits management company (PBM) executes and manages the plan for a fee, typically answering to the plan, which answers to the employer, who foots the ultimate bill. Because of the complex issues and the hands-off position of the human resource staff, the plan often passes on much of the authority and responsibility to the pharmacy benefits manager. PBMs may use a standard template, often based more upon the PBM's needs and financial returns than to the employer's needs and intentions. With some guidance, an astute pharmacy leader can do much to improve upon this typical strategy while enhancing the role of the pharmacist in the process.

Reimbursement Environment and Approach

The prescription drug benefit is simply a subset of health-care and related costs that is comprised primarily of the cost of the drug and dispensing fees as well as the necessary infrastructure and administrative costs. When calculating the overall premium requirements for managed care coverage for a total cost per member per month (PMPM), the plan includes a projected amount for the prescription drug portion, which is a subset PMPM figure. PMPM is the essential financial benchmark for monitoring and assessing the cost of this portion of the benefit and is used as the basis for calculating the rates for the following benefit year.

$$\frac{\text{annual drug costs (all drugs + fees − rebates) + administrative costs}}{12 \text{ (months)} \times N \text{ (members)}} = \frac{\text{drug rider costs}}{\text{PMPM}}$$

Administrative costs typically consist of the costs of claims processing, benefits design and management, and infrastructure costs of the plan for administering the benefit, providing pharmacy clinical management, monitoring, and so forth. Once rates are established, the plan receives approval for the accepted rate for coverage for the plan year, so the revenue per member at that point is predictable. The challenge of managed care then becomes to manage the costs of care, including prescription drugs in this case, for a total equal (and hopefully less) than the quoted rate. If the premium is set at $45.00 PMPM for the year, each member receives their prescription benefit for that amount, whether they receive $10,000 dollars worth of HIV medications or a single prescription for amoxicillin costing $6.00. For a pharmacist accustomed to the hospital reimbursement environment, this is a clear but daunting financial responsibility, not to be taken lightly.

Reimbursement rates for retail pharmacy providers supplying the drugs were briefly discussed earlier in the retail pharmacy section. Such rates are established by the plan, usually with the guidance of the PBM, and are typically driven by the competitive managed care marketplace. It is important to recognize that how AWP and MAC rates are applied and defined can be highly variable, depending on the PBM. Some use MAC rates that are aggressive and broad, covering many products, including some branded products, whereas other plans are more standard and relate primarily to the common generics. AWP rates for some generics are dramatically higher than others, so that the discount from AWP rates can result in widely varying costs for the same drug from a different manufacturer. A sound program administered by a reputable PBM offers a comprehensive MAC program that is clearly defined and fair to provider and payer and an AWP pricing strategy that is thoughtful, fair, and accurate for all concerned. It often takes an astute pharmacist to evaluate these factors to assure the best value for the plan and payer.

The ability to manage the costs of the prescription drug rider depends not just on the reimbursement rates for the providers, which are consistent and aggressive, but on the design details of the benefit and management of the appropriate selection of products by the prescribing physician. For example, the Scott & White managed care pharmacy reported that a 1 percent increase in the use of generic versus branded products was equivalent to approximately a half million dollar reduction in annual cost of the benefit for their population of approximately 185,000 lives.[14] Likewise moving market share within a therapeutic class, such as statin lipotropics, from an expensive brand product with minimal discounts or rebates to an equally effective branded agent can equate to several thousand dollars in savings each quarter for the plan and the payer. Placing the preferred brand in a preferable co-pay status on the formulary saves both the patient and the plan significant dollars. Managed care pharmacy involves the thoughtful use of benefit design, formulary placement, and aggressive contracting to work with the prescribing physician to lower costs in therapeutic classes, while ensuring quality clinical outcomes are considered. Such strategies are analogous to those used in the acute care setting, although the issue of the PBM making this decision and capturing more of the savings is controversial. Today's marketplace is becoming more interested in keeping this within the plan. Thus a major financial opportunity for pharmacy is available in such institutions.

Regulatory Environment and Considerations

Every managed care entity is subject to the insurance regulations of the states within the approved service area. Also in recent years there have been additional mandates and managed care regulations imposed at the federal level, some relate directly or indirectly to the prescription benefit.

Fortunately, most of these regulations relate to the details of operating an at-risk insurance entity and have limited direct implications for managed care pharmacy operations. Most are focused on provider pharmacy contracting, formulary content and changes, and related benefit and coverage issues. Managed care pharmacy services are not typically licensed separately by the state boards of pharmacy as retail pharmacies are, because there is no direct handling of prescription drugs by the plan. The plan may incur significant liability from the actions of their contracted pharmacy network should an error or incident occur. Recent regulations surrounding the Medicare Part D prescription drug program for seniors makes it clear that the prescription plan is ultimately responsible for any misdeeds, fraud, waste, or abuse issues that may occur with their contract providers, including both prescription benefit managers and pharmacies.[15] These liabilities are important financial concerns to consider when developing a managed care pharmacy program and calculating the costs of administration and compliance.

The regulations regarding prescription benefits details both at the state and federal levels should be understood and closely monitored by the managed care pharmacy service to ensure compliance in all areas. The drug rebates from pharmaceutical companies received by the PBMs are being examined more closely, and greater transparency and accountability will be required on the part of all players in the managed care pharmacy business. The Medicare Part D cost reconciliation process also magnifies this concern, because all costs must be reconciled against revenues to determine net loss or gain for the plan year.[16]

Operational Basics and Keys to Success
Financial Analysis—Basic Metrics

To effectively address managed care opportunities within their own systems, hospital pharmacy leaders should develop an understanding of the basics of managed care pharmacy as outlined here. Pharmacy leaders may choose to spend additional time reviewing a basic text or the related journals, attending national meetings such as the Academy of Managed Care Pharmacy (AMCP), or reviewing any PBM reports available from current managed care providers to develop an understanding of the key financial metrics commonly monitored to evaluate performance:

- Drug rider revenue (PMPM)
- Drug rider costs (PMPM) (This may be broken into drug costs vs dispensing costs.)
- Avg. brand prescription cost per Rx
- Avg. generic prescription cost per Rx
- Avg. member co-pay per prescription ($ and %)
- Generic fill rate (% of total prescriptions)
- Formulary compliance rate (%)
- Prior authorizations required (and approved vs denied)
- Average days supply per prescription
- Annual prescriptions per member (and Rx/PMPM)

- Therapeutic class report that includes
  - Top 10 therapeutic classes (by volume and costs)
  - Top 10 drugs within each class (by volume and costs)
  - Average cost/Rx in each of top 10 therapeutic classes
  - Average PMPM cost per therapeutic (a measure sometimes benchmarked)
- Top 200 drug usage report (top down by cost and by Rx volume)
- Trend reports for all these metrics that monitor change (% change from year to year, etc.)

These financial indicators should be routinely available from the provider PBM or claims processing company and can be used to monitor monthly, quarterly, and annual trends. These parameters should be benchmarked against national and regional standards. (Standards are also available from the PBM and from published annual reports available from Novartis, Medco, and Express Scripts, although these annual reports typically lag 12–18 months by the time of publication.)

Financial Analysis—Next Steps

Managed care benchmarks, although important, will vary greatly based upon details of the drug benefit, such as co-pay tiers, benefit caps, formulary coverage, days supply, and so forth. Thus these metrics must be evaluated based upon an in-depth understanding of these factors before actions may be considered.

Routine monitoring of the basic financial indicators as outlined above will help a pharmacy leader to determine the cause of certain trends and outliers and then to seek actions to improve financial performance. Such next steps typically lead to inquiries into other aspects of the prescription benefit that may contribute to the trend, such as:

- Benefit design, including co-pay tiers and differentials, days and quantity supplies, and maintenance drug policies
- Formulary design and product availability, coverage for injections, and so on
- Prior authorization requirements that necessitate medical director approval before dispensing
- Market situations, such as availability of newly released generic products
- Provider pharmacy contract and reimbursement policies
- Pharmacy and Therapeutics Committee guidelines and related medical staff requirements, restrictions, and so on.

Once they become familiar with the basics of managed care and the common indicators and understand these contributing factors, most hospital pharmacy directors and clinical specialists find the financial management of the drug rider to be consistent with similar challenges in the hospital environment. Successful strategies for controlling drug costs while assuring quality care in the hospital, with some adaptation, can become keys to financial success in managed care pharmacy as well. Yet the drug rider and its costs cannot be managed in isolation. Overly aggressive controls or limitations on the availability of appropriate drugs to treat the patient can adversely affect care in other areas, with a negative impact both on care and costs because of rehospitalization and increased emergency department and clinic visits. Effective communication with the prescribing physician is a common denominator in both cases, and a proven clinical pharmacy department usually has great credibility to bring to managed care initiatives.

Areas of Opportunity—Keys to Success

Existing areas of managed care opportunity for pharmacy to consider are likely to reside in one or two key areas: existing managed care organizations either owned or affiliated with the institution and/or the prescription drug benefit provided for employees and their dependents.

Managed Care Organizations—Owned by or Contracted with the Institution

The hospital pharmacy director interested in a possible managed care opportunity must spend sufficient time researching and understanding the existing organization and its current approach to the pharmacy. Once understood, the director must determine if there are areas of concern in the basics of managed care pharmacy that might be better addressed through an integrated pharmacy department with the hospital. Existing pharmacy services often involve outside providers, particularly the prescription benefit management companies (PBM), so there may be political and financial pitfalls to negotiate along the way. Should the opportunity be financially significant, it may be advisable for the director to seek pharmacy leadership with managed care experience to head the initiative. This strategy can expedite the venture, and the new expertise can also mentor the director and others as they learn the managed care pharmacy business.

The savvy and well-established hospital pharmacy director has much to offer the managed care organization in terms of financial expertise and clinical credibility with the Pharmacy and Therapeutics Committee and the medical staff. They can bring their ability to integrate the hospital and managed care pharmacy programs to the organization in ways that will result in superior clinical services and financial returns.

As in the case of the retail pharmacy ventures, important discussions and planning with hospital leadership regarding the appropriate structure and position of managed care pharmacy within the organization is vitally important. This may entail matrix management, new authority structures, and other departures from traditional hospital pharmacy management structures. Such departures can challenge leadership who are less secure, so pharmacy leadership must be steadfast, tactful, and politically astute to negotiate this important key to success.

Employee Prescription Benefit Plan

Almost every health-care institution now offers some form of prescription drug benefit coverage for employees and their dependents. Typically these equate to millions of dollars in employer expenses each year and are rising dramatically faster than other hospital expenses.

Hospital pharmacy directors seeking entrepreneurial opportunities should not overlook this type of managed care opportunity within their institutions.

Suggested strategy for exploring this opportunity should start with a meeting with the benefits manager in the human resources department, with the sanction of hospital leadership. An evaluation of their current benefits situation could include a collaborative and nonthreatening offer to review their basic PBM data for the benefit. This will likely entail their requesting a current report from the PBM. This request may not be met enthusiastically by the PBM but should be pursued regardless.

Once the basic data is received, perform a cursory but thorough review of the details of the prescription drug rider, along with a discussion of recent trends, such as cost versus revenues, increases each year, problems encountered with the benefit design, terms, and financial results. From this analysis, there will likely be target areas in which improvement might be offered in the following ways:

- Improved management of the benefit, contracts, rebates.
- Improved controls on the formulary and coordinating content with leverage of overall institutional formulary and related contracts.
- Improved contracting with pharmacy providers, including mail-order and possible move to in-house pharmacy, where own-use and, in some cases, PHS pricing may offer significant savings.
- Improved rapport and clinical management of the program with the prescribing physician.

In summary, from providing improvements in basic managed care pharmacy to developing innovative programs and bringing prescription volume to in-house retail and/or mail service pharmacy, many opportunities are possible. A successful venture can bring new revenues, reduce costs, improve care, and enhance the image and financial position of the hospital pharmacy in the overall health-care system. So, in spite of the unique challenges and differences between managed care pharmacy and hospital pharmacy, do not overlook the creative possibilities for a successful financial opportunity.

Home Infusion Center Pharmacy

Introduction

Home infusion center pharmacies are specialized pharmacies that primarily mix, prepare, and dispense infusions, injections, and other products for use in the home and other ambulatory settings. These pharmacies represent another key ambulatory service component for potential entrepreneurial consideration by the institutional pharmacy leader. The shortened inpatient length of stay because of DRG pressures has created a need for a higher level of patient care in the home, including intravenous infusions, because patients are going home much sicker and in need of such support. Capitation of payments by managed care and Medicare has further increased the importance of keeping the patient stable at home to avoid the expense of rehospitalization and treatment. Thus the market forces have been in place since the 1980s for home infusion to make economic sense and to offer entrepreneurial opportunities for those able to create the necessary pharmacy services and related home care support required for safe, effective patient care.

Competitive Environment, Financial, and Reimbursement Settings

As the wave of patients moving into the ambulatory and home setting as a result of Prospective Payment reached a critical mass, the home care marketplace quickly geared up to create home care nursing agencies and home infusion pharmacies to address the need. In the beginning the insurance coverage for this expanded setting was poorly defined, ranging from no coverage, to some coverage under major medical with separate deductibles and caps, to more robust coverage for both nursing care and drugs. Because of the lack of definition, the patient's out-of-pocket expenses could range from modest to prohibitive. Charge structures for infusions were poorly defined, and the private sector infusion business unfortunately often maximized their charges in the absence of clear contracts designed specifically for this type of business. To counter this, federal agencies (Medicare and Medicaid), private payers, and managed care eventually moved to rigorous reimbursement contracts and qualification criteria, which dramatically reduced the profit margins for home infusion businesses. Eventually many of the small players who had sprung up experienced severe cash flow problems and went out of business. The players remaining were those who had adequate cash to operate on the smaller margins, capacity and expertise to deal with difficult billing and payment schedules, and the expertise to navigate the reimbursement waters effectively to ensure payment and maximum reimbursement. Many institutions that had quickly developed both home care nursing agencies and home infusion pharmacies experienced the same financial stresses when the margins decreased and found themselves poorly equipped to handle the reimbursement challenges unique to this environment. Some chose to outsource contracts, which limited their business exposure yet provided some options for their patients transitioning into the home environment from the acute care setting. Some of these arrangements have effectively met the patients' needs, but many fall short, particularly in continuity of care with the institution. With a renewed interest in entrepreneurial ventures in the ambulatory setting, home infusion pharmacy is currently experiencing more interest from progressive pharmacy leadership. Today's successful home infusion pharmacy is structured to operate on small margins and to effectively bill to ensure full reimbursement for services rendered. Institutions that can use own-use pricing or 340B appropriately and comply with all regulations have the added leverage of a built-in greater margin that will allow for a better fiscal performance.

Regulatory Environment and Considerations

Home infusion pharmacies are licensed by the respective state boards of pharmacy, as is any other pharmacy. In some states, they come under separate licensure requirements; in others they are licensed as retail pharmacies with additional requirements for licensure and compliance. Any venture should first include a thorough review of state board requirements for home infusion pharmacies and results factored into the financial plans regarding costs of operation, physical requirements, and so forth. In many states, such pharmacies may be required to be licensed and surveyed by the department of health to be able to bill Medicare and Medicaid for home infusion services.

Home infusion pharmacies linked with home health agencies within an institutional structure will likely be required to seek JCAHO accreditation. If so, such standards are a separate consideration from the acute care standards, so the home infusion pharmacist will need to prepare to comply with all such standards.[17] If JCAHO accreditation is not a requirement, it would be recommended that similar standards, such as the NHIA (National Home Infusion Association) home infusion pharmacy accreditation process for operational policies and procedures, particularly regarding patient care records and sterile preparation, be adopted by the pharmacy and closely adhered to through an ongoing quality improvement process. USP 797 standards for sterile preparation areas should also be incorporated into the physical plan and related policies and procedures for patient safety and risk mitigation, whether required by any agency or not.[18] These are not inexpensive requirements and must be factored into any business projections for such services.

Because of the early abuses of some home care and infusion pharmacies, there are strict federal regulations regarding the referral of patients to both home care nursing and infusion services. The patient and family must be allowed a choice of providers, including the institution's own, and there cannot be coercion or any financial kickbacks linked to such referrals, in accordance with federal Medicare guidelines.[19]

In developing the business plan for a home infusion business, the costs of licensing, possible accreditation, and adherence to sterile preparation guidelines should be fully allocated for in the budget process. Because of the risk associated with compounded intravenous medications for this purpose, the legal liability, including additional costs of liability insurance, should also be factored into the business plan.

Operational Basics and Keys to Success

Every hospital pharmacy has an infusion pharmacy located within the main hospital pharmacy. Usually the demands of this service are clinically more complex and trying than the home infusion pharmacy because of the nature of the patients' conditions, the corresponding number and complexity of infusions required, and the 24/7 requirements of acute care. Thus, a home infusion pharmacy venture might be considered an easier version of the hospital operation, and to some degree this is true. However, the incremental challenges come from the demands of working with several different home health agencies, the typical short notice given when patients leave the hospital and must have infusion services in place, and the complexity of assuring appropriate billing and reimbursement for services.

- **Billing and reimbursement challenges**

Billing and reimbursement challenges often require either establishing in-house expertise in the nuances of the billing and reimbursement process or contracting the process through companies with proven ability to bill and to maximize reimbursement. It is not unusual for highly efficient institutional home infusion pharmacies to provide quality services in a cost-effective manner yet fail financially because they do not fully address the reimbursement challenges, or simply try to bill through existing hospital structures and processes.

• **Purchasing leverage**

Because of the aggressive reimbursement environment in home infusion, the cost efficiency of services and the net cost of the drugs will be critical determinants of financial success. Institutions have the potential to use own-use pricing and 340B contracts in some cases, if the project has been carefully structured to meet compliance requirements for such use. This additional margin or purchasing leverage may determine whether such a venture will be financially viable. Thus part of the business plan research must include the careful consideration of such possibilities, including the steps and possible costs to achieve such purchasing leverage.

• **Physician and institutional contacts and credibility**

Continuity of patient care, consistency of approach to drug therapy, and sound planning and communications with physicians, nurses, and discharge planners are all areas in which an infusion pharmacy offered by the institution should have an advantage. Every successful home infusion service has developed a plan for continuity of service to assure policies, approach, and communications work easily and effectively. As stated under regulatory concerns, caution must be taken to assure patient and family choice is protected. However, quality and convenient professional service that works for all parties will sell itself every time, which ensures success of this financial venture.

Long-Term Care (LTC) Pharmacy

Introduction

A long-term care pharmacy is similar in many ways to the traditional hospital pharmacy environment found three or four decades ago. Patients are sequestered in an environment in which they depend on nurses and aides to provide the required level of care, which varies greatly from patient to patient. Most medications administered are oral dosage forms, and the remaining are comprised of injections and infusions. Drugs are often administered by aides or vocational nurses who are conscientious but often lack in-depth understanding of drugs. Reimbursement and regulatory environments are unique and dramatically different from the acute care environment. Most institutions have historically avoided ventures into the long-term care business, but, as the population grows older, we can expect to encounter more opportunities for pharmacy.

Competitive Environment, Including Financial and Reimbursement Approach

Because of the limited number of facilities and provider pharmacies structured to meet their needs, the competitive environment is often restricted by contracts and existing relationships. This makes new entry into the long-term care market difficult. Reimbursement in long-term care is as unique as the care itself. For patients covered by Medicare Part A, the facility receives a per diem rate for all care. This places great financial pressure on the nursing home to control all costs, including medications that can be highly variable. Although some patients take less expensive generic medications, others are prescribed expensive brand name drugs, making per diem costs hard to manage. Furthermore, because the prescribing physicians rarely have connection with the nursing home, the ability to use formularies and other common cost control methods is limited. The emergence of Part D programs brings another factor to reimbursement in this setting. The early months of Medicare Part D—when eligibility and coverage for nursing home patients was often ill-defined—left many homes responsible for paying for their residents' medications to remain compliant with regulatory guidelines. These guidelines state that the nursing facility is responsible for ensuring their patients receive their medications as prescribed, regardless of whether this insurer will pay. Pharmacies need to explore the financial viability of the nursing facility before contracting their services. Pharmacies also need to have an in-depth understanding of reimbursement rules for nursing homes and Medicare Part D to ensure their charges to the facility are compliant and accurate.

Regulatory Environment and Considerations

Long-term care is highly regulated, both on a state and federal level. Restrictive contract arrangements between nursing homes and provider pharmacies in the 1980s brought much-needed scrutiny to such relationships, so transparency is mandatory today. Pharmacies serving long-term care facilities must also meet specific requirements, including 24-hour availability, a delivery service, ability to provide or contract intravenous infusion services, and the creation and maintenance of emergency drug boxes. They must also be able to meet medication packaging requirements. Facilities are all required to have a monthly visit by a consultant pharmacist to review each resident's medications. This pharmacist may or may not be employed by the dispensing pharmacy.

Operational Basics and Keys to Success

Opportunities for institutional pharmacies in long-term care are most likely to come from expanding services to facilities owned or contracted with the institution. A hospital pharmacy director and staff, after performing additional research into the unique needs of these facilities, can develop this service with the same clinical and financial success as traditional hospital services. There are some operational basics to consider for such success, including:

- **Contractual arrangements and reimbursement terms**

    A complete understanding of the long-term care marketplace is essential before finalizing contracts. These contracts must address delivery frequency, day supply dispensed, formulary compliance, payment terms, returns and credits, stat charges, and many other areas. As always, due diligence should be performed to ensure financial integrity, fiscal stability, and legal compliance.

- **Packaging requirements**

Packaging systems designed specifically for this environment are typically required, which include blister packaging in 30-day cards that maintain labeling and integrity of the package while assuring each dose is administered. This requires packaging equipment and manpower to accomplish, which must be factored into the business plan for this venture.

In summary, long-term care facilities are a vital part of the continuum of the care delivery system. Serving their pharmacy needs can be a positive clinical and financial venture for the institutional pharmacist willing to invest the time and resources needed for this unique environment.

Final Thoughts and Suggestions for the Aspiring Hospital Pharmacy Entrepreneur

In summary, here are some key considerations when heading down the entrepreneurial pharmacy adventure trail:

- **Research and background work:** Investing the time, effort, and even expense in thoroughly researching a new pharmacy venture is essential for making a good business decision. Such background work forms the basis for a solid business plan that will ensure approval. The following should be included in this research:
  - Competitive environment and financial setting
  - Reimbursement environment and approach
  - Regulatory environment and considerations
  - Operational basics and keys to success
- **Well-conceived sound business plan with champion(s):** A business plan developed and written in the format preferred by the institutional leadership that predicts capital and operational investment, return on investment (ROI), and timelines is highest priority. This combined with support from one or more champions at the leadership level beyond pharmacy will be critical for success.
- **Critical understandings:** After approval and before the implementation of any new venture, there are some critical understandings that must be agreed upon by pharmacy and leadership, including:
  - **Vision, philosophy, and goals:** An integral part of the business plan and communications with leadership must be the vision, philosophy, and goals for the venture, consistent with overall organizational strategy. If the primary goal is to generate new revenues, that should be understood. If that purpose is combined with a clinical and patient care mission, it also should be agreed upon from the beginning. Explicit buy-in and support, without assumptions of common ground, is essential for success in any venture.
  - **Structure:** Where the new venture will be positioned within pharmacy and within the institution should be evaluated and agreed upon.

- **Basic financial management principles are the same:** Although the setting and many of the variables as described in this chapter are dramatically different, the financial management principles are the same. The basics of budgeting, cost and supply chain controls, tracking and reporting, and constant financial oversight are fundamental to any successful business.

- **Separate cost centers and distinct financial reports:** A separate cost center for the venture, where direct costs, revenues, and indirect costs are budgeted and financial reports are monitored, is essential.

- **Indirect costs:** Hospital accounting charges all areas indirect costs, using various methodologies that can be quite substantial. It is important to budget them into the business plan. A start-up business should be given a reasonable time for business development before such indirect costs are assessed to allow the direct costs and revenues to grow incrementally and in parallel. Often it seems the finance department is overanxious to assign huge indirect costs to new centers, long before they can mature into successful businesses. This can undermine the bottom line and create a negative initial impression in the eyes of key leadership and boards, spelling potential trouble for the long-term success of the venture.

- **Timeline:** Realistic timelines for startup, full implementation, and expectations for breakeven and profit generation should be projected and agreed upon as part of the business and ROI projections.

- **Profits:** Although an integral part of the business plan, it is essential to ensure that leadership understands the expectations for profit and where those are to flow once they become reality. It is far easier to have this discussion before the money begins to flow in than afterward, when the emotions associated with new revenues can cloud the thinking of leadership regarding the initial purpose and intentions for the venture.

- **Existing pharmacy leadership and staff:** Because the new venture falls into a different area of pharmacy, it is easy to forget to include existing pharmacy leadership and staff in the pursuit of a new venture. Failure to do so can threaten the stability of existing pharmacy functions and much-needed support of all the pharmacy team.

Most hospital leadership, including pharmacists, tend to be risk adverse, so anyone electing to propose an entrepreneurial venture will be doing so within that challenging mind-set and environment. Also note that the institutional health-care setting will continue to experience shrinking reimbursement and resulting margins, which makes the search for new financial opportunities essential for economic survival. Pharmacy, because of the common thread of drug therapy that is essential in every area of patient care, has a unique opportunity to pursue entrepreneurial ventures that will help secure the future of the institution and the stability of the pharmacy department. Perhaps the most important factor that will determine success as a pharmacy entrepreneur is not found in following the guidelines outlined in this chapter, even though they are important. Nor will an effective command of the sound financial management principles in this text determine success, although it too is absolutely essential. Rather, the most important factor will be the state of mind of the pharmacy leader, who to be successful must be optimistic, open, and enthusiastic about new ideas and able to embrace change and implement innovation. This leader must also have the capacity to listen well and to learn, to visualize a new idea and lead others to it, and to accept reasonable risk as a necessary part of the equation for success. Most of all, this pharmacy leader must see an entrepreneurial opportunity as a professional challenge and a fun experience instead of as another task on an endless to-do list. The factors that will influence the success of the pharmacy entrepreneur are changing constantly, so that some of the details mentioned in this chapter will likely be no longer relevant in ten years, five years, or even one year. However, this entrepreneurial spirit and state of mind, combined with a sound command of pharmacy financial principles and management, will allow the pharmacy leader to envision the opportunity that hugs the edge of chaotic change, seizing today's and tomorrow's opportunities with predictable success regardless!

References

1. Woodward BW. Contributions of pharmacy management to systems' success: Scott & White Hospital, Clinics, & Health Plan. *Am. J. Health Syst. Pharm.* 1996; 53: S13–S18.
2. Scott & White Dept. of Pharmacy Internal Reports. 2003.
3. Scott & White Dept. of Pharmacy Internal Annual Reports & Budget. 2003.
4. National Association of Chain Drug Stores (NACDS) Industry Facts. 2005. http://www.nacds.org/wmspage.cfm?parm1=507 (accessed 2007 February 15).
5. Ibid.
6. Novartis Pharmacy Benefit Report, 2006 Edition. East Hanover, NJ, Novartis Pharmaceuticals Corporation, 2006.
7. U.S. Federal Government. Nonprofit Institutions Act, 15 U.S.C. 13a (NPIA). www.ftc.gov (accessed 15 February 2007).
8. U.S. Federal Government. Public Law 102-585, the Veterans Health Care Act of 1992, Section 340B of the Public Health Service Act. www.hrsa.gov/opa/introduction.htm (accessed 15 February 2007).
9. Woodward BW. Contributions of pharmacy management to systems' success: Scott & White Hospital, Clinics, & Health Plan. *Am. J. Health. Syst. Pharm.* 1996; 53: S13–S18.
10. Novartis Pharmacy Benefit Report, 2006 Edition. East Hanover, NJ, Novartis Pharmaceuticals Corporation, 2006.
11. Specialty Pharmacy Trends & Management Strategies Report. Exhibit 1. Pharmaceutical Care Management Association (PCMA). www.pcmanet.org/research (accessed 15 February 2007).
12. Specialty Pharmacy Trends & Management Strategies Report. Exhibit 4. Pharmaceutical Care Management Association (PCMA) www.pcmanet.org/research (accessed 15 February 2007).
13. Scott & White Health Plan Internal Reports—Employee Drug Plan. 2003.
14. Scott & White Prescription Services PBM Summary Report. 2003.

15. U.S. Federal Government. Federal Register Part V Social Security Administration 20 CFR Part 418 Medicare Part D Subsidies; Final Rule. www.ssa.gov/legislation/medicare/medicare part D.pdf (accessed 15 February 2007).

16. See 14 above.

17. Joint Commission on Accreditation of Healthcare Organizations (JCAHO). About JCAHO Home Infusion Pharmacy Accreditation. www.nhianet.org/ppopresources/ JCAHOinfusion facts.pdf (accessed 15 February 2007).

18. What Is USP 797? www.USP797.org (accessed 15 February 2007).

19. U.S. Federal Government. Federal Register/ Vol 67, No. 186/ Wednesday, Sept. 25, 2002. Proposed Rules. www.oig.hhs.gov/fraud/docs/safe harbor regulation/medica (accessed 15 February 2007).

Glossary

Academic medical centers—Similar to community not-for-profit facilities, academic medical centers are generally organized as tax-exempt under Internal Revenue Service regulations (501 (c)(3)). Their primary purpose is to provide community benefit through various programs and services. Access to capital is mainly through donations (which are usually tax-deductible to the donor), bonds and other debt instruments, and efficient operations. A major part of their mission is teaching new health-care professionals and funding research. These additional activities carry a higher cost structure, which is often partly offset by other funding sources such as grants, state legislative funding, and so forth.

Accounting methods—The three basic accounting methods used by health-care organizations are cash basis, accrual basis, and fund accounting.

Accrual basis accounting—Used for most businesses, this method seeks to "accrue" revenues and expenses to the proper period in which they are earned.

Activity matrix—A matrix of prioritized activities, resources, and costs for pharmacy services to be delivered in an institution.

Acuity—A measure of severity of illness.

Administrative data—Payment, cost, and activity data generated anytime a patient has an encounter with a provider or facility when reimbursement is sought for those services.

Administrative fees—Fees paid by the hospital for its membership to belong to a GPO and to access the contracts the GPO offers, or fees paid by the manufacturer or supplier of the product. Administrative fees typically range from 1 to 3 percent of the purchase price of the product, and they must be disclosed in an agreement between the GPO and each participating member.

Advance beneficiary notice (ABN)—A written notice (on form CMS-R-131) given to a patient before that patient receives items or services, notifying the patient that Medicare may deny payment for that specific procedure or treatment, and that the patient will be personally responsible for full payment if Medicare denies payment.

The ABN explains alternative treatment options, quality-of-life issues, and the patient's obligation to pay for the therapy if the claim is not approved by CMS. The ABN must be signed by the physician providing services and by the patient. The patient must disclose any coverage or financial assistance from secondary insurance providers, medication assistance programs, patient assistance programs, or charities.

Ambulatory payment classification(APC)—The APC outpatient prospective payment system (OPPS) is a reimbursement method that categorizes outpatient visits into groups according to clinical characteristics, typical resource use, costs associated with the diagnoses, and procedures performed. An APC is a diagnostic classification analogous to an outpatient diagnosis–related group.

Balance sheet—Lists assets owned by the organization on the left side of the report, and the liabilities owed and the equity of the organization on the right side of the report. Assets must equal liabilities plus equity (or net assets).

Benchmarking—The continuous process of measuring products, services, and practices against the company's toughest competitors, or against those companies identified as industry leaders, so as to find and implement best practice.

Board of trustees—All hospital operations are governed by a board of trustees that commonly consists of members of the hospital's senior management team and representatives from the medical staff and the community.

Budget—A plan for future expenses and revenue, typically over a 12-month period. A budget does not represent the actual amount of money available to be spent, but is a plan based on history and on an understanding of the future. The pharmacy budget is designed to be a thoughtful, data-driven forecast of future expenses and revenue, and a yardstick for measuring financial performance over the course of the financial year.

Budget variance—The difference between the budgeted amount and the actual amount spent for a period. Variances can be described as positive (expenses lower than forecast; revenues higher than forecast) or negative (expenses higher than forecast; revenues lower than forecast). Variances can also be absolute: the total actual amount is higher irrespective of volume, or volume-adjusted.

Bundled contracts—Contracts for multiple products produced by a single manufacturer. This type of contract is usually anchored by a key product in a competitive market, along with several other products for which the manufacturer has competition from other suppliers.

Business plan—A document with a standard format and structure that clearly explains the what, why, when, who, and how of the project. It is a comprehensive explanation of the opportunity, the people involved, the money required to implement the plan, where the resources will come from, and what financial results the opportunity is likely to produce.

Capital budget—Typically comprises items that cost more than a fixed threshold amount (e.g., an expense greater than $5,000) and that have a useful life greater than a specified number of years (e.g., five years). Capital expense budgets are typically set several years in advance. Pharmacy examples include installing new IV admixture hoods, remodeling a pharmacy, or building a new pharmacy satellite.

Case mix index (CMI)—Indicator of acuity to recognize the additional cost and resources required to care for more seriously ill patients.

Cash-basis accounting—Recognizes income and expense only when cash is received or disbursed. It ignores liabilities for purchases made but not yet received, and for assets earned but not yet collected. Cash-basis accounting is typically limited to individuals or small community organizations.

Centers for Medicare and Medicaid Services (CMS)—A federal agency in the US Department of Health and Human Services (DHHS) that administers the Medicare program and works with state governments to administer Medicaid and the State Children's Health Insurance Program (SCHIP). CMS establishes program policies in accordance with congressional mandates through regulations, transmittals, and directives to fiscal intermediaries.

Clinical decision-support system (CDSS)—A centralized data warehouse to analyze combined administrative, clinical, and financial data.

Community-based (or not-for-profit) facilities—Generally organized as tax-exempt under Internal Revenue Service regulations (501(c)(3)). Such facilities provide community benefits through various programs and services, and they are funded mainly through donations, bonds, other debt instruments, and efficient operations.

Compensation philosophy—A pay and benefit structure and philosophy developed to attract, retain, and motivate employees, while allocating available funds in the most effective manner.

Competitive environment analysis—Research report that includes an overview of the pharmacy's competitors, their nature, the number, and their advantages and vulnerabilities. This research also considers the overall size of the market in terms of gross dollars and net profits, clients and customers, and growth trends over the past three to ten years. The analysis should include any external or internal trends that would affect the potential for success or failure, as well as how this proposed venture would succeed in such an environment.

Continuing education—Instruction that is beyond the requirements for entry into a profession. Continuing education may include courses, programs, or organized learning experiences.

Continuous Quality Improvement (CQI)—A management philosophy that asserts that most things can be improved upon. CQI is an approach to quality that builds upon traditional quality assurance methods by emphasizing the organization and systems. CQI emphasizes process improvement and supports the use of objective data to assess and improve processes.

Contract purchase—Purchases made through membership in a GPO.

Contribution margin—The amount by which total departmental revenue exceeds total departmental expenses.

Cost accounting system—(or cost-allocating system, or decision-support system) A process that uses information from the hospital's general ledger system applied to individual patient accounts from the hospital's billing system to perform detailed data analysis. Used to allocate the hospital's total cost to the patient database with no comparisons to budget, or a standard cost.

Cost-containment plan—Documents areas in which targeted interventions may improve quality and reduce cost.

Data element—A reported metric (e.g., volume statistic, expense, revenue, etc.) within a productivity monitoring system.

Delphi process—A structured process for collecting and compiling knowledge and developing consensus in a group through a series of questionnaires with a feedback process through which agreed-upon values are developed with the help of a facilitator.

Departmental outsourcing—The outsourcing of the management of the entire pharmacy department.

Diagnosis related group (DRG)—A system used by Medicare to classify inpatient hospital services in which hospitals are paid a fixed rate for specific diagnoses. A DRG is expected to have consistent hospital resource use. DRGs were developed for Medicare as part of the prospective payment system. A DRG is assigned based on diagnoses, procedures, age, sex, and the presence of complications or comorbidities.

Direct expenses—Expenses that can be clearly identified as having been incurred in the operation of a department of the hospital.

Direct time study—A series of direct observations of a task to determine the average time required to complete the task and to assign a standard deviation to the average measurement.

Disproportionate share hospital (DSH) program pricing—(or 340(b) drug pricing program) A federal program for eligible safety net providers that gives discounts on the cost of pharmaceuticals; typically, to qualify for 340(b) pricing, a hospital must provide care to a certain percentage (>11.75%) of low-income individuals.

Earnings Before Interest, Deductions, Taxes and Amortization (EBIDTA)—Net revenue less operating expenses equals earnings before depreciation, interest, taxes, and amortization (EBIDTA for for-profit reporting) or the excess of revenues over expenses (for not-for-profit reporting).

Expense—A payment made by the health system to others for value received. Pharmacy expenses can be divided into three categories: supplies, human resources, and other expenses.

Fiscal intermediaries—(FI) Fiscal intermediaries are regional and state Medicare contractors that provide reimbursement review and medical coverage review. Medicare fiscal intermediaries are private insurance companies that serve as the federal government's agents in the administration of the Medicare program, including the payment of claims.

Fiscal services—The collective name for a number of different departments often led by the chief financial officer. Fiscal services can sometimes simply refer to the accounting department.

Fixed expenses—Expenses that do not fluctuate as volumes in the hospital change. Examples include the monthly lease payment for office space or equipment and core staffing levels in some revenue-producing departments and such overhead departments as administration, human resources, and fiscal services.

Flexible budget—An interactive budget that adjusts the static budget based on the actual volume and mix for a period of time.

For-profit facilities—Generally organized as taxable entities. Besides their organizational mission, their primary focus is on generating a return for the shareholder or owner(s). Access to capital is mainly through the sale of stock, debt instruments, and efficient operations.

FTE—A full-time equivalent employee, computed by dividing the number of man-hours for the period by the number of man-hours a full-time employee would be paid for that period.

Functional outsourcing—The outsourcing of a specific function within the pharmacy, such as nuclear radiopharmaceuticals, intravenous compounding, clinical services, packaging services, and after-hours order entry.

Fund accounting—Typically used by governmental entities and academic medical centers, fund accounting establishes specific funds for a variety of uses, such as the equipment replacement fund and the general fund. The general fund serves as the operating fund for the entity.

Gap analysis structured method—Used to document the difference between where a particular department or process is versus where it should be.

Gross revenue—The total amount of revenue billed, based on the established charging structure.

Group purchasing organizations (GPOs)—Organizations whose primary service is developing purchasing contracts for product and nonlabor service agreements that their membership can access. By pooling the purchases of their member hospitals, GPOs can negotiate lower prices from suppliers and manufacturers.

HCPCS coding—The process of organizing data into meaningful categories for analysis. The HCPCS code set is one of the standard code sets used for this purpose. The HCPCS is organized into two principal subsystems, referred to as level I and level II of the HCPCS. Level I of the HCPCS comprises the CPT (current procedural terminology), a numeric coding system maintained by the American Medical Association (AMA). The CPT is a uniform coding system comprising descriptive terms and identifying codes used primarily to identify medical services and procedures. Level II of the HCPCS is a standardized coding system used primarily to identify products, supplies, and services not included in the CPT codes.

High-priority medications—A list of 60 to 80 drug products that represent as much as 80 percent of total annual medication expenditures. *Compare* **Low-priority medications.**

Home infusion center pharmacies—Specialized pharmacies that primarily mix, prepare, and dispense infusions, injections, and other products for use in the home and in other ambulatory settings.

Hospital profit box—A hospital financial model that focuses on the income statement.

Human intellectual capital (HIC)—The value of the collective experience, wisdom, education, and other factors that represent an institution's population.

Human resource expenses—Consist of the salary and benefit costs for pharmacists, pharmacy technicians, pharmacy managers, and others.

ICD-9-CM classification system—The International Classification of Diseases, ninth revision, clinical modification (ICD-9-CM) is a coding system based on the World Health Organization's ninth revision, International Classification of Diseases (ICD-9). ICD-9-CM is the official system of assigning codes to diagnoses and procedures associated with hospital care in the United States. The ICD-9-CM is designed for the classification of morbidity and mortality information for statistical purposes, for the indexing of records, and for ease of data storage and retrieval. The ICD-9-CM classification for diagnoses and injuries is grouped into 17 chapters that are typically arranged by body systems. These codes can be up to five digits in length, permitting detailed descriptions.

Implementation plan—A plan with a timetable indicating key milestones.

Income statement—(or operating statement, or statement of revenues and expenses) Reports financial performance of the organization for a designated period of time. It details revenues earned and related expenses incurred in the operation of the organization.

Indirect expenses—Expenses such as employee benefits, or depreciation, that are similar in nature to revenue deductions in that they require an allocation to be made.

Institutional review board (IRB)—An institutional review board (IRB) is a committee formally designated to monitor, review, and approve biomedical and behavioral research involving humans. The IRB focuses on the protection of the rights and welfare of research subjects.

Integrated delivery networks (IDNs)—Networks of facilities and providers, usually anchored by one or two large hospitals (many times teaching hospitals), and several smaller community or rural hospitals, clinics, and other alternate sites of care, that work together to provide care to a specific market or geographic area.

Intermediate Product (IP)—Represents the standard costs associated with dispensing one unit of a drug. These costs include all resources of the institution related directly and indirectly to the drug.

Internal benchmarking—(i.e., internal productivity monitoring) A process of measuring current department performance against performance over time, comparing current and future department performance against prior department performance.

Key indicators—List of performance measures used to monitor changes in financial operations over time; reviewed at least annually to be sure that the reports and ratios focus on the current main issues.

Letters of commitment (LOCs)—Letters that the pharmaceutical supplier requires the provider to sign in order to access the program. LOCs may be managed by the GPO to track membership enrollment in the program, or by the pharmaceutical supplier, in which case the GPO may not be able to reliably track which members have enrolled in the program.

Local coverage determinations (LCDs)—(or local medical review policies) A local coverage determination (LCD), as established by Section 522 of the Benefits Improvement and Protection Act, is a decision by a fiscal intermediary whether to cover a particular service on an intermediary-wide or carrier-wide basis in accordance with Section 1862(a)(1)(A) of the Social Security Act (i.e., a determination as to whether the service is reasonable and necessary).

Long-term care pharmacy—A pharmacy designed specifically to meet the needs of those in long-term care. Most medications administered in such a pharmacy are oral dosage forms, and the remaining comprise injections and infusions.

Lost charges—Patient-chargeable items for which pharmacy appears to have provided a dose through the first dose process or cart fill, when a second replacement dose is requested by nursing because the initial dispensed dose cannot be located. The replacement dose is then billed back to the HCO for chargeback to the department in which the loss occurred.

Low-priority medications—A large number of medications that represent a small proportion of the entire medication budget. *Compare* **High-priority medications.**

Mail-service pharmacy—A pharmacy that mails drugs to patients. Such a pharmacy is often a cost-saving alternative to the traditional retail pharmacy.

Managed care—A highly competitive arena in which the primary strategy is to offer a comprehensive bundle of health-care services for a set fee over a specific amount of time, using principles of health management and financial control. Managed care is a risk-based business and a form of insurance.

Market competitive clause—A clause that often exists in generic pharmaceutical contracts to allow for price reductions if competitors within the generic class offer a lower price to GPO members.

Market—Group of customers with a set of common characteristics, who want to buy the service.

Marketing plan—A plan to inform potential customers of the new service and ongoing marketing efforts. A marketing plan should include an overall strategy and may include tactics for each target group. Collateral materials and media should be described to provide additional insight on how the new service will be promoted. The plan should include a schedule for introducing the new service and for promoting, as well as a general plan for tracking results of the marketing effort.

Medicaid Program—Title XIX of the Social Security Act is a Federal/State entitlement program that pays for medical assistance for certain individuals and families with low incomes and resources. This program, known as Medicaid, became law in 1965 as a cooperative venture jointly funded by federal and state governments to assist states in furnishing medical assistance to eligible needy persons. Medicaid is the largest source of funding for medical and health-related services for America's poorest people.

Medicare Coverage Advisory Committee (MCAC)—The MCAC reviews and evaluates medical literature, reviews technical assessments, and examines data and information on the effectiveness and appropriateness of medical items and services covered or eligible for coverage under Medicare. The MCAC is also responsible for advising on the scope of medical coverage provided and for the rationale for clinical decisions, as well as for recommending the compendia that are used to support medical decisions.

Medicare Program—A Federal entitlement program that provides access to and pays for medical care for people age 65 or older, for people under age 65 with certain disabilities, and for people of all ages with end-stage renal disease.

Medicare Prospective Payment System (MPPS)—The MPPS was introduced by the federal government in October, 1983, as a way to change hospital behavior through financial incentives that encourage more cost-efficient management of medical care. Under PPS, hospitals are paid a predetermined rate for each Medicare admission. Each patient is classified into a diagnosis-related group (DRG) on the basis of clinical information. Except for certain patients with exceptionally high costs (called outliers), the hospital is paid a flat rate for the DRG, regardless of the actual services provided. MPPS introduced the fixed-price payer into the hospital profit box.

Medicare's limited income subsidy (LIS) benefit—Federal assistance that can increase a patient's cost savings by paying part of his or her monthly premium, annual deductibles, and monthly prescription copayments under the Medicare Part D program. This extra assistance can be worth as much as $3700 annually for an individual patient.

Medication budget—The health system's plan for medication expenditures during the budget period. The medication budget is the sum of the high-priority, new medication, nonformulary, and low-priority budget components, minus the savings identified in the cost-containment plan.

Medication therapy management services (MTMS)—Services provided by the pharmacy, which optimize therapeutic care (including managing and monitoring drug therapy in patients receiving treatment for cancer or chronic conditions such as asthma and diabetes, consulting with patients and their families on the proper use of medication, conducting wellness and disease prevention programs to improve public health, and overseeing medication use in a variety of settings, such as home care settings, hospitals, ambulatory care settings, long-term care facilities, clinics, and intensive care units).

Minibid—A bid conducted for a specific drug or contract if the awarded supplier decides it cannot continue to be price competitive.

Monthly operating statement—A monthly accounting of expenses and revenues prepared by the finance department. The monthly operating statement details the pharmacy's performance against revenue, expense, workload, and additional selected indicators.

Net revenue—Gross revenue less deductions for negotiated discounts, mandated contractual adjustments, and the write-off for charity care. It is the real measure of the revenue earned by the hospital.

Nonacute care facility—Medical treatment facility that does not address urgent or severe needs. A nonacute care facility may include physician offices, retail pharmacies, clinics, long-term care facilities, home care agencies, and other alternate sites of care.

Noncontract purchase—Occurs when a pharmaceutical purchase is made though neither the GPO nor an individual member contract.

Nonformulary agents—Those drugs not found on a hospital or health plan's approved drug list; such drugs may not be covered or may result in a higher copayment.

Normalization—A movement or transfer of reported costs, volumes, and hours from one department to another for the purpose of assuring that those data are reported and combined in the same way by each participating hospital. Normalizations are meant to allocate specific expenses into the most appropriate operational department across all organizations, and they thus enable more accurate comparisons among dissimilar organizations.

Off contract purchase—Occurs when the member hospital does not purchase through the GPO agreement but through an individual contract with the supplier or another GPO or distributor agreement with the supplier.

Operating budget—A forecast of the daily expenses required to operate the pharmacy, including labor, drugs, supplies, and other support below the capital expense threshold.

Operational benchmarking—(also commonly referred to as external benchmarking and external productivity monitoring) A system whereby hospitals submit department-level data (usually on a quarterly cycle) into a vendor-managed financial and operational comparative database to compare departmental operational and financial performance to peer organizations.

Order management—Everything the pharmacy does to understand, translate, perfect, and prepare the physician's order for fulfillment. Order entry, or order review, usually comprises a large part of this process.

Outlier payments—Provisions within the Medicare Act provide for Medicare payments for cases that incur extraordinarily high costs (outliers). These payments are made to Medicare-participating hospitals in addition to the basic prospective payments.

Outsourcing—A contract between a health system and an outside company to provide pharmaceutical services or management.

Overhead—Cost of the indirect services that support the pharmacy, but are not directly paid by the pharmacy. These include housekeeping, heat and air-conditioning, electricity, health system administration, health system purchasing, information systems support, human resources, finance, and others.

Patient assistance programs (PAP)—Patient assistance programs are run by pharmaceutical companies to provide free medications to people who cannot afford to buy their medicine. PAPs provide opportunities for individuals with no insurance or prescription coverage to receive low-cost or free pharmaceuticals.

Patronage fees—The portion of the administrative fees returned to a GPO's membership each year. Most GPOs subtract operating expenses from the administrative fees and return the remainder of the fees to their membership each year. The percentage returned to the member hospitals varies among GPOs.

Pay-for-performance (P4P)—Compensation for high-quality care, based on established quality indicators.

Peer group—A grouping of like hospitals or hospital departments.

Per diem rate—Fixed-price per patient day; most favored payment methodology of health insurers.

Per member per month (PMPM)—A fixed payment per month that is received for providing services to a member.

Percentile—A relative ranking of performance versus a compare (peer) group. In operational benchmarking, percentiles range from 0 to 100 percent, and better performance is typically signified by a lower percentile ranking.

Performance agreements—Contract agreements designed to reward hospitals for increased use of a specific product within a therapeutic class. Performance agreements typically have multiple tiers, each of which is associated with a product price. Tiers are differentiated based on a market share percentage scale, the total number of units purchased, the total of dollars spent, or a combination of these attributes. The price a member pays for a contracted product decreases as the market share percentage for the product increases, the total units purchased increase, or the total dollars spent increase. Performance agreement calculation of market share is usually based on a market basket of competitive products, whereby the contracted product usage is divided by overall usage of all other products in the market basket.

Pharmacy informatics—The effective acquisition, storage, organization, analysis, management, and use of information in the delivery of pharmaceutical care and the delivery of optimal medication-related patient care and health outcomes.

Prescription drug benefit—A contract that defines the benefits, including formulary coverage, co-pays, deductibles, and caps according to the specifications of the employer, who is picking up most of the expenditures. The prescription drug benefit portion is often defined by the plan and priced on a per member per month (PMPM) basis.

Procedure analysis report—Depicts the current price, current month and year-to-date volumes, and gross charges for each procedure code in the pharmacy and includes departmental totals of volumes and revenue. (PS ref: chapter 2, page 10, para 1)

Productivity ratio—A measure of productivity (output/input). Productivity ratios are often divided into *labor productivity ratios* (e.g., hours worked or paid per unit of output, hours worked per 100 orders processed, doses dispensed per hour worked) and *cost-based productivity ratios* (e.g., expense per unit of output, drug cost per 100 orders processed, total pharmacy cost per patient discharge).

Rebates—A percentage of the total purchase cost of the product returned to the purchaser. Rebates are meant as an incentive to purchase more product. Rebates are also used to hide the actual price of the product either from the pharmacy distributor or from other competitors.

Regulatory environment investigation—Research such as a regulatory environment investigation considers the unique regulatory issues associated with the pharmacy business. Such research must be thorough and is as important to success as any other financial factor in the project evaluation.

Reimbursement analysis—A research report that considers the reimbursement issues unique to the business venture, outlining any advantages, leverage, or limitations to be considered. The reimbursement analysis should include a realistic appraisal of how reimbursement issues will affect the project and its chances for success. Strategies for maximizing any advantages and for dealing with the challenges should be a part of this research, and they should become a fundamental component of the final business plan.

Relative value unit (RVU)—Depending on the cost type, this RVU can be the actual cost per unit, labor minutes per unit, or a weighting factor that helps distribute the cost accordingly.

Replacement cost—The resources and monies expended to replace a separated employee. These resources include the cost of identifying and attracting applicants, conducting screening interviews, testing or other assessment of competency, preemployment administrative expenses, travel and moving expenses, and recruitment or other incentive payments.

Responsibility accounting—Responsibility reports show the department manager his or her responsibility in the financial picture. The report presents *only* those items that the manager is, or should be, directly responsible for in his or her department. The most common responsibility accounting report is the monthly department operations report.

Retail pharmacy—A community pharmacy in which drugs are sold to patients.

Return on investment (ROI)—A structured calculation of the operating cost and revenue changes that the health system will incur with the new capital expense. ROI calculations are often stated in the number of months or years that a capital purchase takes to pay back its purchase cost.

Revenue—Money received for products or services provided to customers. Pharmacy revenues consist primarily of patient charges, which may arise from doses administered in an inpatient setting or from prescriptions dispensed in an outpatient setting.

Reverse auction—A bid process where multiple suppliers bid for a contract through an electronic auction process. Through the auction process, the price is driven down rather than driven up (hence the term *reverse auction*).

Salary accrual—An estimate of the amount of salary and wage expense incurred between the end of the last pay period of the month and the end of the month used to properly match expenses to revenue.

Self-reporting—Relies on staff to document the amount of time required to perform an activity. Self-reporting studies are best conducted in situations of low to moderate activity volume with easily definable start and stop times with little variation in activity interpretability.

Specialty pharmacy—A pharmacy that stocks, prepares, and dispenses drugs to patients, primarily to those in the home or in other outpatient settings. The drugs dispensed are limited in number, but they tend to be expensive, and they frequently require administration by self-injection. These drugs are often not routinely stocked in a neighborhood pharmacy.

Staff development—A structured development plan created between the staff member and the department manager to improve performance. Staff development is another plan for the career growth of particular individuals within the department. Formal education may be included, such as the Master of Business Administration (MBA) or other specialized education programs. In some organizations, a formal mentoring program may be available for managers or for peak performers who wish to advance.

Staffing plan—A plan that creates an optimal relationship between the available resources (hours of pharmacist and technician work time) and the coverage hours and activities of the pharmacy and that seeks to achieve the greatest utility and output while meeting the human needs of staff. The basis for a staffing plan includes the scope of services of the pharmacy, practice standards and regulatory requirements, the leverage provided by the skills and competencies of the pharmacy staff, the capabilities of automation and technology, and an understanding and acknowledgement of the support needs at practice interfaces with physicians, nurses, and others who work in the medication use process.

Standard cost accounting, product costing— Process of determining the price of a product by examining the various expenses accumulated in the development and sale of that product.

Statement of cash flows—Final financial statement. It identifies the sources and uses of cash in the organization. The statement must tie to the cash balance reported on the balance sheet.

Statement of owner's equity or fund balance— Provides a detailed account of the equity balance at the beginning and end of the reporting period. The net income or loss (excess of revenues over expenses, in the case of a not-for-profit organization) is often the most significant transaction. Net income increases equity on the balance sheet; net losses decrease equity.

Static budget—Snapshot of expected costs; not adjusted or altered after the budget is submitted.

Stepwise analysis—Method of variance analysis that lines up all the factors being analyzed, starting with all factors at their budgeted level. At each step in the analysis, one of the factors is shown at its actual level rather than at its budgeted level.

Stop loss provision—Contract provisions in which additional payments to the hospital are generated from the insurer when an individual admission reaches a certain charge level (similar to outlier payments). These additional payments can take any form (per diem, case rate, percentage of charges), with percentage of charges being preferred by the hospital financial manager.

Strategic plan—A document describing the resources required, the costs incurred, and the benefits realized in acquiring those resources to achieve long-term goals.

Strategic pricing—A pricing method that analyzes each procedure code by payer source (charge-based or cost-based). Strategic pricing places as much of a price increase as is possible on procedures with high usage by charge-based payers and as little as possible on procedures with a high usage by cost-based payers generating a higher net return for the hospital.

SWOT (strengths, weaknesses, opportunities, and threats) analysis—A structured strategic planning method that results in a report that enables the pharmacy to evaluate how to enhance strengths, mitigate or eliminate a weakness, and capitalize on an opportunity, and that helps the hospital plan how to deal with threats.

Tax Equity and Fiscal Responsibility Act of 1982 (TEFRA)—Changed the Medicare program from a cost-based payer to a fixed-price payer for inpatient acute care admissions, leaving outpatient, physical rehabilitation, transplant, and behavioral health services as cost-based payers. TEFRA resulted in the implementation of the Medicare prospective payment system and introduced the fixed-price payer. Under TEFRA, hospitals in the same geographic area are all paid the same base rate for each admission. This base rate is then multiplied by the program-determined cost weight for the DRG to determine the actual payment by Medicare to the hospital.

Therapeutic interchange—To modify the market share of drugs in a specific therapeutic class by moving market share toward one product in a class by deeming products therapeutically equivalent to the medication prescribed. Examples of therapeutic categories in which interchange programs may be considered include antiemetics, antimicrobials, and erythropoietic growth factors.

Time standard—The mean time required to perform a task.

Variable expenses—Expenses that fluctuate as volumes in the hospital change. Pharmacy drug cost is an example of a variable expense—the more patients the hospital has, generally the higher the total drug cost, and the fewer patients a hospital has, the lower the drug cost.

Variance—Differences between the budget and actual expense expressed in absolute dollars and as percentage differences.

Volume budget—The number of admissions, patient days, CMI, outpatient visits, emergency department visits, and other activities for the budget year; prepared by the CFO.

Volume indicator—The frequency with which activities occur, often reported as a mean frequency when nonautomated sources are used to provide the frequency.

Weighting—A method used to recombine a department's varied work outputs equitably to produce a single figure that represents the department's entire output. Weighting can also be defined as a measure of time to perform one unit of each department output.

Work sampling—A method to estimate the percent of time that staff spend on various activities; an indirect method of establishing time require-ments. The work sampling method of measurement is best for measuring the relative frequency of all tasks staff perform, and for measuring intermittent activities that are not closely structured in time, that occur infrequently, and for which data would thus require an inordinate amount of time to collect through direct observation.

Workload unit—A unit of measure to monitor financial performance. On the inpatient side patient days, number of admissions, and number of discharges are common measures. On the outpatient side patient visits, such as emergency room or clinic visits, are common indicators. For those organizations that provide traditional retail prescription services, prescription volume is also a common measure.

Technical terms outlining the function of Medicare, Medicaid and other reimbursement and financial functions of the Department of Health and Human Services and the Centers for Medicare and Medicaid Services (CMS) were researched and validated at the time of publication. Readers are referred to these web sites to ensure that their understanding of the terms, and that use and function of these terms are current. Web Sites: www.cms.hhs.gov, www.cdc.gov, www.hhs.gov, www.medicare.gov.

Index